The End of Alzheimer's PROGRAMME

The Practical Plan to Prevent and Reverse Cognitive Decline at Any Age

Dr Dale Bredesen

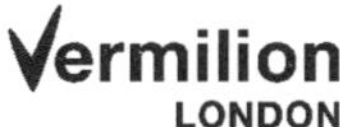

LONDON

1

Vermilion, an imprint of Ebury Publishing
20 Vauxhall Bridge Road,
London SW1V 2SA

Vermilion is part of the Penguin Random House group of companies
whose addresses can be found at global.penguinrandomhouse.com

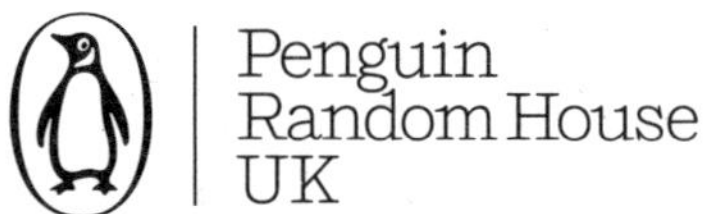

Illustrations by Joe LeMonnier

First published in the UK in 2020 by Vermilion
First published in the US in 2020 by Avery, an imprint
of Penguin Random House LLC, New York

www.penguin.co.uk

A CIP catalogue record for this book is available from the British Library

ISBN 9781785042270

Printed and bound in Great Britain by Clays Ltd, Elcograf S.p.A.

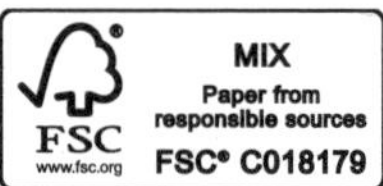

Penguin Random House is committed to a sustainable future for our business, our readers and our planet. This book is made from Forest Stewardship Council® certified paper.

This book is dedicated to Julie G. and the 3,000+ members of ApoE4.Info, who embrace the twenty-first-century approach to health and are together offering hope to the more than one billion people at high risk for Alzheimer's disease worldwide.

Contents

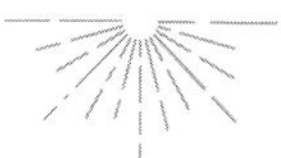

Visit endofalzheimersprogram.com to see every reference in this book.

Foreword

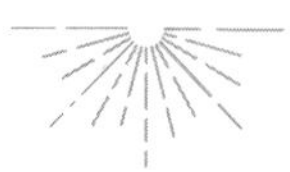

At every crossway on the road that leads to the future, each progressive spirit is opposed by a thousand men assigned to guard the past.
—MAURICE MAETERLINCK

NEVER BEFORE HAS THE practice of medicine been as polarized by the dichotomy between reductionism and holism as exists today with relation to the treatment of Alzheimer's disease.

Reductionism, as it is applied to the practice of medicine, takes the position that in order to best understand a disease process and ultimately formulate and implement an appropriate therapeutic intervention, both the disease and the intervention need to be reduced to the simplest operative parts and mechanisms. Many have credited the sixteenth-century French philosopher René Descartes with codifying this paradigm. Descartes, in Part V of his *Discourse*, described the world as being nothing more than a clockwork machine that could be understood in its entirety through an exploration of its individual components. And clearly the progress of the science of medicine historically and in the present is deeply punctuated by landmark advances characterized by dedication to this approach.

Whether we are speaking of Antonie Philips van Leeuwenhoek, using a single-lensed microscope to discover *animalcules* (microbes), or the sequencing of the human genome, the underpinnings of

Western medicine continue to honour the notion that looking deeper and deeper at constituent parts will ultimately provide a knowledge base that will reveal sought-after solutions to challenging disease processes.

To be sure, microscopy led to an understanding of pathophysiology that directly resulted in wondrous advances leveraged for salubrious outcomes. But myopically engaging a philosophy centred on drilling down to unity in terms of parts and processes inevitably segues to sanctioning a therapy equally centred on the validation of the singular. Simply stated, embracing reductionism in medicine supports the ideology of monotherapy, the idea that the goal of modern medical research should be the development of single, magic bullets that are designed and marketed to counter single diseases.

As Harvard physician Dr Andrew Ahn put it in a paper exploring the limits of reductionism in medicine:

> Reductionism pervades the medical sciences and affects the way we diagnose, treat, and prevent diseases. While it has been responsible for tremendous successes in modern medicine, there are limits to reductionism, and an alternative explanation must be sought to complement it.

As of this writing, no disease process highlights the limitations of a reductionist approach as it relates to therapy more than senile dementia of the Alzheimer's type. To be sure, the deep dive to unravel the etiology of this now-epidemic disease has been under way for decades and underwritten by hundreds of millions of dollars. Applying a reductionist approach has indeed revealed fascinating mechanisms that are likely involved in what ultimately manifests as this disease that now affects 5.5 million Americans. But alas, no single or combination pharmaceutical therapy has any effect whatsoever on modifying the inexorable course of Alzheimer's disease.

As a testament to the tenacity of the pharmaceutical industry, several drugs are marketed to Americans and indeed globally with the idea that they somehow "treat" Alzheimer's disease. But while these medicines may minimally affect Alzheimer's *symptoms*, again they provide no benefit whatsoever with respect to actually improving the ultimate outcome. As Dr Michal Schnaider-Beeri recently revealed in an editorial in the journal *Neurology*: "Despite great scientific efforts to find treatments for Alzheimer disease (AD), only 5 medications are marketed, with limited beneficial effects on symptoms, on a limited proportion of patients, without modification of the disease course."

More recently, the concern for the lack of efficacy of these medications was overshadowed by a report appearing in *The Journal of the American Medical Association* revealing that not only do the commonly prescribed Alzheimer's drugs lack efficacy, but their utilization is actually associated with *more rapid cognitive decline.*

In contradistinction to reductionism, holism places more value on exploring the forest as opposed to focusing on the single tree. To be sure, a holistic approach to health and disease absolutely embraces the discoveries of deep scientific pursuits, but the fundamental difference in comparison to reductionism is found when examining how science is utilized as it relates to actually treating a malady. Whereas reductionism looks for the one home-run solution, holism considers any and all options available if there's something positive to offer.

As you will soon discover in the pages that follow, for the first time ever a therapeutic intervention has been developed that successfully treats Alzheimer's disease. The protocol developed by Dr Bredesen is by definition holistic. His programme incorporates the discoveries of research across a multitude of disciplines that have bearing on Alzheimer's pathogenesis. Our most highly respected scientific research has clearly delineated the specific mechanisms whereby a vast array of seemingly unrelated processes contributes to the ultimate manifestation of this disease. And it is precisely because Alzheimer's disease manifests from the confluence of multiple factors that its remediation requires the orchestration of diverse instruments.

Although the source of the quote "The definition of insanity is doing the same thing over and over again and expecting a different result" has been questioned, its relevance to the pursuit of a single drug approach to the treatment of Alzheimer's disease is unquestionable. Sanity now prevails with Dr Bredesen's challenge to the status quo that may well bring an end to Alzheimer's disease.

David Perlmutter, MD

Naples, Florida

January 2019

PART ONE

ALZHEIMER'S: The Final Generation?

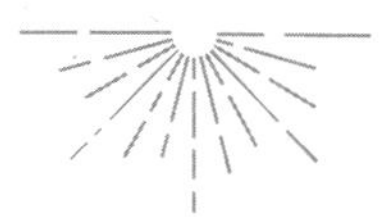

CHAPTER 1

A New Kind of Vaccine

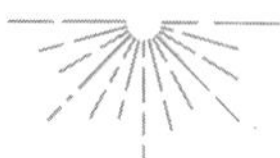

Knowing is not enough; we must apply.

Being willing is not enough; we must do.

—LEONARDO DA VINCI

ALZHEIMER'S DISEASE SHOULD BE—AND *shall* be—a rare disease. Remember polio? Remember syphilis? Leprosy? These were all scourges at one time or another, and Alzheimer's disease shares features with all of them. How many people do you know who suffer from polio or syphilis or leprosy today? There was a time when the word *polio* struck fear into the hearts of many, including my mother. It was the 1950s, I was a nursery school pupil, and people would, out of nowhere it seemed, rapidly become paralyzed. Some died, some lived with severe disabilities, and iron lungs proliferated. My mother explained to me that an expert had suggested that polio might be carried by flies, so I should try to avoid flies—not an easy thing to do for a little kid, running around the playground and through the woods!

Thankfully, polio turned out to be completely preventable by vaccine. Now we need a vaccine to prevent Alzheimer's disease. However, the "vaccine" for twenty-first-century diseases such as Alzheimer's looks quite different from the polio vaccine—it is not an injection, it is an "unjection."* It is a personalized programme, derived from many inputs measuring all of your critical parameters—from genome to microbiome to metabolome to exposome—contributing to cognitive decline, using a computer-based algorithm to identify the type of Alzheimer's (yes, there is more than one type, and that's important to know for effective prevention and treatment) and generate an optimal programme to prevent or reverse the problem. If you are insulin resistant, for example, as nearly half of Americans are, then you are at increased risk for Alzheimer's disease, but this can be reversed. If you have unrecognized chronic inflammation, as millions of Americans do, then you are at risk for Alzheimer's disease, but this can be identified and mitigated. If you are deficient in zinc, as a billion people are globally, or in vitamin D, then you are at increased risk for cognitive decline, but this can be addressed. If you have an occult infection with *Babesia* or *Borrelia* or *Ehrlichia* from a tick bite, or viral infections such as *Herpes simplex* or HHV-6, or unrecognized exposure to mycotoxins (poisons produced by some moulds), then you are at increased risk for cognitive decline, but this can be treated. Most important, if you are genetically predisposed to Alzheimer's disease, as over 75 million Americans are, you can now adopt a programme to avoid it or resolve it, as we have published repeatedly over the past several years.

So that's what a twenty-first-century "vaccine" for Alzheimer's looks like—no injection needlestick, no thiomersal, no mercury, no Guillain-Barré (paralysis) risk, but in some ways even more effective than the old-fashioned vaccines. Just as there were global projects to vaccinate against smallpox, so should there be global projects to prevent and reverse cognitive decline, utilizing the twenty-first-century "vaccine." This is the way to eradicate the very illnesses that are killing us today—complex chronic diseases such as Alzheimer's, Parkinson's, macular degeneration, cardiovascular disease, hypertension, type 2 diabetes, cancer, and on and on. These should *all* be—and all

* The term "unjection" has been trademarked by Pfizer.

can be—rare diseases, instead of the ubiquitous contributors to our ill health that they represent today.

Nina came to see me "for prevention of Alzheimer's disease," she said—her grandmother had developed dementia in her 60s, and her mother had been only 55 when she began to struggle to find the right word while speaking and lost her ability to do simple calculations, such as working out a tip. She deteriorated and was diagnosed with Alzheimer's disease, something that Nina wanted to avoid, if possible. She had been given the standard line by the expert she had consulted earlier, that "there is nothing that prevents, reverses, or delays Alzheimer's disease."

She carried a single copy of the common Alzheimer's risk gene, ApoE4, just as 75 million Americans do. Her ApoE4 gene was likely passed down from her mother and grandmother, and was probably the major genetic contributor to their development of dementia. She also had a past history of a borderline low vitamin B_{12} and low vitamin D.

Although she was only 48 years old and had essentially no cognitive complaints—she thought she was one of the "worried well"—she scored poorly on her MoCA test (MoCA is an abbreviation for Montreal Cognitive Assessment), which is a simple, quick screening test that samples various types of brain function, such as memory, organization, calculation, and verbal ability. Most of us should score anywhere from 28 to 30 out of the total of 30 possible on the MoCA test, but Nina scored only a 23, indicating that she already had mild cognitive impairment (MCI), a pre-Alzheimer's condition. Additional neuropsychological testing confirmed her MCI diagnosis—she was already well on her way to the dementia that her mother and grandmother had unfortunately developed.

She began on the programme that my research group and I developed, called ReCODE (for reversal of cognitive decline), and after several months, she noticed a major change: she said, "I had no idea how bad things were with my thinking until I got better." She scored a perfect 30 on the MoCA, and has sustained her improvement since then. She emailed me: "Thanks so much for the opportunity to participate in this programme. It has been a life saver for me, and for that I am forever grateful."

You may be thinking, "Sure, Nina improved, but she was still at a relatively early stage of cognitive decline. What if she had had late-stage Alzheimer's disease?"

Let me tell you about Claudia.

> Claudia is a 78-year-old woman who developed cognitive decline and progressed to having severe Alzheimer's disease. Her MoCA score was zero. She was unable to speak except for an occasional yes or no. She was unable to ride her bicycle, unable to dress herself, and unable to care for herself. She was evaluated and began on the protocol, personalized for her own cognitive decline inducers. Her evaluation indicated several contributors that had not been identified previously, including mycotoxins produced by moulds. She was negative, but showed insulin resistance. She was treated by an outstanding physician, Dr Mary Kay Ross, who is an expert in treating patients with biotoxin exposure. Claudia had ups and downs as she removed her exposure, optimized her detoxification, adjusted her diet, and started on the different synaptic supports. However, over the next four months, she began to improve, regaining her ability to speak, beginning to email again, dressing herself in the basics, riding her bicycle, and even dancing with her husband.
>
> Her husband wrote: "Tonight we went for a nice walk and she thanked me for getting her out so she could observe things. She pointed out a number of things, including the pink-lit clouds caused by the setting sun. Later we sat together and talked, and I read each one of the blog posts to her, explaining what's been happening each step of the way. And she said, 'It seems to me that I'm going to be all right, and that I'm going to be able to enjoy things again.'"

I hasten to add that Claudia is the exception, not the rule—in general, the earlier you start the protocol, the more likely you are to have a positive outcome and the more complete the response is. Nonetheless, as Claudia's case illustrates, some people even very late in the course have indeed shown marked improvement. Furthermore, such improvement—indeed, any improvement at all—was unthinkable even a few years ago, and is still unthinkable to many who are pursuing standard single-drug approaches.

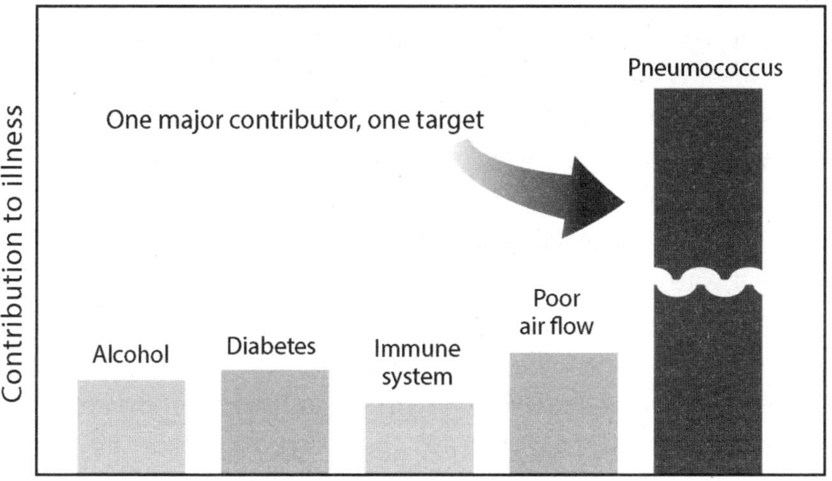

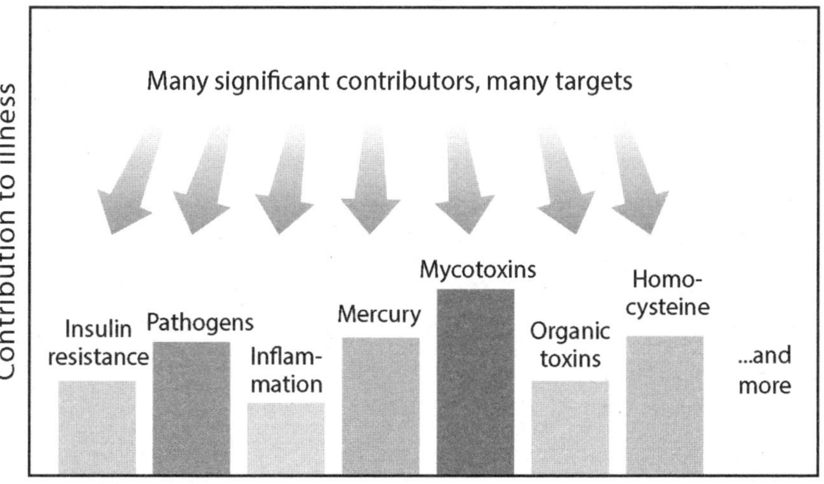

Simple illnesses such as pneumonia versus complex illnesses such as Alzheimer's. Simple illnesses may have many contributors, but a single one is far and away the dominant, and therefore a single drug, such as penicillin, is often curative. In contrast, complex illnesses typically have many contributors, but no single contributor is the clear dominant, and therefore identifying and addressing multiple contributors with a precision protocol is the most effective approach to treatment.

But let's get back to Nina—Nina remains on the twenty-first-century "vaccine" for Alzheimer's disease, a personalized, precision medicine programme, analyzing and addressing the biochemical parameters that contribute to Alzheimer's. This twenty-first-century "vaccine" works not only for prevention but also for early reversal, something that the twentieth-century injectables did not. But that's not all: beyond prevention and reversal is *enhancement* of cognitive ability at every age. Whether you are a 40-something or 80-something or even a 20-something, using the protocol described here should enhance your cognitive ability, optimize your focus and work, sharpen your memory, and improve your speaking.

Nina's history demonstrates one of the important lessons: cognitive decline often sneaks up on you. Indeed, the Nobel laureate Richard Feynman—the Einstein of the latter half of the twentieth century—developed cognitive decline, which turned out to be due to a subdural haematoma (a blood clot pushing against his brain). When the haematoma was removed and his brilliance had returned, he commented on the lack of insight one has into one's own cognitive compromise. Thus these complex chronic illnesses are like a boa constrictor: as they take hold of you, for years you do not feel the squeeze . . . they wrap their coils around you, and you might feel a senior moment or two, or perhaps forget where you parked, but you think, *Doesn't everyone do that?* Even the doctor cannot see the creeping constriction. Until it is too late and you have an advanced-stage terminal illness. Here's the great news, though—the Achilles' heel of all of these complex chronic illnesses is that we can see them coming for *years* ahead of time, thus giving us plenty of time for prevention (okay, so boa constrictors don't have heels, I get it, but you see the point—we can conquer these diseases early on). All we have to do is bother to look.

Unfortunately, however, that is exactly what is not happening.

Wait, what?! We can address a trillion-dollar global health problem, save millions of lives, prevent the absolute horror of dementia, keep countless families intact, avoid care homes, and enhance global health—but we are not bothering to detect or address the constrictive coils as they are tightening around us for years? How can this be? Tragically, this has happened for several reasons. As one US healthcare executive put it, "Why would we help our competitors? Most patients are not on our health plans for too many years before switching to another plan, so if we institute prevention, we are simply helping our competition, and we are not about to do that." Somebody forgot to tell this greedy bottom-feeder that the enemy is the disease, not another healthcare company. Imagine sitting in your expensive corner office and making a decision that you know will result in unnecessary suffering for thousands of families, just to make a few more bucks. I don't think that most of us could do that.

But that's not the only reason that Alzheimer's sneaks up on so many of us. GP visits limited to 5 minutes, lack of the key tests needed, minimizing testing to save costs, and lack of teaching of new principles of medicine are all important contributors. As the leader of one of the most respected medical schools in the United States told me, "We'd like to teach these new approaches to the medical students, but we can't do that until they are accepted by all doctors." And of course they won't be accepted by doctors until they are taught in medical school. Catch-22. So while Silicon Valley is leading us towards the twenty-second century, the medical establishment is leading the way back to the nineteenth. . . .

There was a hilarious skit on the US satirical programme *Saturday Night Live* years ago, in which the CEO of USAir addressed the various problems that had occurred with the beleaguered airline, concluding with the upbeat, reassuring tag line, "USAir—we learn something from *every crash*!" The idea that an airline would not focus on *preventing* crashes, and would instead focus on learning *after* its own crashes, sounded outrageous—truly dark humour—but it's exactly the approach healthcare uses on us, its victims . . . *er*, I mean patients. We now have the ability to prevent and reverse cognitive decline, as well as other complex chronic illnesses, and we must make this the standard of care if we are to keep our own cognition and prevent a huge strain on the healthcare systems, among many other important outcomes.

So if our doctors fail to do the appropriate tests to predict and prevent cognitive decline, and we fail to take the critical steps to prevent it, then many in the US and around the world—about 45 million of the currently living Americans—will go on to develop Alzheimer's disease, which, unsettlingly, has become the third leading cause of death.[1] As we become symptomatic, we will likely seek evaluation from an expert, who will tell us "It's Alzheimer's disease." This is like taking your car in to a mechanic because it is not functioning well and having the mechanic say, "Oh, we know exactly

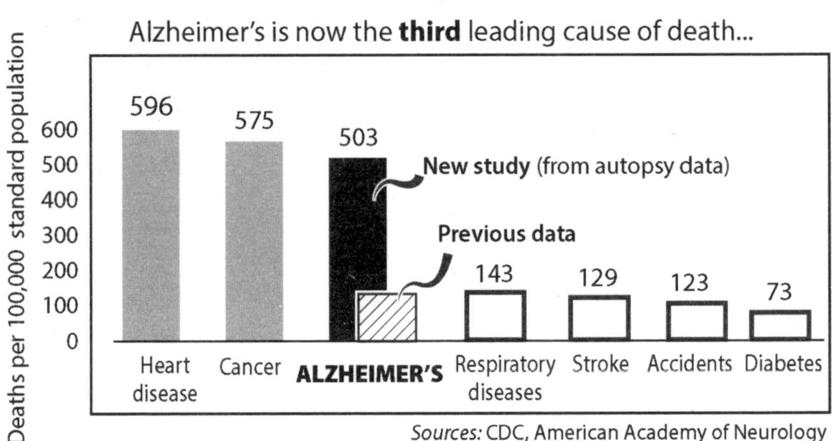

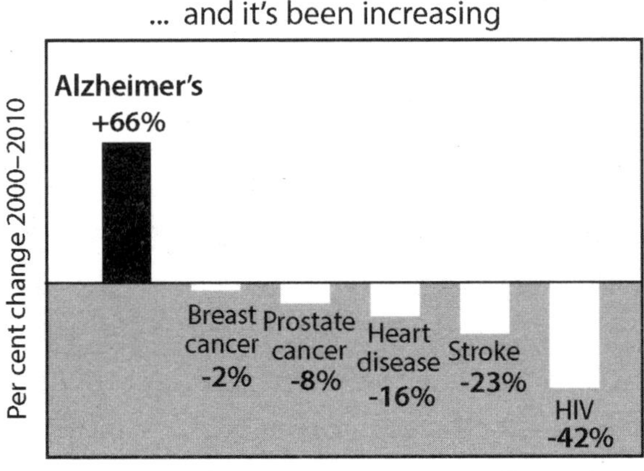

Alzheimer's is now the third leading cause of death in the United States. Furthermore, whereas other common diseases such as heart disease and stroke are on the decline, Alzheimer's disease is on the rise.

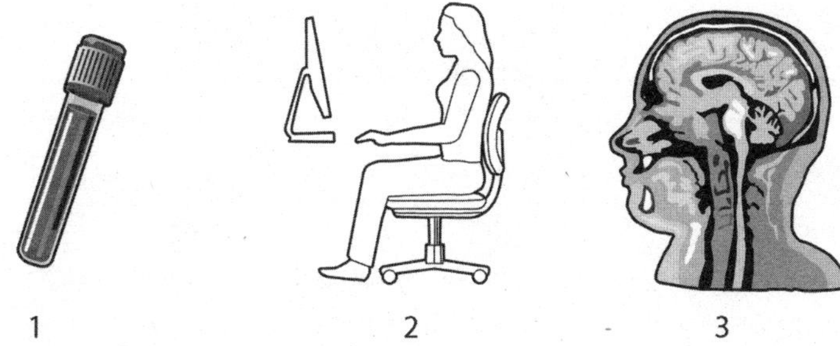

A "cognoscopy" includes a set of blood tests that reveals risk for Alzheimer's; a simple online cognitive assessment that takes only about 30 minutes; and an MRI scan with volumetrics (the MRI is optional for those who have no symptoms, but is recommended for those who already have symptoms of cognitive decline).

what this is, we see it all the time—it's called car-not-working syndrome. It tends to happen in older cars. There is no known cause, and no cure—your car is going to die." When you knit your brow and ask the expert whether he or she is planning to do tests that might identify the root cause of the problem, the response is "No, we don't do those tests—they are not reimbursed." This is why I recommend that, just as we all know to get a colonoscopy when we turn 50, we should get a "cognoscopy" when we turn 45 (or as soon as possible thereafter)—a set of blood tests and a simple online cognitive assessment, so that we'll know what to do to prevent cognitive decline—so that we can indeed make Alzheimer's a *rare* disease, just as it should be.

So now let's look at what Alzheimer's disease actually *is*: how we can truly understand it, why it is so common, and most important, how we can prevent it and actually reverse cognitive decline, sustaining the improvement, just as we have now done for hundreds of patients.[2] This is what my laboratory colleagues and I have researched for thirty years. In 2011, we proposed the first comprehensive trial for Alzheimer's disease, based on our research findings, which showed us that we must evaluate and target dozens of contributing factors if we are to address the underlying drivers of the disease, instead of employing the usual single-drug (monotherapy) approach, which has failed repeatedly. Unfortunately, the trial was denied by the US Institutional Review Board (IRB), which felt that it was too complicated

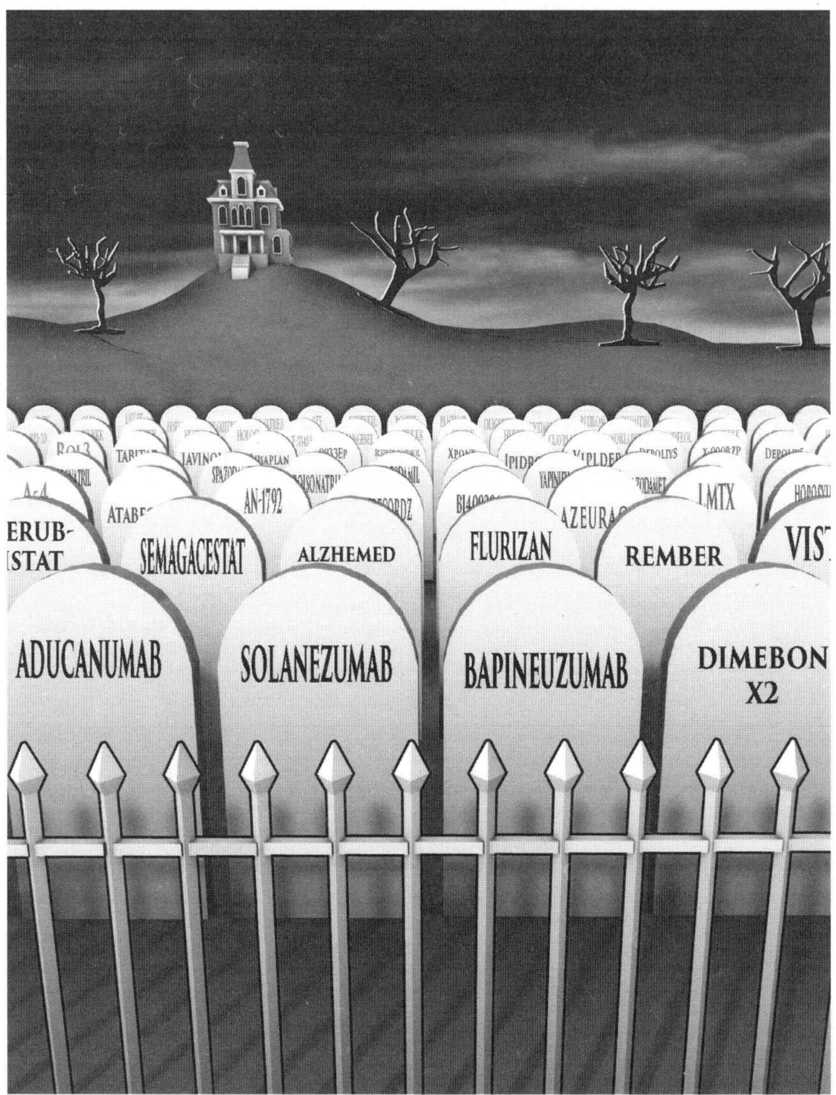

***Game of Throwns.* Monotherapies (single drugs) for Alzheimer's and other complex chronic illnesses have failed repeatedly—more than 400 times. Even the "successes" do not improve cognition sustainably or alter the cognitive decline.**

and that it did not conform to the usual standard in which each trial evaluates only a single drug or treatment. Of course our response was that Alzheimer's disease is not a simple single-variable disease and therefore does not lend itself to the standard, single-drug treatment. Unfortunately, our response fell on deaf ears.

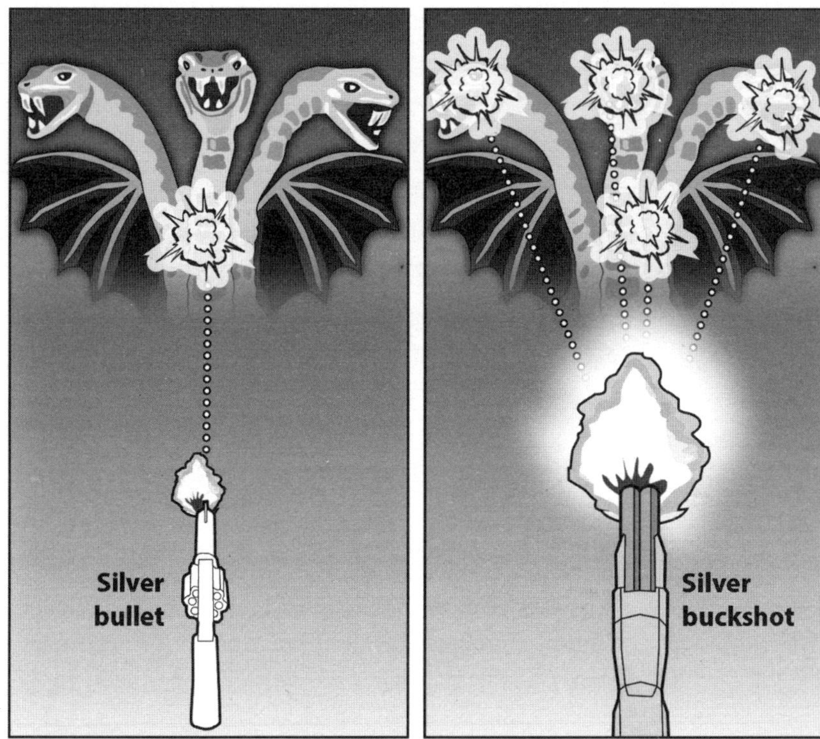

Whereas the "silver bullet" approach has failed, a "silver buckshot" approach has provided the first successes in reversing cognitive decline.

Why did our years of laboratory research dictate such an atypical approach? Because what we had discovered suggested a true paradigm shift in the way we prevent and reverse cognitive decline (and by extension, other neurodegenerative diseases, and indeed most chronic complex illnesses)—not a silver bullet, but rather *silver buckshot*.

Here's how it all works: there have been many, many theories of Alzheimer's disease—it has been suggested to be due to free radicals or calcium or aluminium or mercury or amyloid or tau or prions (replicating proteins) or diabetes of the brain ("type 3 diabetes") or membrane damage or damage to mitochondria (the energy centres of cells) or brain ageing, and on and on—but *no single theory* has led to an effective treatment, despite billions of dollars of clinical trials and drug development.

In contrast, what we discovered reveals how to prevent and treat Alzheimer's: at the heart of Alzheimer's disease sits a switch called APP, the amyloid precursor protein, which protrudes from your brain cells. APP responds in two opposing ways, depending on its environment. It's as if you are the president of the country MyBrainistan. When things are good, the treasury is full, there are no ongoing wars, there is no runaway inflation, and no major pollution to clean up; you decide that it is a propitious time to build and to maintain the infrastructure of your country. So you send out the appropriate orders, and new buildings are constructed, new interactions occur, and the country's network becomes more extensive. That is what is happening in your brain moment by moment when you have optimal levels of nutrients, hormones, and growth factors (i.e. the treasury is full), there are no pathogens or associated inflammation (i.e. no ongoing wars), you have no insulin resistance (i.e. no runaway inflation), and you have no major exposure to toxins (i.e. no major pollution). Therefore, your APP signals growth, and it does this by being cut by molecular scissors called proteases, at a specific site called the alpha site, thus fragmenting into the two growth and maintenance pieces (called peptides), sAPPα (which stands for soluble APP fragment cleaved at the alpha site) and αCTF (the carboxyterminal fragment—that is, the back end of the APP protein—from the alpha site cleavage). This results in synaptoblastic signalling (from the Greek word for "germinate" or "produce")—making the very synapses (connections) in your brain that are needed for memories and overall cognition.

Now imagine that, in your second term as the president of MyBrainistan, things change. The treasury is no longer full, so you can no longer build and fix the infrastructure; invaders cross your borders, and so you deploy napalm to kill the advancing enemy; inflation has occurred during the good years, so it takes more from the treasury to fund any growth; and the weak infrastructure has led to severe pollution, so you must begin to clean up the pollution. This is what happens to your brain in Alzheimer's disease and in the years of cognitive decline that lead up to full-blown Alzheimer's: a lack of support from nutrients, hormones, and trophic factors requires

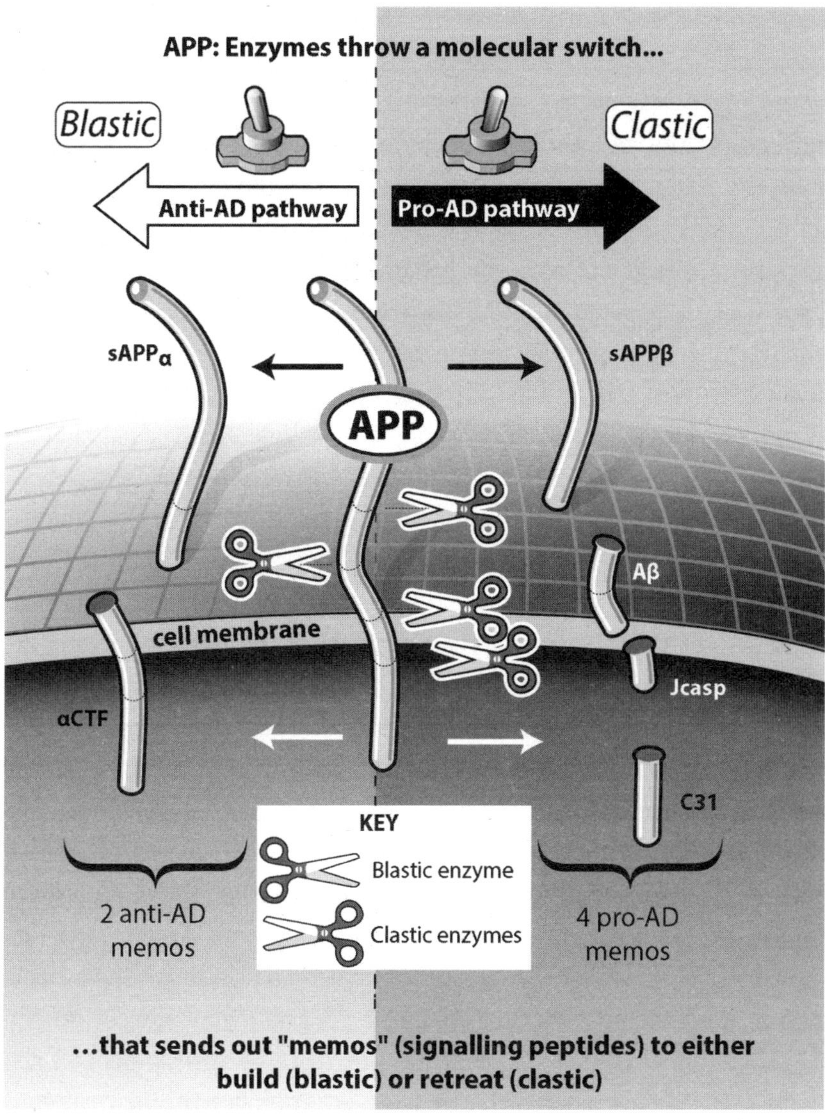

APP (amyloid precursor protein) is a molecular switch that may be cleaved to produce two fragments (peptides) that mediate synaptic growth and maintenance—synaptoblastic signalling—or, alternatively, to produce four fragments that mediate synaptic loss and neurite retraction—synaptoclastic signalling.

downsizing; microbes and inflammatory fragments are fought with the very amyloid that we associate with Alzheimer's disease,[3] which is very much like napalm; insulin resistance means that the insulin secreted is simply not as effective at keeping neurons alive (insulin is normally a potent supportive molecule for brain cells, and indeed, when you grow brain cells in a dish, insulin is essential for their health and vitality); and toxins such as mercury are bound up by the amyloid. In order to address these various insults, the APP is cleaved at different sites—not at the alpha site, which occurs when things are good, but rather at three sites, the beta, gamma, and caspase sites, producing 4 fragments: sAPPβ (soluble APP cleaved at the beta site), Aβ (the amyloid peptide we associate with Alzheimer's disease), Jcasp (the juxtamembrane piece that is cut at the caspase site, which is near the end of the protein), and C31 (the final 31 amino acids of the protein). As you can imagine, these four fragments—the "four horsemen" (by analogy with the Four Horsemen of the Apocalypse)—signal downsizing instead of growth. This is called synaptoclastic signalling (from the Greek word for breaking)—removing synapses.

Now let's go back to MyBrainistan one more time, and imagine that you have just been elected to a third term as president (yes, you actually can serve three terms in MyBrainistan!), but your country has split into North MyBrainistan and South MyBrainistan, so you may be the leader of either one—which one will it be? North MyBrainistan is a bellicose nation, one that has decided to put its resources into defence (and offence), whereas South MyBrainistan focuses its resources on research and development. Each, therefore, has specific advantages and disadvantages. That is the way your genetics influence your risk for Alzheimer's: although there are dozens of genes that play a role in your risk, the most common genetic risk is via a single, truly remarkable gene called ApoE, for apolipoprotein E. You have two copies—one from your mother and one from your father—and so you may end up with no copies of the high-risk version of ApoE, which is ApoE4, or with one copy, or with two. Nearly three-quarters of the population have zero copies (most of us are ApoE3/3, so we have two copies of ApoE3 and zero copies of ApoE4)—and our lifetime risk for Alzheimer's is about 9 per cent. However, about a quarter of us have a single copy of ApoE4, which carries a lifetime risk of approximately 30 per cent. Finally, a small number of us—only about 2 per cent, carry two copies, and our lifetime risk is very high—well over 50 per cent—so it is more likely that we will develop Alzheimer's than that we will avoid it. In part 2 of this book, you'll hear directly from Julie, who has two copies of ApoE4 and experienced significant symptoms of cognitive decline but has recovered so beautifully that she has been an invaluable contributor to this book.

If you carry ApoE4, you are the ruler of North MyBrainistan—you have put your resources into defence, and therefore you are resistant to invaders. Those of us who carry ApoE4 resist parasites and other infections, and therefore have an advantage in squalid conditions. In fact, it has been suggested that this ApoE4-related resistance was one of the major factors that allowed our ancient ancestors, the early hominids, to come down from the trees and walk along the savannah, puncturing their feet but limiting life-threatening infections. This fits well with the fact that ApoE4 was the primordial ApoE for hominids. Our ancestors were all ApoE4/4 until just 220,000 years ago—in other words, for 96 per cent of our evolution as hominids—when ApoE3 appeared. However, since we develop a brisk inflammatory response, which is great for eating raw meat and surviving wounds but takes its toll on our bodies over the years, we have increased risk for inflammation-related conditions such as Alzheimer's disease and cardiovascular disease.

If you do not carry ApoE4, you are the ruler of South MyBrainistan—you have put your resources into research and development (i.e. less inflammation, more efficient metabolism, more longevity). Those of us who do not carry ApoE4 are more susceptible to invasion by predators such as parasites, but if we can avoid these, our lower level of inflammation is associated with a lower risk for Alzheimer's and cardiovascular disease, and on average a few years longer lifespan.

You can see now that what we call Alzheimer's disease is actually *a protective response* to these different insults: microbes and other inflammagens, insulin resistance, toxins, and the loss of support by nutrients, hormones, and growth factors. It is a *protective downsizing programme.*

In other words, Alzheimer's is a brain in retreat—a *scorched earth retreat*—suffering its own collateral damage while pulling back, and its cognitive decline can be prevented or reversed by addressing the very factors contributing to this imbalance between the synaptoblastic signalling and the synaptoclastic signalling. Indeed, we recently

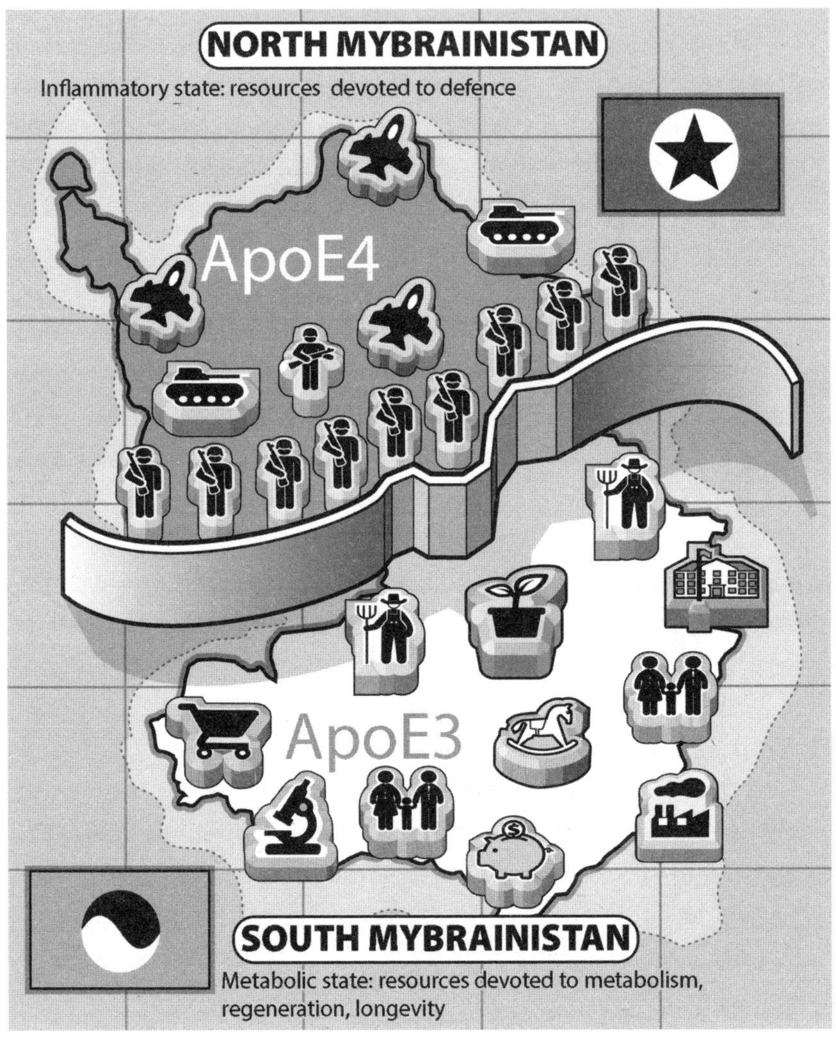

North MyBrainistan vs. South MyBrainistan. North MyBrainistan puts its resources into defence and warfare, and thus is analogous to ApoE4-positive cells and individuals; whereas South MyBrainistan puts its resources into research and development, and thus is analogous to ApoE4-negative individuals.

published a medical paper describing a hundred patients, some with Alzheimer's and others with pre-Alzheimer's, all of whom showed documented, quantified improvement.[4] Not only was cognition improved, but some patients also underwent quantitative EEGs (these measure brain-wave speed, which typically slows with dementia), which also showed amelioration, or volumetric MRI scans (which detect shrinkage in various brain regions), which also demonstrated improvement. This is not to say that every person who undertakes the protocol responds, because that is not the case, but we have documented unprecedented improvements, and most important, *sustained* improvements, by using this targeted, programmatic approach.

So how exactly does one go about translating these concepts into an actionable plan that each one of us can use? That's precisely what this book is all about. You shall read all of the details necessary to adopt your own personalized, targeted programme to enhance cognition, whether you choose to do so with your doctor or health coach or other health professional or on your own.

In my previous book, *The End of Alzheimer's,* I outlined the scientific research that led to our development of the ReCODE protocol, and described the first version of ReCODE and its success. In the more than eight years since the first patient began this protocol in 2012, we have learned a tremendous amount about what it takes to optimize the approach and all of the components; we have trained over 1,500 doctors from ten countries and all over the United States; the book has appeared in thirty-one languages; and we have received over 40,000 questions and comments. One of the most common suggestions was that we provide further details, as well as updates, on the protocol. Therefore, the current book is replete with details, websites, resources, work-arounds for roadblocks, and new information, all with the goal of giving each of us the best chance for cognitive success and with the goal of reducing the global burden of dementia and enhancing global cognition for those who do not suffer from dementia.

So let's get started with the basics. If you are experiencing or are at risk for cognitive decline, or if your goal is to enhance your cognition, then you simply want to increase all of the contributors to your synapto*blastic* signalling and reduce all of the contributors to your synapto*clastic* signalling. To do this, you'll want to know about the potential contributors:

- **Do you have ongoing *inflammation*?** This is easy to check. You'll want to know your hs-CRP (high sensitivity C-reactive protein). You can also get an idea from your A/G ratio (albumin to globulin ratio). If inflammation is present, you'll want to know *why*—what is causing it? This is critical, since your best results will be achieved by removing the cause or causes of the inflammation. Beware—although some of us have symptoms of inflammation such as arthritis or inflammatory bowel disease, many of us have no symptoms until cognitive decline or heart attack or stroke occurs. One of the most common causes of chronic inflammation is leaky gut—the leaking of bacteria, fragments of bacteria, other microbes, incompletely digested food molecules, and other molecules, which enter the bloodstream and incite an inflammatory response. Another common cause is metabolic syndrome, which is a combination of hypertension (high blood pressure), high cholesterol, high glucose (diabetes or pre-diabetes), and inflammation, associated with a diet high in sugars or other simple carbohydrates.[5] A third common cause is poor dentition—periodontitis (inflammation around the teeth) or gingivitis (inflammation of the gums).
- **Do you have *insulin resistance*?** Also easy to check—you'll want to know your fasting insulin level, and you can get some complementary information from your haemoglobin A1c and fasting glucose. If diabetes runs in your family, you may wish to add one final test—the most sensitive—which is an oral glucose tolerance test with insulin levels.
- **Do you have an optimal level of *nutrients, hormones,* and *trophic factors* (growth factors)?** We can determine most of these with simple blood tests such as vitamin B_{12}, vitamin D,

homocysteine, and free T3, all part of the "cognoscopy" that we recommend for everyone who is 45 or over. While there are not yet good clinical tests to determine brain levels of most trophic factors, we nonetheless have methods to improve these. Finally, it's very helpful to make sure that your oxygen and glucose are not dropping too low at night, and you can check your oxygen with an oximeter (which your doctor can lend you or you can purchase) and your glucose with a glucose monitor, such as the FreeStyle Libre by Abbott Labs.

Table 1 lists the target levels of various nutrients, hormones, and toxins. Your health practitioner may wish to order additional tests, based on your presentation and results. (In the UK, you may have to pay for these tests since many are not available through the NHS.)

TABLE 1. TARGET VALUES OF BIOCHEMICAL AND PHYSIOLOGICAL TESTS ASSOCIATED WITH COGNITION.

	CRITICAL TESTS	TARGET VALUES	COMMENTS
Inflammation, protection, and vascular	hs-CRP	<0.9 mg/dL	Systemic inflammation
	Fasting insulin Fasting glucose Haemoglobin A1c HOMA-IR	3.0–5.0 µIU/mL* 70–90 mg/dL 4.0–5.3% <1.2	Glycotoxicity and insulin resistance markers
	Body mass index (BMI)	18.5–25	Weight (lbs) µ 703/ height (inches)^2
	Waist to hip ratio (women) Waist to hip ratio (men)	<0.85 <0.9	
	Homocysteine	≤ 7µmol/L	Reflects methylation, inflammation, and detox
	Vitamin B_6 Vitamin B_9 (folate) Vitamin B_{12}	25–50 mcg/L (PP) 10–25 ng/mL 500–1500 pg/mL	Improve methylation and reduce homocysteine

(Table continues)

	CRITICAL TESTS	TARGET VALUES	COMMENTS
	Vitamin C Vitamin D Vitamin E	1.3–2.5 mg/dL 50–80 ng/mL 12–20 mg/L	
	Omega-6 to omega-3 ratio	1:1 to 4:1 (beware that <0.5:1 may be associated with bleeding tendency)	Ratio of inflammatory to anti-inflammatory omega fats
	Omega-3 index	≥10% (ApoE4+) 8–10% (ApoE4-)	Proportion of anti-inflammatory omega-3 fats
	AA to EPA ratio (arachidonic acid to eicosapentaenoic acid ratio)	<3:1	Ratio of inflammatory AA to anti-inflammatory EPA
	A/G ratio (albumin to globulin ratio) Albumin	≥1.8:1 4.5–5.4 g/dL	Markers of inflammation, liver health, and amyloid clearance
	LDL-P Small dense LDL Oxidized LDL	700–1200 nM <28 mg/dL <60 ng/mL	LDL-P is LDL particle number
	Total cholesterol HDL cholesterol Triglycerides TG to HDL ratio	150–200 mg/dL >50 mg/dL <150 mg/dL <1.1	
	CoQ10	1.1–2.2 mcg/mL	Affected by cholesterol level
	Glutathione	>250 mcg/mL (>814 μM)	Major antioxidant and detoxicant
	Leaky gut, leaky blood-brain barrier, gluten sensitivity, autoantibodies	Negative	
Minerals	RBC-magnesium	5.2–6.5 mg/dL	Preferable to serum magnesium
	Copper Zinc	90–110 mcg/dL 90–110 mcg/dL	
	Selenium	110–150 ng/mL	
	Potassium	4.5–5.5 mEq/L	
Trophic support	Vitamin D	50–80 ng/mL	(25OH-D3)
	Oestradiol Progesterone	50–250 pg/mL 1–20 ng/dL (P)	Women; age dependent

	CRITICAL TESTS	TARGET VALUES	COMMENTS
	Pregnenolone Cortisol (AM) DHEA-S (women) DHEA-S (men)	100–250 ng/dL 10–18 mcg/dL 100–380 mcg/dL 150–500 mcg/dL	Age dependent
	Testosterone Free testosterone	500–1000 ng/dL 18–26 pg/ml	Men; age dependent
	Free T3 Free T4 Reverse T3 TSH Free T3 to reverse T3 Anti-thyroglobulin antibodies Anti-TPO	3.2–4.2 pg/mL 1.3–1.8 ng/dL <20 ng/dL <2.0 mIU/L >0.02:1 Negative Negative	mIU/L = μIU/mL
Toxin-related	Mercury Lead Arsenic Cadmium	<5 mcg/L <2 mcg/dL <7 mcg/L <2.5 mcg/dL	Heavy metals
	Mercury Tri-Test	<50th percentile	Hair, blood, urine
	Organic toxins (urine)	Negative	Benzene, toluene, etc.
	Glyphosate (urine)	<1.0 mcg/g creatinine	Herbicide
	Copper to zinc ratio	0.8–1.2:1	Higher ratios associated with dementia
	C4a TGF-β1 MMP-9 MSH	<2830 ng/mL <2380/mL 85–332 ng/mL 35–81 pg/mL	Associated with inflammatory response
	Urinary mycotoxins	Negative	May include contributions from inhalation, ingestion, and infection
	BUN Creatinine	<20 mg/dL <1.0 mg/dL	Reflects kidney function
	AST ALT	<25 U/L <25 U/L	Reflects liver damage
	VCS (visual contrast sensitivity)	Pass	Failure associated with biotoxin exposure
	ERMI test	<2	Mould index from building

(Table continues)

	CRITICAL TESTS	TARGET VALUES	COMMENTS
	HERTSMI-2 test	<11	Index of most toxic moulds
Pathogen-related	CD57	60–360 cells/μL	Reduced with Lyme
	MARCoNS	Negative	
	Antibodies to tick-borne pathogens	Negative	*Borrelia, Babesia, Bartonella, Ehrlichia, Anaplasma*
	Antibodies to *Herpes* family viruses	Negative	HSV-1, HSV-2, HHV-6, VZV, EBV, CMV
Neurophysiology	Peak alpha frequency on quantitative EEG	8.9–11 Hz	Slows with cognitive decline; useful for following progress
	P300b on evoked response testing	<450 ms	Delayed with cognitive decline; useful for following progress
Other tests	MoCA (Montreal Cognitive Assessment)	28–30	
	Nocturnal oxygen saturation (SpO_2)	96–98%	Affected by living at high altitude
	AHI (apnoea-hypopnea index)	<5 events per hour	>5 indicates sleep apnoea
	Oral DNA	Negative for pathogens	*P. gingivalis, T. denticola*, etc.
	Stool analysis	No pathogens or dysbiosis	
	ImmuKnow (CD4 function, indicated by ATP production)	≥525 ng/mL	Indicates function of helper cells of the cellular arm of the adaptive immune system

Abbreviations: AA, arachidonic acid; AHI, apnoea-hypopnea index; ALT, alanine aminotransferase; AST, aspartate aminotransferase; BMI, body mass index; BUN, blood urea nitrogen; C4a, complement split product 4a; CD57, cluster of differentiation 57; CMV, cytomegalovirus; CoQ10, coenzyme Q10 (ubiquinone); DHEA-S, dehydroepiandrosterone sulfate; DNA, deoxyribonucleic acid; EBV, Epstein-Barr virus; EEG, electroencephalogram; EPA, eicosapentaenoic acid; ERMI, Environmental Protection Agency relative mould index; HERTSMI-2, Health Effects Roster of Type-Specific Formers of Mycotoxins and Inflammagens – 2nd Version;

HHV-6, *Human herpesvirus* 6 (A and B); HOMA-IR, homeostatic model assessment of insulin resistance; hs-CRP, high-sensitivity C-reactive protein; HSV-1, *Herpes simplex virus* 1; HSV-2, *Herpes simplex virus* 2; LDL, low-density lipoprotein; MARCoNS, multiple antibiotic-resistant coagulase negative *Staphylococcus*; MMP-9, matrix metalloproteinase-9; MoCA, Montreal cognitive assessment; MSH alpha-melanocyte stimulating hormone; P300b, positive wave at 300 milliseconds (event-related potential), component B; PP, pyridoxal phosphate; RBC, red blood cell; SpO2, peripheral capillary oxygen saturation; T3, triiodothyronine; T4, thyroxine; TG, triglycerides; TGF-β1, transforming growth factor beta-1; TPO, thyroid peroxidase; TSH, thyroid-stimulating hormone; VZV, varicella zoster virus.
***For those who are insulin sensitive, with fasting glucose <90 mg/dL, fasting insulin of <3.0 is still in a healthy range.**

- **Do you have *specific pathogens***—microbes that cause your brain to respond by producing the amyloid of Alzheimer's disease? These may be spirochetes (spiral-shaped bacteria, which are relatives of the organism that causes syphilis) such as *Borrelia* (the Lyme disease spirochete), viruses such as *Herpes* (especially *Herpes simplex-1*, HSV-1, or HHV-6A), parasites such as *Babesia* (a relative of the malaria parasite, one that many of us contract from tick bites), bacteria such as *Porphyromonas gingivalis* (which is associated with poor dental hygiene), or other pathogens. While there is no simple way currently to find out, if for any given person, these pathogens are hiding out in amyloid plaques in our brains, we can check blood tests to determine if we've been exposed to these microbes, and therefore get an idea about which are most likely contributing.

- **Are you immunosuppressed?** If your immune system is not working well, then these very infectious agents—viruses, moulds, bacteria, parasites, and spirochetes described above—are able to survive in your body and gain access to your brain. Your brain then protects itself by making—you guessed it—the amyloid that we associate with Alzheimer's. So it's helpful to know if your immune system is indeed functioning optimally, and again, some simple blood tests such as immunoglobulins, the ImmuKnow test, and lymphocyte subsets can let us know.

Lola is a 58-year-old woman who had six years of progressive loss in her ability to organize, calculate, find words, and read, all of which began with a bout of depression. Her MoCA score was 0. Her MRI showed generalized atrophy, and a diagnosis of Alzheimer's disease was made. She was ApoE4-negative. Her ImmuKnow test, which assesses a key part of the immune system (cellular immune system helper cells), was markedly abnormal at 206 ng/ml (normal is >525), and her urine revealed extremely high levels (25 to 100 times the typical toxic level) of three mould toxins that suppress the immune system: ochratoxin A, zearalenone, and mycophenolic acid.

- **Do you have exposure to toxins,** such as mercury or mycotoxins (mould-produced toxins)? These can be identified readily by blood and urine testing, and removing these toxins can be very beneficial to cognition.

There are several ways to obtain these tests: your doctor can order them (in the UK you may well have to seek out a private clinic or practitioner), you can seek out a practitioner trained in our ReCODE protocol, or you can get these directly from the website, MyRecodeReport.com. Once you have an idea about your risk factors, you can address each one. In chapter 2, I'll describe how to target these various contributors to cognitive decline successfully, and then in chapter 3, explain the most important points we have learned in years of working with patients with cognitive decline, using ReCODE.

CHAPTER 2

An Inconvenient Sleuth

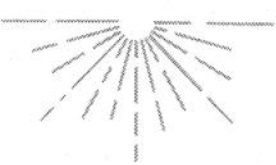

Mediocrity excels at but one endeavor:

protecting its own interests.

—R. F. LOEB

THE FAMOUS BASKETBALL COACH, player, and executive Pat Riley exhorted his players to adopt the following attitude when the game is on the line: "Imagine that your head is underwater and you will not be able to breathe again unless you win." That is some motivation indeed! And it is the attitude we must have about Alzheimer's disease as well, and in fact about neurodegenerative diseases as a whole—these have all been untreatable terminal illnesses, and if we do not approach them as a societal emergency we will see 13 million demented Americans by 2050, their families destroyed, Medicare bankrupt, and a multi-trillion-dollar global burden of dementia (In an already-overburdened NHS in the UK this issue will have similar results.). Yet our "standard of care" is to treat without determining the cause of or contributors to Alzheimer's, to limit our treatment to a drug or two, to avoid targeted programmes of treatment, to refuse clinical trials of multifaceted therapeutics, and to repeat the same old tired, ineffective approaches again and again. Where is the innovation? Where is the inspiration? Perhaps we need a pep talk from Pat Riley?

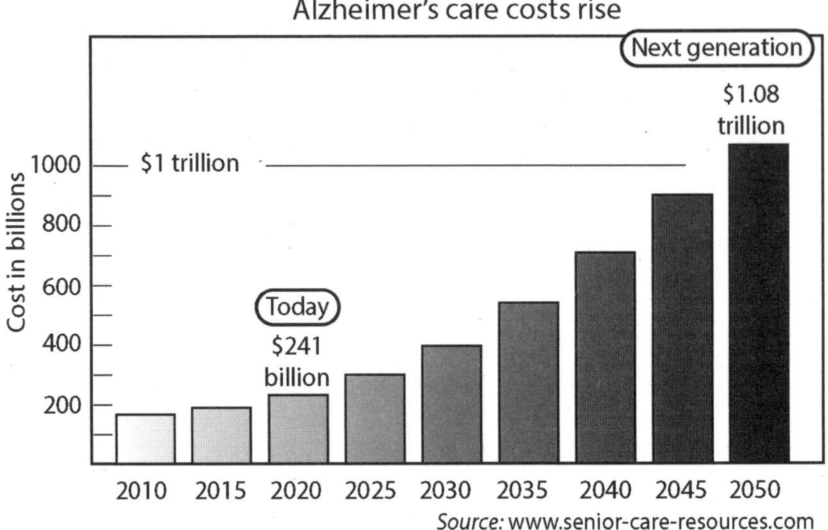

Alzheimer's costs are staggering, and they are on the rise.

Therefore, please don't be concerned if you get your tests, take them to your doctor, and he or she is sceptical. If you ask your doctor to obtain these tests, don't be surprised if he or she brushes you off with an all-knowing smile or even a look of disdain. As they say, "An expert is someone who does not want to be told anything new in his or her field of expertise." This personalized approach to cognitive decline is a twenty-first-century approach, not yet in practice by the vast majority of doctors. As one neurologist said, "I wouldn't order these tests because I would not know how to interpret them." Another doctor said, "These tests don't tell you whether you have Alzheimer's or not." True; what they tell you is *why* you have cognitive decline (or risk for decline)—what all of the contributors are. Determining if you have Alzheimer's does not help you to avoid it or reverse it; determining *why* is the key. Most people who already have Alzheimer's disease or MCI (mild cognitive impairment, the harbinger of Alzheimer's) or SCI (subjective cognitive impairment, which precedes MCI) turn out to have between ten and twenty-five contributors, and these are identified by the tests so that each can be addressed therapeutically.

So let's summarize the treatment and prevention plans here, and then I'll include the various details in the Handbook sections that follow. The idea is straightforward: practitioners have attempted to treat dementia for thousands of years without knowing what *caused* it or contributed to it, but now, for the first time, we can actually treat the underlying mechanisms. Of course, when Ayurvedic doctors treated dementia thousands of years ago, they did not refer to it as Alzheimer's disease—it was not until 1906 and 1907 that Dr Alois Alzheimer published his famous papers—but Ayurvedic doctors clearly described and attempted to treat dementia, and what we now call Alzheimer's disease is the most common syndrome of dementia.

Twenty years ago, our laboratory research led us to identify the APP switch I described earlier, and when we began to look at what factors flip this switch towards the Alzheimer's side—the synaptoclastic side—we found that there are different groups of factors, and thus there are actually different *types* of Alzheimer's disease. These types align with the very tests I listed in chapter 1:

- **Type 1 Alzheimer's is *inflammatory*, or hot,** so if you have ongoing inflammation, you are increasing your risk for Alzheimer's disease. In fact, one of the major mediators of the inflammatory response is called NFκB (nuclear factor kappa-light-chain enhancer of activated B cells), and this increases the production of the very molecular scissors that produce the amyloid from APP, so there really is a direct link from inflammation to Alzheimer's.

- **Type 2 Alzheimer's is *atrophic*, or cold,** so if you have suboptimal levels of nutrients, hormones, or trophic factors (cell growth factors like NGF, nerve growth factor), you are increasing your risk for Alzheimer's disease. Simply put, you do not have the support necessary to maintain the five hundred trillion (500,000,000,000,000) synaptic connections in your brain. On the positive side, optimizing those same nutrients, hormones, and trophic factors offers you the best chance for optimizing your memory and overall cognitive function.

- **Type 1.5 Alzheimer's is *glycotoxic*, or sweet,** so if you have high blood sugar or high fasting insulin, as 80 million Americans do, you are increasing your risk for Alzheimer's disease. We call this type 1.5 because it has features of both type 1 and type 2: chronic inflammation (type 1) occurs because the glucose actually attaches to many of your proteins, like remoras to a shark, causing an inflammatory response to these altered proteins (such as haemoglobin A1c, which is haemoglobin with a glucose stuck to it, and hundreds of other proteins). Reduced trophic support (type 2) occurs because your insulin—which is a critical growth factor for your brain cells—has been high chronically, causing your cells to lose their sensitivity to insulin.

Sammy is a 68-year-old man who developed progressive memory loss. On testing, he was unable to name the day, month, or year. His MoCA score was only 12 out of 30 (the average for full-blown Alzheimer's disease is 16.2, so he was already more advanced than the typical Alzheimer's patient), and his MRI showed brain atrophy (shrinkage). His body mass index (BMI, which should be 19–25 for a male) was 31.7, indicating obesity. His fasting insulin was high at 14, his fasting glucose was high at 102, and his haemoglobin A1c was high at 5.8, indicating that he had pre-diabetes. His inflammatory and toxic markers were negative. A diagnosis of type 1.5 Alzheimer's disease (glycotoxic) was made.

- **Type 3 Alzheimer's disease is *toxic*, or vile,** so if you have exposure to toxins such as mercury, toluene, or mycotoxins (toxins made by certain moulds such as *Stachybotrys* and *Penicillium*), then you are increasing your risk for Alzheimer's disease. Since we are exposed to hundreds of toxins—from the mercury in seafood and dental amalgams to air pollution to the benzene in paraffin candles to the trichothecenes from the black mould growing in water-damaged homes, and on and on—we all experience this risk to a greater or lesser degree, so the key is to minimize exposure, identify the toxins to which we are exposed, and increase excretion and metabolism of the toxins.

- **Type 4 Alzheimer's disease is *vascular*, or pale,** so if you have cardiovascular disease, you are at increased risk for Alzheimer's disease. Indeed, vascular leakiness represents one of the earliest changes identified in Alzheimer's disease.
- **Type 5 Alzheimer's disease is *traumatic*, or dazed,** so if you have a history of head trauma—whether from a traffic accident or a fall or even repeated minor head injuries during sports—you are at increased risk for Alzheimer's disease.

You can see from these different types of Alzheimer's disease we identified, and the causes of each one, that virtually all of us are at some risk for Alzheimer's, and indeed, this is one of the reasons that it is such a common disease. With the many toxins to which we are exposed, the processed foods, the high-carbohydrate and unhealthy fat content of the SAD (standard American diet and that of the UK), the leaky gut so many of us have, and the lipid abnormalities ("cholesterol," although the cholesterol itself is actually not the problem), most of us have a significant risk for Alzheimer's disease. The good news is that nearly all of us can avoid or reverse the problem, now that we understand the contributors. To do that, we simply need to address the underlying drivers of the disease process—it's like patching thirty-six holes in your roof—the same ones that we profile in the subtyping described above, and the earlier we do this, the easier it is to achieve success. The overall goal of treatment can be summarized as *removal*, *resilience*, and *rebuilding*: *removal* of the exposures contributing to cognitive decline, *resilience* resulting from optimal health support, and *rebuilding* of the neural network. Here's how we do that:

- **First, we want to address insulin resistance**—in other words, we want to become insulin sensitive. Insulin is a hormone made in your pancreas, and it has several different jobs. It is a major player in metabolism—it binds to its receptor, which induces glucose entry and fat storage, thus reducing the glucose in your blood. However, it is also a key growth factor for neurons, so losing sensitivity is a very significant problem.

Virtually everyone with Alzheimer's has indeed lost sensitivity to insulin and become resistant, at least in the brain.[1] Eighty million Americans are insulin resistant and this is an increasing problem throughout the developed and developing world. When your insulin has been elevated for years—just as it has for most of us who have eaten a standard Western diet—the molecular composition of the signalling pathway actually changes, its phosphorylation pattern modified. So it's as if you were living for years in such strong sunlight that you kept very dark sunglasses on at all times; with the light now dim, you cannot see anything. Indeed, the insulin-resistant cells no longer respond appropriately to normal levels of insulin, which means that your neurons no longer have the support needed for survival and interaction.

This insulin resistance is the same phenomenon that occurs in type 2 diabetes, so Alzheimer's and diabetes are relatives. Indeed, some have suggested that Alzheimer's disease be called "type 3 diabetes,"[2] but as you can see from the many other contributors to cognitive decline (pathogens, toxins, etc.), it is not quite that simple.

Restoring insulin sensitivity can be achieved by combining the KetoFLEX 12/3 diet and lifestyle (explained in detail in chapter 4), optimizing key nutrients such as zinc (which is involved in multiple steps of insulin secretion and effect), exercising regularly, reducing stress, treating sleep apnoea if present, and if needed, taking a supplement such as berberine, cinnamon, alpha-lipoic acid, or chromium picolinate. Virtually all of us can become insulin sensitive using this approach.

In order to give you the best results for your insulin sensitivity and glucose levels, there is a convenient new method that helps to optimize the various steps you are doing. It is called continuous glucose monitoring (CGM), and you can do this with FreeStyle Libre, a wearable patch for your upper arm that monitors your glucose continuously for two weeks, so that you can see what may be spiking your glucose and what may be leading to glucose that is too low (hypoglycaemia). Both spikes and dips may contribute to cognitive decline, so smoothing those out is an effective approach.

- **Second, we want to get into ketosis**—in other words, burn fat. Alzheimer's is associated with reduced ability to utilize glucose in the brain, in an L pattern, affecting the temporal lobe (running horizontally along your temple) and the parietal lobe (running vertically up behind your ear). For many, this decreased glucose utilization, which is driven by the insulin resistance described immediately above, is ongoing for more than a decade before cognitive decline. Ketones can bridge the energy gap, and have been shown to improve cognitive decline.[3] When you combine the ability to utilize ketones with the insulin sensitivity mentioned, you have a powerful weapon against dementia—*metabolic flexibility*, that is, the ability to burn either ketones or glucose. We have found, after studying many patients on our protocol, that those who develop ketosis in the range of 1.0 to 4.0 millimolar beta-hydroxybutyrate (BHB) level tend to do the best, although if you are without any symptoms yet, it may be enough to be in the 0.5 to 1.0 range. You can use a simple, inexpensive ketone meter to measure your ketones (details in the Handbook section in part 2).

  Getting into ketosis is straightforward in theory (see the details in the Handbook section), but not as easy in practice, since the insulin resistance that is so prevalent in Alzheimer's and pre-Alzheimer's actually inhibits fat metabolism and thus prevents our production of the very ketones we need (as well as perpetuating sugar craving, thus creating a metabolic dementia cycle). In order to terminate the cycle, we recommend a three-pronged approach: a plant-rich, fibre-rich, low-carbohydrate diet, high in healthy fats; fasting overnight for at least 12 hours; and exercising regularly. Your body will respond by breaking down fats, turning them into ketones. Many people find that just getting into ketosis gives them more mental clarity, improves their memory, enhances alertness and focus, and gives them more energy.

There are two caveats to the advantages of ketosis: one is *how* you get there, and the other is *when* you get there. For *how* you get there, many people think about bacon immediately when they hear the word *ketosis*, but the brain-friendly ketosis is plant-rich, not bacon-rich! (Bacon has its own toxicity issues, in part from its toxic nitrate preservatives, toxins introduced in feed, and its saturated fat, among other liabilities.) In the Handbook section of this book, you'll have details of the optimal diet and nutrition for cognition and reversal of cognitive decline, which is called KetoFLEX 12/3.

One more point on *how* you get into ketosis: for many of us, we'll be able to produce ketones from the burning of our own fat (which is preferable), but for some of us (especially those who are very thin—see pages 97–98 "Excessive Weight Loss"— and thus have little body fat to burn), we'll need some help initially to produce enough ketones to meet the needs of our brains. We can get this help from taking MCT oil (medium-chain triglyceride oil) or from taking ketones themselves, either as ketone salts (e.g. Perfect Keto) or ketone esters (e.g. KetoneAid). Each of these helpers has its advantages and disadvantages. If you take MCT oil (for example, as caprylic acid, or less desirably, as I'll explain later, coconut oil), you can take up to 1 tablespoon three times per day, and this should increase your ketone level to the optimal range. However, since MCT is a saturated fat, it may increase your cholesterol, so it's a good idea to check your LDL-P (LDL particle number; target = 700–1200 nM), which is a much more important indicator of vascular risk than total cholesterol is.

Now, about *when* you get into ketosis: if you take ketone salts or ketone esters, these will increase your ketone level rapidly, but they have a relatively short-term effect of a few hours. The ketone esters don't taste very good, but increase ketone level more markedly than the ketone salts, which are more palatable but do not cause the major bump in ketone level. The advantage of these "exogenous ketones" is that they do not cause the increase in cholesterol that may occur with MCT oil.

Irene is a 69-year-old woman who developed trouble with organizing, calculating, following directions, and remembering. She was ApoE4-positive, and scored only 18 out of 30 on the MoCA test, indicating that she had Alzheimer's disease or late-stage MCI (mild cognitive impairment) on the brink of Alzheimer's disease. Her tests indicated both type 2 (atrophic) and type 3 (toxic) Alzheimer's. She began the ReCODE protocol and included ketone salts in order to raise her ketone level to 1.5 millimolar BHB, which she and her husband checked with a ketone meter. Over the next nine months, her MoCA score increased from 18 to 27, her symptoms improved, and she has sustained her improvement over the past year.

- **Third, we want to optimize all nutrient, hormone, and trophic (growth factor) support.** In other words, we want to create resilience, optimize our immune systems, support our mitochondria, and begin to rebuild our brains' synaptic networks. One of the major unanswered questions is how long—how late into the process of Alzheimer's disease—can we rebuild? How late can we still re-establish the lost connections in our brains? Well, you can think of the loss of functional connections in Alzheimer's as being something like the loss of mobile phone connection. The most mild problem is that the signal is poor, but both phones are still working fine. The more severe problem is that the phone is actually turned off, so you won't be able to call until the phone is turned back on. The most severe problem is that the phone is actually destroyed. In an analogous fashion, the early changes of Alzheimer's jam the communication between brain cells without destroying the physical connections or killing the cells; as the disease progresses, the connections are lost but the cells are still alive; and finally, the neurons themselves perish, often by suicide.

Therefore, it is perhaps not surprising that we are finding that when someone is in the earliest stages, it is very common to achieve and sustain improvement, whereas the longer the disease progression continues and the more severe it is, the more difficult it is to turn it around. So what is needed for rebuilding when so many synapses and neurons have been lost? Stem cells? Trophic factors? Stimulation by light, electricity, or magnetism? We have indeed seen some improvement with stem cells, and this represents a very promising area for therapeutics. In fact, there are ongoing trials of stem cells for Alzheimer's disease. However, these trials typically use stem cells alone, without addressing what is actually causing the cognitive decline, so it may turn out to be a bit like trying to, in effect, rebuild the house as it is burning down. In other words, we need to determine whether stem cell treatments work better after the various factors that are contributing to cognitive decline are targeted and the progression halted.

No matter where we are in the development of cognitive decline, we want to optimize the nutrients, hormones, and trophic factors (growth factors) supporting the brain. Indeed, low levels of many of these—such as vitamin B_1 (thiamine), vitamin B_{12}, vitamin D, testosterone, oestrogen, and nerve growth factor—are associated with cognitive decline. So we want to optimize all of these biochemicals that provide support—not just bring them to the low end of "normal," which is often suboptimal, but ensure there is enough for the best functioning of the nervous system. These include the fat-derived ketones described earlier, the insulin to support the insulin sensitivity described earlier, and other nutrients such as the B vitamins, vitamin C, vitamin D, vitamin E, vitamin K_2, omega-3 fats (such as DHA, the docosahexaenoic acid utilized for synapse formation), choline and other neurotransmitter precursors, key metals such as zinc, magnesium, copper, and selenium, and other nutrients. How to get these will be described in detail in the sections on the KetoFLEX 12/3 diet (chapter 4) and on supplements (chapter 21).

In addition to nutrients, we want to make sure to optimize our hormone levels, since these are critical for making and maintaining synapses. For many of us, optimal nutrition and lifestyle will lead to optimal hormone production, but for others of us, we'll want to support our brain function by achieving the most effective levels of thyroid, pregnenolone, oestradiol, progesterone, testosterone, DHEA (dehydroepiandrosterone, a stress hormone), and cortisol. Beyond these hormones, although the jury is still out, there is scientific rationale to suggest that increasing growth hormone, which can be achieved using supplements called secretagogues, may support synaptic rebuilding. A trial using growth hormone as a monotherapy failed to slow decline in 2008,[4] but in that trial none of the other potential contributors to cognitive decline was addressed, so this approach has never been tested as part of a targeted, multicomponent protocol.

Finally, in addition to nutrients and hormones, support for our 500 trillion brain synapses is provided by neurotrophic factors such as NGF (nerve growth factor), BDNF (brain-derived neurotrophic factor), and NT-3 (neurotrophin-3). We can increase some of these by various means, such as exercise (which has been shown to increase BDNF) or brain training or by taking whole coffee fruit extract or 7,8-dihydroxyflavones (which can substitute for BDNF by activating its receptor, as described by my colleague, Professor Keqiang Ye).[5]

- **Fourth, we want to resolve and prevent inflammation.** The amyloid that we associate with Alzheimer's disease is actually a part of the inflammatory response; as noted earlier, it is protective, killing pathogens such as bacteria and fungi. So as long as there is ongoing inflammation, you can expect ongoing amyloid production and Alzheimer's. What we want to do, therefore, is to *remove the cause* of the inflammation, *resolve* the inflammation, then *prevent* future inflammation.

  The most common cause of chronic inflammation is leaky gut (increased permeability of the small intestine to bacteria, bacterial fragments, and food particles), which can be caused by stress, sugar, alcohol, processed foods, aspirin and related anti-inflammatories (e.g. ibuprofen), soft drinks, PPIs (proton-pump inhibitors used to treat acid reflux, or heartburn), and other damaging agents, so we want to know our gut status. We can do this with the GI Effects test from Genova Diagnostics, or with the Cyrex Array 2, or the Vibrant Wellness Gut Zoomer, or with other gut tests. Cyrex testing in the UK is available through Regenerus Labs, and only a healthcare professional registered in the UK or Ireland can order these tests.

  For the many of us with leaky gut or with dysbiosis (a change in the normal microbes in our gut, which can occur if we have taken antibiotics, for example), there are several ways to heal the gut and then bring our microbiomes back to normal. After eliminating the causes listed above (such as processed foods), some like to use bone broth (which you can buy or make yourself), while others like slippery elm or DGL (which is a licorice derivative available over the counter) or ProButyrate or powdered collagen or L-glutamine. After your gut has healed for a few weeks, probiotics (from fermented foods such as kimchi, sauerkraut, or in capsules) and prebiotics (from foods such as Mexican yam, Jerusalem artichoke, raw leeks, raw garlic, banana, or in capsules with the probiotics) help get your gut microbiome back to optimal. This is a critical goal, because good gut bacteria and other microorganisms work tirelessly for your health, aiding your digestion, preventing disease-related bacteria and fungi, supporting a healthy immune system, reducing inflammation, and helping with detoxification.

If you have inflammation but no leaky gut, then you may have periodontitis (infections around your teeth) or gingivitis (infection of your gums) from suboptimal dental hygiene, or an infection of a root canal in your mouth, or a chronic sinus infection, or infection with a chronic pathogen such as *Borrelia* (Lyme disease), or metabolic syndrome (insulin resistance, high blood pressure, high triglycerides, and inflammation, often accompanied by obesity), or exposure to inflammatory substances from air pollution or mould toxins (mycotoxins).

Once the cause of the inflammation has been determined, this should be removed, then the inflammation should be resolved, for which you can use specialized pro-resolving mediators (SPM) or high doses (1 to 3 grams) of omega-3 fatty acids. After the inflammation is resolved, which may take several weeks, you should prevent further inflammation. There are several excellent anti-inflammatories for this, such as curcumin, fish oil or krill oil (omega-3 fats), ginger, and cinnamon (and for those of us with low pregnenolone, simply bringing this back to normal is anti-inflammatory). Please avoid aspirin and other non-steroidal anti-inflammatory drugs (NSAIDs) if at all possible, since they cause leaky gut, erode the stomach lining, and may damage your kidneys or liver.

- **Fifth, we want to treat chronic pathogens.** In other words, if you have a chronic undiagnosed infection, it is likely to be contributing to cognitive decline, so let's identify it and target it (and similarly, anyone who has begun to improve can expect a setback when an infection occurs, such as the flu or a urinary tract infection). The old-fashioned view of infections is that you are either infected—"sick"—or uninfected—"well." However, it has turned out to be much more complicated than that, and we'll delve into the microbiome and the microbes that affect cognition in chapter 20. The bottom line is that we are all living, every day, with more than a thousand different species of microbes! In our mouths, large intestines, and sinuses; on our skin; and somewhat unbelievably, apparently even in our brains! The brains of patients with Alzheimer's disease may harbour bacteria, viruses, spirochetes (spiral bacteria, such as those causing Lyme disease), fungi, or parasites. It is the protective response to these that causes the very changes we call Alzheimer's disease, so we want to target such agents so that our brains will not have to produce the protective amyloid, since that same protective agent leads to the downsizing of our neural connections that causes our cognitive decline.

Now that we understand that we live with microbes every day—they are part of us, which gives a whole new meaning to the term I!—it becomes clear that optimal health is not simply about getting rid of a bad germ. Instead, it is about getting the right balance of germs. The good germs actually help keep the bad germs at bay (as well as working with you to optimize your metabolism), so you must be very careful about taking antibiotics and wiping out both good and bad indiscriminately. This is why it is so important to have a healthy gut microbiome, and the same goes for your mouth, sinuses, and skin. It is not yet clear whether there constitutes a normal microbiome for the brain or whether the reality is that any organism in the brain will always be abnormal—this is currently being researched. As noted earlier however, numerous pathogens have been identified in Alzheimer's brains, and these same are absent in the vast majority of non-Alzheimer's brains, so there is either infection or an alteration in the microbiome of the brain in Alzheimer's disease. Whichever way it turns out, we need to target these contributors to Alzheimer's, since as long as they are present, the brain will continue to produce the amyloid in an attempt to combat them, and this will contribute to the progression of Alzheimer's disease.

It is somewhat surprising to think of harbouring infectious agents in the body for many years without them being recognized; this is very different from developing pneumonia, for example, in which symptoms occur very quickly. In contrast, the agents associated with Alzheimer's disease essentially wage a cold war with our brains and bodies, so symptoms may be minimal or absent until, after what may be a decade or two, one develops Alzheimer's disease. These agents may be from tick bites, such as *Borrelia*, *Babesia*, *Bartonella*, *Ehrlichia*, or *Anaplasma*. Ticks may carry dozens of different organisms, so it is common to find people who have been treated for Lyme disease but are still infected with one of these other organisms, leading to chronic inflammation.

Viruses may also live within us for decades, as the *Herpes* viruses do, and these also may incite inflammation and cognitive decline. In fact, a recent study showed that those who had treated known outbreaks of *Herpes* with antivirals such as valacyclovir had a much lower incidence of dementia.[6] *Herpes* family viruses that infect humans include HSV-1 (which typically affects lips), HSV-2 (which is usually genital), varicella zoster (which causes chicken pox and the painful rash of zoster), HHV-6A and HHV-6B (these may infect the brain for years), HHV-7, HHV-8, CMV (cytomegalovirus, which is global but especially common in Asia), and EBV (Epstein-Barr virus, which is associated with mononucleosis and with some cases of chronic fatigue). This does not mean that every person infected with any of these *Herpes* viruses will develop dementia; it simply means that these viruses may be one source of chronic inflammation, which in turn elevates the risk of cognitive decline.

The brains of patients with Alzheimer's disease may also contain oral bacteria, such as *P. gingivalis* or *T. denticola* or *F. nucleatum*, which are associated with poor dental hygiene, or fungi such as the yeast *Candida*. Moulds such as *Penicillium*, *Aspergillus*, and *Stachybotrys* (black mould), as well as the toxins they produce, are also of concern, since they may colonize sinuses or the gastrointestinal tract.

So the key for pathogen treatment involves three steps:

- Step 1: Determine whether you have any of these pathogens, using blood tests.
- Step 2: Support your immune system (details in chapter 20 on microbes).
- Step 3: Target the specific pathogen(s) identified (many people turn out to have more than one), with the appropriate antibiotics or antivirals or antifungals, whether this involves specific drugs or non-pharmaceutical treatment or a combination. If you do end up needing antibiotics, remember that they affect your gut microbiome, so you'll want to restock your microbiome afterward, once again using probiotics and prebiotics.

- **Sixth, we want to identify and remove toxins**—metals such as mercury, organics such as toluene and benzene, and biotoxins such as mould toxins (mycotoxins). For years, we have tested for and tried to avoid carcinogens in our food, health products, and other products to which we are exposed, and thanks to the Ames test, we have largely been able to do this. But what about dementogens? These are not listed on any labels of any products we buy. However, many different chemicals can contribute to cognitive decline, either directly or indirectly. In fact, it is relatively common for multiple chemicals to conspire to compromise cognition.

Fabiana is a 53-year-old woman known for her brilliance and scientific knowledge. She sat down to play cards with her family and was unable to remember how to play. She developed a progressive dementia with features typical of type 3 (toxic) Alzheimer's: non-amnestic onset, executive dysfunction (problems with organizing), dyscalculia (problems with calculating), ApoE4-negative (she was ApoE3/3,), and amyloid PET scan positive. She lived in a mouldy setting—her ERMI score (the Environmental Relative Mouldiness Index, which is zero for an average home and considered high if over 2) was very high at 12—and a test for mycotoxins in her urine identified high levels of multiple toxins: ochratoxin A, trichothecenes, gliotoxin, and aflatoxins, indicating that she was harbouring toxins from different moulds such as *Stachybotrys*, *Penicillium*, and *Aspergillus*. With detoxification, she began to improve.

These toxins can be identified by lab tests described fully in chapter 19 on dementogens, which include tests for metals, organic toxins, and biotoxins. If toxins are indeed present, then detoxification is paramount, and the protocol will depend on which toxins are present. Two recent excellent books on detoxification are worth reading: *The Toxin Solution* by Dr Joseph Pizzorno, which is especially helpful for those with chemotoxins such as toluene or formaldehyde; and *Toxic: Heal Your Body from Mold Toxicity, Lyme Disease, Multiple Chemical Sensitivities, and Chronic Environmental Illness* by Dr Neil Nathan, which is especially helpful for biotoxins such as the mould toxins that affected Fabiana.

- **Finally, we want to rule out sleep apnoea, and optimize sleep.** I am not sure that I can state this strongly enough: *everyone* who has cognitive decline or is concerned about risk for cognitive decline should be checked for their oxygen at night. This is relatively easy to do—your doctor can lend you, or you can purchase, an oximeter, which you simply wear on your finger overnight, or you can have a sleep study. Both of these will tell you whether your oxygen levels are dropping dangerously low while you sleep. Optimally, your oxygen saturation at night should remain in the 96 to 98 per cent range, and if you are slipping down into the 80s or plummeting down into the 70s, you are doing your brain a

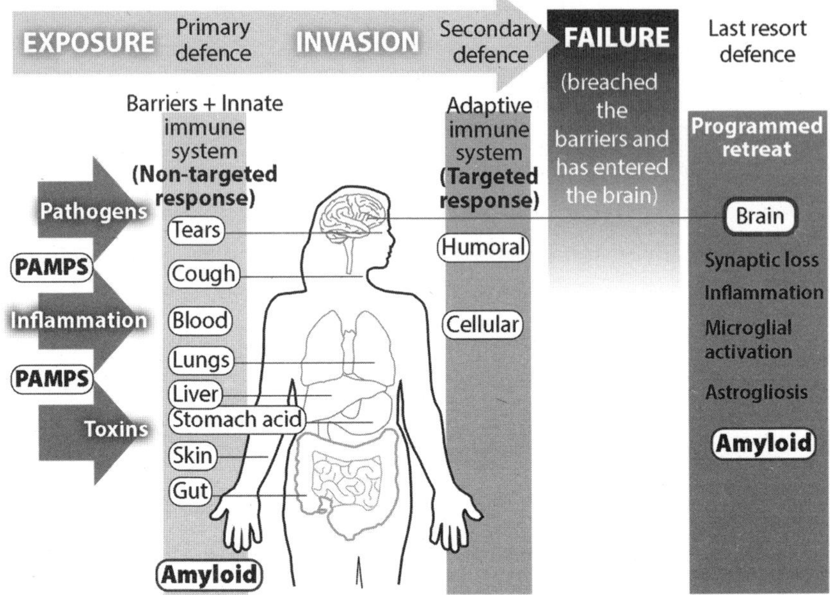

The amyloid-beta that is associated with Alzheimer's disease is part of the innate immune system's response to numerous infectious agents and other inflammatory processes that breach our barriers and other defences and reach the brain (PAMP, pathogen-associated molecular pattern).

disservice. If so, this is often from sleep apnoea, but you don't necessarily have to have sleep apnoea to have these "desaturation" events, so the key is to know whether your oxygen is dropping at night. If it is, this is an important contributor to cognitive decline or risk for decline, and it is easily addressed. You can try a dental device to improve breathing, or you can use a CPAP device (continuous positive airway pressure); in fact, many people will improve simply by reducing inflammation and weight. Whatever technique you choose, the key is simply to ensure that your oxygenation did indeed respond. In other words, as for all of these interventions in the programme, the goal is outcome, not method—whatever works! One additional note on CPAP—please make sure that the settings on the CPAP are optimized for your oxygenation, since, for example, inhalation and exhalation pressures may affect the efficacy of the CPAP.

Beyond sleep apnoea and nocturnal desaturation events, optimizing sleep preparation, timing, and quality is critical, and details are included in chapter 14. Furthermore, some of us also experience poor oxygenation during the day—especially if we live at high altitude or have lung disease—and this may also contribute to cognitive decline. This is easily checked with the same oximeter as used at night and can be addressed with EWOT—exercise with oxygen therapy.

You can now see, with all of the many potential contributors to the cognitive decline of Alzheimer's disease—from insulin resistance to the many different pathogens and toxins to the lack of support from nutrients, hormones, and trophic factors to leaky gut to sleep apnoea to high stress and more—why it is so important to identify these various contributing factors and address them with a personalized, targeted protocol. In this way, we are treating the factors that actually cause our cognitive decline instead of allowing the contributors to continue to degenerate our brains while we blindly take a drug that does not alter the underlying cause of the decline. In fact, future drug trials may be more successful if performed in combination with a personalized programme that addresses the disease mechanisms.

So let's sum up the approach to treatment, remembering that it will be different for each person, depending on what contributors we identify:

- We want to become insulin sensitive: fasting insulin <5.5 microIU/ml, haemoglobin A1c 4.0–5.3%, fasting glucose 70–90 mg/dL.
- We want to get into ketosis (and in the long run, become metabolically flexible, able to generate our own ketones by burning our fat), in the range of 1.0 to 4.0 mM BHB, and include a minimum of 12 hours of overnight fasting (minimum of 14 hours if you are ApoE4-positive).

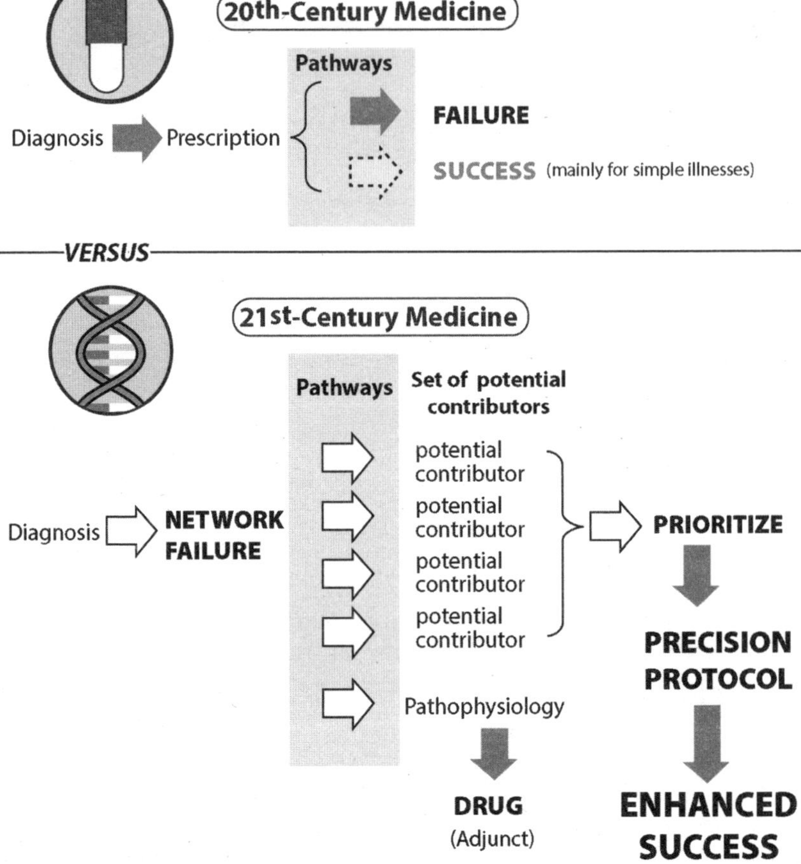

Twentieth-century medicine treats a disease with a medication that has nothing to do with the root-cause contributors to the disease, and therefore has been largely ineffective in complex chronic illnesses such as Alzheimer's disease. In contrast, twenty-first-century medicine is systems-based precision medicine in which a diagnosis identifies a network failure, from which potential contributors can be identified and targeted.

- We want to optimize nutrients, hormones, and trophic factors, including oxygenation as well as support for mitochondria and the immune system.
- We want to resolve inflammation, remove its source(s), heal the gut, heal periodontitis, and optimize the microbiome both for the gut and mouth.

- We want to treat identified pathogens.
- We want to identify toxins—metals such as mercury, organics such as toluene, and biotoxins such as trichothecenes—then detoxify.
- We want to resolve sleep apnoea if present, maintain oxygen saturation at 96 to 98 per cent while sleeping (and ensure it is not low during the day), and optimize sleep hygiene.

Together, these tip the scale from synapto*clastic* signalling to synapto*blastic* signalling and provide the building blocks required; these therapeutic steps constitute *removal, resilience,* and *rebuilding.*

We are now in the midst of the first clinical trial in history in which each patient has his/her *causes* of cognitive decline identified, and then each contributing factor is addressed with a personalized, precision medicine programme. In contrast, all previous trials have predetermined a treatment, typically a single drug, and have therefore not addressed what factors are actually causing the cognitive decline.

It has now been eight years since ReCODE was developed and the very first patient improved her cognitive status. She was unable to continue the programme on four occasions due to travel, viral infection, running out of some of the components, and deciding she might not need it anymore, and each time she began to decline again after ten to fourteen days. Each time she reinstituted the programme, she began to improve again. Eight years in, she is doing very well, still working and cognitively sound.

During these eight years, we have learned many lessons about what is required to optimize outcome and where the pitfalls lie, and these lessons are discussed in the next chapter.

CHAPTER 3

Man Bites Dogma: Lessons Learned

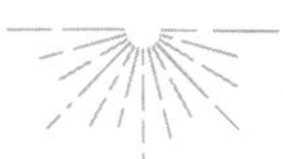

There are certain life lessons that can only be learned in the struggle.
—IDOWU KOYENIKAN

THERE ARE FEW WORDS that characterize Alzheimer's disease more accurately than *struggle*—a struggle for the patients trying to survive it, a struggle for the families trying to cope with it, a struggle for the doctors trying to treat it, a struggle for the scientists trying to understand it, and a struggle for society trying to defeat it.

Now that we have begun to understand the mechanisms involved, the many contributors, and finally how to prevent and treat it successfully, it is still a struggle to optimize prediction, prevention, and reversal of cognitive decline. But we are learning. Especially from the patients who show the greatest improvement, and those who follow the protocol but show the least effect. With each lesson learned, we are able to add many more people to the list of those who can be helped. So here are some of the key lessons learned, and questions answered, in the eight years of the ReCODE protocol:

- **Most people who develop cognitive decline have more than one subtype of Alzheimer's disease.** Although there are occasional people who truly have a pure type 1 (inflammatory) or type 2 (atrophic), or a pure version of one of the other types, most people have contributions from multiple subtypes, although one subtype is often dominant and therefore most important on which to focus. For example, many patients have high fasting insulin characteristic of type 1.5, but also have low vitamin D characteristic of type 2, and may also have mycotoxin exposure characteristic of type 3. Therefore, it is important to address these various contributors to achieve the best outcome.

- **The protocol may be difficult at first for those who are underweight.** If you are thin—for example, if your BMI is <18.5 (see table 1)—then you may have some initial difficulty generating ketones from your own fat, in part because you may not have much fatty tissue.[1] Furthermore, you may lose weight initially on the KetoFLEX 12/3 diet (as many people do), which may cause you to become even thinner and to feel out of energy and even less sharp mentally. There is an excellent description in chapter 7 to help you with this. You can increase fat consumption, add resistant starches (see chapter 9), or generate ketones from MCT oil (up to one tablespoon three times per day) or ketone salts or esters. Follow your ketone levels, and keep the ketones up in the 1.0–4.0 mM BHB range (in the long run there are some advantages to generating them from your own body, but don't worry about that initially). You can also liberalize your diet once or twice per week, with some sweet potatoes or other starchy vegetables or some additional low-glycaemic fruits like strawberries, so that you will not lose weight. Please be sure that your gut is working well and you have probiotics and prebiotics, as well as digestive enzymes if needed, since poor nutrient absorption is one problem that may be present in those who are very thin.
- **Beware the diagnosis of pseudodementia.** Pseudodementia is a false dementia that is simply the result of depression

(some people with depression appear to be demented, since they are poorly and inaccurately responsive but clear when the depression lifts). This is a fairly common diagnosis and is meant to relieve one's worries, but it is turning out that depression (which itself is often associated with systemic inflammation) is actually a relatively common harbinger of dementia, especially type 3 (toxic) Alzheimer's disease.

> A 54-year-old man complained of difficulty thinking and said that it felt as if the inside of his head was "on fire." He lost his job and became depressed. He was evaluated by a neurologist specializing in Alzheimer's disease, who made a diagnosis of pseudodementia due to depression after noting that the MRI showed no brain atrophy (shrinkage). He was treated with an antidepressant, which helped very little, and over the ensuing two years his cognitive decline worsened. His MRI once again showed no atrophy, but his cerebrospinal fluid revealed abnormalities compatible with Alzheimer's disease. He was placed on donepezil and memantine, which had little effect. As he continued to decline, further evaluation showed him to be ApoE4/4, to have severe sleep apnoea, and to have marked cerebral atrophy by MRI. His MoCA score at that point was only 11.

The correct diagnosis and appropriate treatment of this patient were delayed by at least two years because of the suggested diagnosis of "pseudodementia." Furthermore, the MRI atrophy did not appear until well after cognitive decline, so using a "negative" MRI as evidence for "pseudodementia" is a concern.

- **Beware those who tell you to "come back next year, you are not that bad yet."** It is relatively common to be told that you have MCI, not yet Alzheimer's, and that since donepezil is actually approved for dementia (Alzheimer's but not MCI), you should return in a year and see where things stand. This is of course the opposite of what you should be doing. If you have not already undertaken a prevention programme, and you now have cognitive decline, the earlier you start a programme to reverse the decline, the better off you are. I cannot tell you how often I have heard from people who were told that they should "come back in a year" and then, a year later, that "it's too late now, what you have is not treatable."

> Kerwin is a 55-year-old man who was told to come back in a year because he had "only MCI," with a PET scan suggesting early Alzheimer's. Fortunately he did not wait, and his evaluation showed that he had type 3 (toxic) MCI, well on his way to Alzheimer's disease. With detoxification, he improved and sustained that improvement.

- **Nearly everyone with any degree of cognitive decline has at least one of the most common contributors:** (1) insulin resistance; (2) mycotoxin exposure (from moulds such as *Penicillium* or *Aspergillus*) or mercury exposure; (3) reduced oxygen while sleeping (whether from sleep apnoea or other causes); (4) leaky gut; (5) poor dental hygiene; (6) chronic infections with viruses such as *Herpes simplex* or tick-borne pathogens such as *Borrelia* or *Babesia*; (7) nutritional deficiencies such as vitamin B_{12} or vitamin D; (8) vascular disease. Therefore it is critical to test for these contributors, and treat any that are identified.
- **You don't necessarily need to patch all of the many identified contributors to cognitive decline in order to achieve success.** The very first patient was only able to address twelve of a few dozen contributors to her cognitive decline, but she improved and has sustained her improvement for more than eight years now. For each person, there is a threshold—some will need to do more, some less—that we need to exceed to achieve improvement, so please keep optimizing until you get results, and then continue to tweak in order to see further improvement.

- **Although the earlier the treatment the better the outcome (and prevention is best), we have seen clear improvements with MoCA scores as low as 0.** The probability and completeness of improvement are highest with the earliest cases of cognitive decline, and we therefore recommend that everyone practise prevention or early reversal. For those in the later stages, some improve and some do not, and therefore we recommend that their children adopt preventive measures.

- **Although it generally takes three to six months for improvement, we have seen improvement in as little as four days.** There are some factors that can be addressed rapidly, such as exposure to inhaled toxins, but in general, you need to "live the protocol" for at least three to six months to see results. Please keep optimizing for best results.

- **Although the ApoE4-positive group (which represents two-thirds of patients with Alzheimer's) has been most difficult to treat in most drug trials, these patients tend to respond better than ApoE4-negative patients to ReCODE, although both may respond.** It is not yet clear why this is, but it may be because those who carry the ApoE4 allele are more prone to inflammation, which is reduced by the protocol. In contrast, those who are ApoE4-negative tend to have more toxin contribution (and therefore often present as type 3), which takes longer to treat successfully.

- **Just as for cardiovascular disease, there is a threshold for improvement.** One must get over this threshold to begin to see improvement. There is no simple way, unfortunately, to know where this threshold is, so it works best to continue to address the contributors to cognitive decline until the decline stops, and then improvements begin. This threshold is easier to reach the earlier on in the degenerative process you start the protocol.

- **Improvement typically occurs in three phases.** First, the decline slows and then stops. Second, small improvements are noticed, such as improved engagement with loved ones or less confusion associated with simple tasks. Third, more significant improvements are noted, such as improved memory, vocabulary, facial recognition, and organization. These should all be sustained as long as the protocol is sustained, although there are often setbacks with stress or infections (e.g. influenza or urinary tract infection) or loss of sleep. One of the common reasons for setback is a new exposure. For example, when someone with type 3 (toxic) Alzheimer's is sensitive to mycotoxins (produced by some moulds), a new water leak at home or work may cause re-exposure and therefore lead to a resumption of decline.
- **For laboratory tests, beware the term *WNL*—"within normal limits" (some people jokingly refer to WNL as "we never looked") or "in the normal range."** These values have absolutely nothing to do with what is optimal for function—in fact, only one in twenty people will be outside the "normal range." The "normal range" is statistical, not physiological, and not necessarily optimal for brain function. You want to be in the best range, not simply the "normal range." As an example, homocysteine, which is associated with Alzheimer's, brain atrophy, inflammation, and cardiovascular disease, has a "normal range" up to 12 micromoles per litre, but as it rises above 6, it is increasingly associated with brain atrophy. Therefore, if you want to do everything possible to prevent or reverse cognitive decline, why would you leave your homocysteine at 12? Better to be down below 7.
- **It is critical to continue to optimize all parameters—don't assume that the initial treatment is optimal.** As the biochemistry goes, so goes the cognition. Please remember that the underlying processes leading to cognitive decline go on for years, so it takes time to address all of the contributors.

For best results, please keep tweaking—this is an ongoing process, not a single prescription.

- **If there is continued decline, then in most cases something has been missed or the compliance is poor.** If you are following the various parts of your personalized programme, it should address the underlying contributors to your cognitive decline, and within three to six months, you should witness the beginning of some improvement. If decline continues unabated, then typically something has been missed—such as a chronic infection or toxin exposure or leaky gut or sleep apnoea—or the programme has not been followed. Admittedly, this process can be complicated, so you can take it one step at a time. For example, if you haven't got into the optimal ketone range of 1.0–4.0, then it should help to focus on that. Please take a look at chapter 22, on troubleshooting, if things have continued to decline after six months on the protocol.

- **Improvements are sustained unless there is a change in compliance or exposure.** This is an important point—with other treatments, even brief improvements are followed by a return to decline. However, when you are actually addressing the underlying causes of the cognitive decline, then the improvements are sustained. The longest anyone has been on the protocol is eight years now, and the improvement has been sustained, except for four brief periods when she discontinued the protocol and noted decline within one or two weeks, with improvement once again when she restarted.

- **Identifying pathogens and toxins and optimizing immune status are critical for best outcomes.** It is a wonderful idea to start with the basics—KetoFLEX 12/3 diet, exercise, sleep optimization, stress reduction, and brain training, along with supplements and herbs (and in some cases, hormones) as indicated. What is sometimes missed, however, are specific microbes, toxins, and support for the immune system, so please work with your health practitioner to address these items as well.

- **Improvements can be enhanced with repeated optimization.** Please keep optimizing! Many people find that as they begin to optimize more parameters, they continue to see enhancements in their cognitive abilities. They continue to score better and better on their brain training and get sharper and sharper in their day-to-day interactions. You'll hear from Marcy later, who went from having a memory that her significant other described as "disastrous" to one that was "just plain lousy" and finally to having "a mind like a steel trap." Therefore, please remember that this is not like taking penicillin for an infection—you don't do it and then stop. It is a process of continued tweaking for the best outcome. Please don't worry if it looks daunting to get started. Just start with the basics, then add over time, working with your practitioner and health coach.

- **As a general rule, those with higher levels of ketosis (BHB = 1.0–4.0 mM) show better cognitive improvement than those with lower levels (especially BHB <0.5 mM).** Ketone energetic support for your brain is very important, so if you are able to achieve ketosis—which you can measure with a ketone meter (Precision Xtra or Keto-Mojo or Keto Guru)—without using MCT oil or ketone salts or esters, that is preferable. However, if you cannot, then you can increase ketone level with MCT oil (you can use up to 1 tablespoon three times per day, but start slowly and work up so that you don't develop diarrhoea) or with ketone salts or ketone esters.

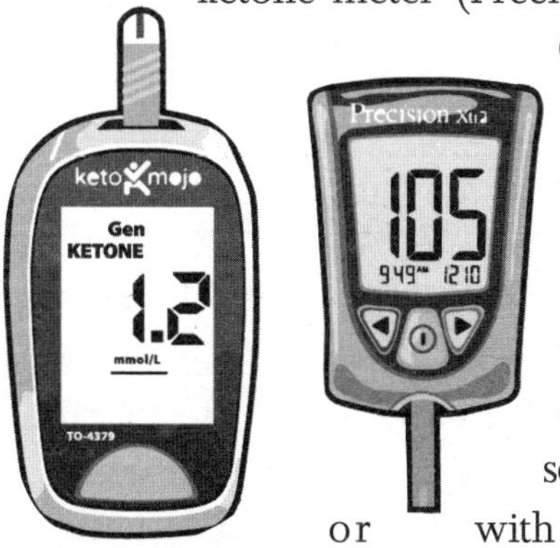

Examples of ketone meters. These can determine both ketone level and glucose level.

- **Many find that some form of stimulation, as part of the overall protocol, enhances improvement.** This may be with light stimulation (photobiomodulation) or magnetic stimulation (e.g. with MeRT, magnetic e-resonant therapy), and of course brain training represents a distinct form of stimulation.

- **The long-term pro-inflammatory state and interaction associated with Alzheimer's disease may require "rebooting" or "resetting" to enjoy sustained improvement.** This may involve dynamic neural retraining (see chapter 16) or neural feedback or polyvagal stimulation or other forms of neuro-immune modulation.

- **After addressing pathogens, toxins, insulin resistance, inflammation, gut leak, trophic and nutrient support, and so forth, if damage prior to treatment initiation has been extensive, please consider stem cells.** There are ongoing clinical trials of stem cells for Alzheimer's disease. My concern about using stem cells as the *sole* therapy, without addressing the contributors to the disease, is that this is akin to trying to rebuild a house as it's burning down—it may make more sense to put out the fire first and then rebuild. However, I do think it likely that stem cells will ultimately play an important role in the reversal of cognitive decline, especially for those who do not reverse the decline in its earliest stages.

- **Since neurodegenerative diseases such as Alzheimer's and Lewy body disease are ongoing for years or even decades before diagnosis, these may affect many relationships prior to any clear symptoms of dementia.** I often wonder how many of the domestic disputes, political squabbles, international incidents, misunderstandings, and just plain bad moods are actually the result of early symptoms and pathological processes associated with neurodegenerative diseases.

Perhaps even more commonly, the symptoms may be associated with underlying processes that never lead to a diagnosis but nevertheless, in the early stages, affect behaviour, mood, or performance. Perhaps the most well-recognized example is the aggression and depression that are so common in CTE (chronic traumatic encephalopathy, as seen in the movie *Concussion*), the brain damage that results from head trauma, but this represents only a small fraction of the behavioural changes associated with neurodegeneration.

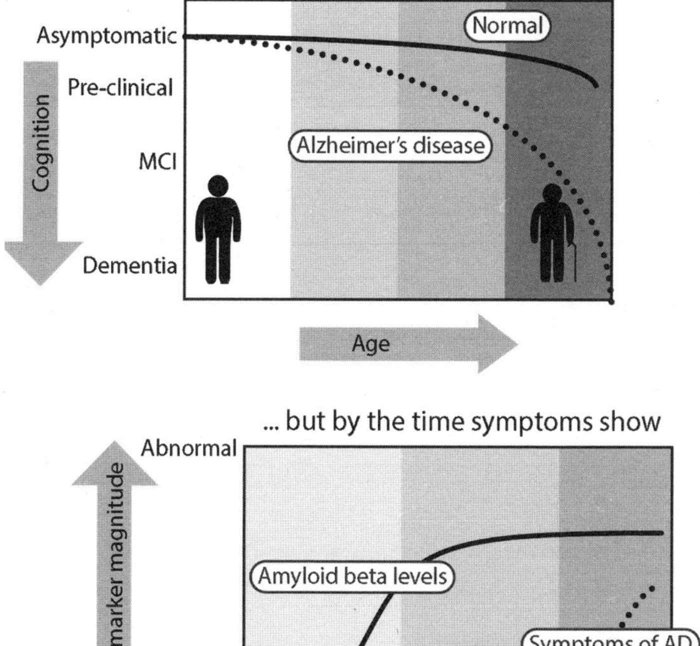

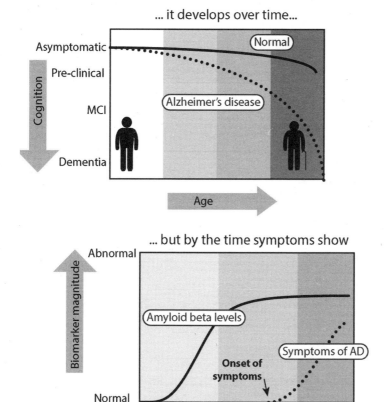

By the time a diagnosis of Alzheimer's disease is made, the underlying pathophysiology has been ongoing for many years.

Very frequently, clinicians hear about "inexplicable behaviour" in someone years before a dementia diagnosis is made. Therefore, please consider this possibility in patients and loved ones, especially now that prevention and early reversal are readily available.

> Bradley was an even-tempered 85-year-old professor who had lived his life as a family man and gentleman when, after fifty years of a loving and stable marriage, he began to argue with his wife more frequently and vehemently. During one argument, he hit her, something that was completely out of character for him and which he had never done before. On questioning, it turned out that he had also begun to notice memory problems, and his evaluation ultimately revealed that he had early Lewy body disease.

You may have seen the television commercial claiming that the first survivor of Alzheimer's disease is "out there somewhere" . . . and if you'll just "donate to our organization, we'll make it happen." Well, that is quite misleading, because it's not someday, the first survivors are already here, they are well documented, and their cases are published in medical journals.[2] Now, in the chapters that follow, you'll hear in detail how so many people are achieving success.

PART TWO

THE HANDBOOK SECTION 1: Reversing Cognitive Decline

with Julie Gregory and
Aida Lasheen Bredesen, MD

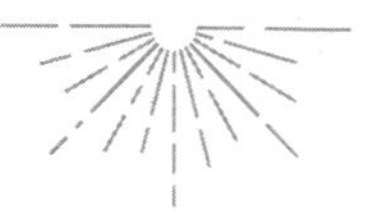

I hear and I forget. I see and I remember.
I do and I understand.
—CONFUCIUS

THERE IS AN OLD joke that illustrates what we are trying to do here: a farmer was concerned about decreasing milk production at his farm, so he contacted the local university to see if academic experts could help. The university sent a problem-solving team, led by a brilliant theoretical physicist, and collected data for two weeks. Crunching all of the data led to gigabytes of output. The physicist returned to the farmer and said, "Well, we have calculated a solution to your problem. Unfortunately, it applies only to a spherical cow in a vacuum." Of course real cows are not spherical and don't live in a vacuum, so all of that nice theoretical work did not help the farmer. We have a similar situation in neuroscience: lots of interesting brain research on cells in petri dishes and worms and fruit flies, but it is extremely difficult to translate the results into effective solutions for human diseases such as Alzheimer's, Lou Gehrig's disease, and Huntington's disease. In fact, virtually all of the attempts to translate results in lab animals to effective treatments for human neurodegenerative diseases have failed. So that's what this section is about—translating the results we obtained over thirty years of laboratory research into workable, effective solutions for Alzheimer's, pre-Alzheimer's (MCI and SCI), and the prevention of Alzheimer's, and providing specific details on every aspect needed for success in improving cognition.

As a physician scientist, I may be able to *tell* you what will be most helpful, but for you to *see* and *remember*, and ultimately *do* and *understand*, there is nothing better than having someone who is living the protocol every day—someone who has actually *felt* what it is like to reverse cognitive decline—give you experience-based practical solutions. Therefore, for this part of the book (section 1 of the Handbook), I've teamed up with Julie Gregory and my wife, Dr Aida Lasheen Bredesen. Since Julie, who is ApoE4/4 (homozygous), has reversed her own cognitive decline, she's amassed a wealth of experience in translating research into practical application. Her keen observations provide a level of vigilance that she applies daily and generously shares with us. Julie is the founder and president of ApoE4.Info, a grassroots non-profit organization that supports ApoE4 carriers. My wife, Dr Aida Lasheen Bredesen, is a doctor with an integrative approach honed from her early years spent in developing countries, where the chronic illnesses of Western civilization are much less common. Each of us brings a complementary background and skill set. Together we form a unique team that offers you the best methods for prevention and reversal of cognitive decline. Indeed, I am not aware of any other book that combines the expertise of a neuroscientist, a clinician, and a patient to offer the most efficacious solutions for cognitive decline. As you'll see, there are many practical solutions, hints, tricks, and work-arounds, a combination of which maximizes your chance for great success. So I offer my sincere gratitude to Julie and Aida. Let's all get to work!

CHAPTER 4

Enhancing Cognition with KetoFLEX 12/3

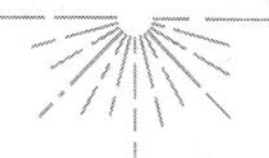

Healing doesn't mean the damage never existed.
It means the damage no longer controls your life.
—NATIVE AMERICAN WISDOM

OUR GOAL IS TO empower *you*. If you've ever asked your doctor for help with neuroprotection, you've likely received a blank stare, condescension, or even outright criticism in response. One couple emailed me that they had handed a copy of my book to their GP, who scowled and said tersely, "Doctors don't have time to read." *Yikes*. You may have seen in some doctor's surgery the coffee mug reading: "Please do not confuse your Google search with my medical degree." Fair enough, perhaps, but to date a medical degree has not offered an effective solution for cognitive decline. Patients who are at risk report their neurologists telling them to "Wait for it" or "Good luck with that," offering no hope whatsoever. To the millions of us who are at high risk or are already experiencing symptoms, this is unacceptable, especially since Alzheimer's is now one of the leading causes of morbidity and mortality in the world. We have a wealth of published peer-reviewed medical literature that demonstrates the efficacy of the enabling strategies that we'll describe. Sadly, effective patient education can't be accomplished in a typical five-minute office visit. It's much easier to write a prescription for one of the two types of FDA- or NICE-approved drugs for Alzheimer's, which does *nothing* to change the trajectory of the disease (or perhaps less than nothing—recently it has been found that the use of these drugs for Alzheimer's is actually associated with more rapid decline, offering only temporary symptomatic relief[1]). That's a point worth repeating: using a drug to fight Alzheimer's does not stop the decline—you may get a temporary improvement, but then you'll go right back to declining—whereas when you target the *cause* of the problem—with the very programme we are describing here—then the improvement is *sustained* (and in fact there are people who have sustained their improvement on our protocol for more than eight years now, long after they would otherwise have likely been in a nursing home). That's why you need to become your own advocate and begin taking charge of your cognitive health today. The sooner you start, the better chance you'll have of preventing cognitive decline as you age, enhancing your current cognitive ability, or reversing symptoms if they've begun.

The pace at which you institute these suggested changes depends upon many individual factors, such as your metabolic state (especially insulin resistance); your ability to move, sleep, and deal with stress; and your support systems to help you to initiate and maintain change. They can be implemented slowly over weeks, months, or all at once. Those making the transition quickly have the opportunity to promote healing more rapidly, but should also be aware of the possible, though usually mild and transitory, side effects that can result, which we'll discuss below with strategies to help you reach success.

Critics of this approach say it's too expensive or too complicated. Our goal is to make this approach accessible and affordable for everyone. At every opportunity, we'll share inexpensive alternatives for implementing this lifestyle and overall protocol. We know the pathology that leads to Alzheimer's takes a decade or more before definite symptoms appear, so it's vital to intervene as early as possible to change the trajectory of this disease process. The first step is to change the false paradigm that Alzheimer's is hopeless into one of accurate information. We want to educate you as part of a healthcare revolution that puts the power in your hands so that you can protect your cognitive health and enjoy a long and vibrant health span.

GETTING STARTED

What kind of a crazy name is KetoFLEX 12/3, and what the heck does it mean? As described in *The End of Alzheimer's*, *keto* refers to *ketosis*, a natural process by which your liver produces ketone bodies (aceto-acetate, beta-hydroxybutyrate, and acetone) by breaking down fat, providing an excellent fuel for cognition and increasing the production of brain-derived neurotrophic factor (BDNF) for neuronal and synaptic support.[2]

FLEX refers to two different facets of the approach: one, it promotes metabolic *flexibility*, restoring your body's innate ability to metabolize either fat or glucose as fuel while maintaining insulin sensitivity to maximize the fuel supply for your brain. Two, while the diet is heavily plant-based, it allows for the *flexibility* to include animal products (or not) based on your preference and unique needs. Lastly, 12/3 refers to the amount of time that you'll spend fasting every day—at least twelve hours between the end of dinner and the start of breakfast or brunch or lunch, and at least three hours between dinner and bedtime.

Implemented correctly, it's more than a diet; it's a *lifestyle*, with nutrition being one of several key components. You'll be combining our dietary recommendations with fasting and exercise to restore or maintain *metabolic* health. Metabolic is a term that refers to the many chemical reactions that keep us alive, including the ingestion of food, breaking it down and creating energy and cellular components. A healthy metabolism optimizes overall health and provides steady fuel for your brain.

Our goal is to transform your relationship with food from one of dependence to one of sustainable nourishment without hunger. You'll spend less time in the kitchen, be less dependent on frequent meals, and have more time to spend outdoors being active and meaningfully socially engaged. Our clean, nutrient-dense, heavily plant-based,

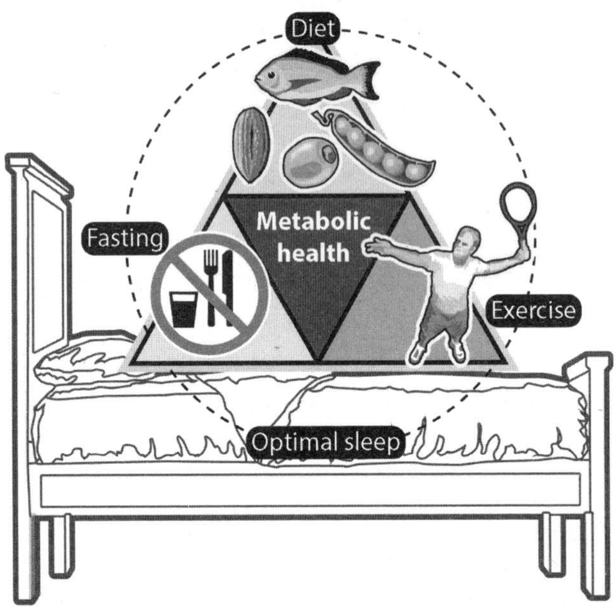

The KetoFLEX 12/3 diet and lifestyle combine fasting, exercise, and a plant-rich, mildly ketogenic diet with optimal sleep to create a foundation that supports cognition.

wholefood diet provides a satiety that processed foods simply can't provide. You'll find that optimal nutrition for your brain is delicious and satisfying, making this new way of eating and living joyful and easy to sustain.

To summarize, the three components of the KetoFLEX 12/3 lifestyle are diet, fasting, and exercise (on a foundation of quality sleep, which we'll discuss in chapter 14). When these are combined, they heal metabolism and provide clean sustainable fuel for your brain. Practising these three strategies concurrently yields a synergistic effect that promotes more rapid healing than employing any one of them alone. Additionally, you needn't restrict as many carbs, fast as long, nor exercise as hard to create ketones. Score! It's the combination of the three that leads to optimized health and avoidance of the chronic diseases rampant throughout modern civilization, from dementia to metabolic syndrome to hypertension. In the next several chapters, we'll take a deeper dive into the dietary recommendations.

We'll cover the importance of fasting when we break down the food pyramid. (Sneak preview: It's the base of the pyramid. Yes, it's that important!) Exercise will be discussed below. Don't lose track of the concept that each of these strategies is equally important, and together they comprise the KetoFLEX 12/3 approach.

KetoFLEX 12/3 specifically focuses on the mechanisms known to contribute to cognitive decline. This lifestyle will:

- Create critical insulin sensitivity
- Reduce inflammation
- Address neuronal fuel reduction and mitochondrial deficiency
- Increase circulation and optimize blood pressure
- Provide raw materials for synaptic support
- Protect against nutrient deficiencies associated with cognitive decline
- Promote cellular autophagy and beta-amyloid clearance
- Promote detoxification
- Protect against muscle and bone loss associated with cognitive decline.

What makes the KetoFLEX 12/3 approach unique is that we encourage you to use actual data to help you optimize your health to achieve improved (and sustained) cognition. You needn't *wonder* if you're on the right track. You can track and tweak the effect your choices are having based on real-time data, periodic assessments, and laboratory testing.

Dietary Confusion: Infobesity!

> Georgia is 58 years old and suffered from arthritis, high cholesterol, prediabetes, low thyroid function, obesity, and poor memory. She was eating a standard American diet. I suggested to her that she read a few of the excellent books on nutrition by the experts, such as Dr Joel Fuhrman's *Eat to Live*, Dr Mark Hyman's *Eat Fat, Get Thin,* and Dr Steven Gundry's

> *The Plant Paradox*. She began to change her diet. She lost 45 kg, her cholesterol came down to normal, her arthritis disappeared, and her prediabetes abated. She became energetic and started to ride her bicycle. Her memory improved. She started to read voraciously about nutrition and health, but began to note that different books and articles suggested very different diets. This was confusing to her—which one was right? She asked me if there is a word to describe being overwhelmed with nutritional information, and I responded, "I guess you could call it 'infobesity.'"

We'll try to avoid "infobesity" here, and instead focus on useful, specific, and actionable advice for enhancing cognition.

Diet is often the biggest stumbling block for anyone wanting to prevent or remediate cognitive decline. The advice from experts is often wildly contradictory, leading many people to feel confused about the best dietary path. The KetoFLEX 12/3 approach breaks through the confusion by focusing on specific mechanisms that promote neuroprotection, providing a clear path to optimize cognition and overall health.

Why does the dietary advice for neuroprotection vary so dramatically? There's a huge void in nutritional science as it relates to cognition, for multiple reasons. The biggest issue is the lack of well-constructed longitudinal studies. First, long-term clinical trials are expensive, and few sources of finance are willing to put up large sums of money without the opportunity for a return on their investment. Second, there are so many confounders, providing potentially false associations. In free-living human subjects—each of whom has a different genome (genetics) and epigenome (the dynamic modulation and control of the reading of your DNA, which is affected by your environment, among other influences), providing variability at the outset—it's practically impossible to ensure that everyone is following a prescribed diet or accurately reporting what he or she has eaten on food frequency questionnaires. Other behaviours or stressors can easily have a confounding effect that is independent of diet alone. Third, so much of accepted nutritional science is based on epidemiological evidence, which reveals association but not necessarily causation. For instance, think about the many positive health outcomes associated with the Mediterranean diet from epidemiological observation. One could argue that this is *proof* that wholegrains, a component of the diet, are healthy. Without specifically testing that assertion by using a control group that adheres to the Mediterranean diet *without* wholegrains, that claim doesn't hold up to scientific scrutiny. How do we know that it isn't the *other* components of the diet or the lifestyle that provide the health benefits? With a lack of definitive proof that one diet as opposed to another will help to protect cognition, you'll find it hard to feel assured that you're on the right path.

We want to take away the fear that you're eating the wrong thing or that you've done irreparable harm up until this point. We encourage you to do the best that you can moving forward. We understand that it's not always possible to follow each aspect of the diet perfectly, but we'll help you identify foods and eating patterns that make you feel better as opposed to those that are having a harmful effect. Over time, you will find it easier to identify healthier foods and to incorporate the many changes that we're recommending because you'll feel and look so much better. It's really simple. When you put your brain first, everything else follows.

Most important, the "side effects" of this diet and lifestyle approach are virtually all positive: increased energy, weight loss (if that's a goal), reduced blood pressure, stabilization of blood sugar, reduction in coronary artery disease risk, enhanced mood, improved skin, and a reversal of biological age, leading to cognitive improvement and longevity.

IS NUTRITIONAL KETOSIS RIGHT FOR EVERYONE?

Not necessarily! That's the beauty of personalized medicine. To clarify, nutritional ketosis refers to a specific dietary pattern, using fewer carbohydrates and more fat to generate ketones. You'll

(continued)

recall, the goal of the KetoFLEX 12/3 lifestyle—fasting, exercise, and diet—is to restore metabolic flexibility, the ability to burn both glucose and fat as fuel, in those who've become insulin resistant. Interestingly, research suggests that everyone with Alzheimer's has brain insulin resistance and therefore an urgent need for fuel, even if peripheral (body) symptoms and markers are absent.[3] Nutritional ketosis can be very helpful for those with insulin resistance or for anyone who has symptoms of cognitive decline.

Be aware that as you heal, your need for dietary fat may change over time. Many find that as their daily fast extends and they exercise more, those strategies will naturally lead to ketosis without needing as much fat as they initially required. Also, once insulin resistance is healed and metabolic flexibility restored, you can experiment with adding more resistant starches while recording the effect on your cognition. Some people find that once they are healthier, they no longer need higher levels of ketosis. This is a personalized programme. Let your biomarkers (fasting glucose, insulin, and haemoglobin A1c, as well as cognitive performance) guide your dietary choices. Your goal is to attain metabolic flexibility, insulin sensitivity, and cognitive clarity.

What about younger people or those who come to the programme concerned about prevention, who are already insulin sensitive and metabolically healthy? This group may not need to focus as much on increasing dietary fat, but rather on preventing insulin resistance by implementing a daily fast, adding exercise, and otherwise partaking of the nutritional food choices in our pyramid. Simply avoiding the foods not in the pyramid—sugar, refined carbohydrates, and unhealthy oils—will be very helpful for this group.

Because ApoE4 carriers demonstrate an asymptomatic mild reduction in glucose utilization (a neuronal fuel shortage) as early as age 20, they may want to consider measuring their ketone levels.[4] Beta-hydroxybutyrate (BHB) levels as low as 0.4–0.5 mmol/L can effectively address this deficit.[5] It's very easy to achieve these lower levels with the strategies outlined in the

KetoFLEX 12/3 lifestyle. As ApoE4 carriers age, they'll need to monitor for symptoms of insulin resistance more aggressively and may want to consider raising their BHB goals.

Additionally, those with vascular dementia or known heart disease should prioritize healing their underlying insulin resistance before implementing nutritional ketosis. See page 127 in chapter 8.

KETOSIS

Let's take a deeper dive into ketosis. The very word strikes fear into the hearts of many because it's often confused with *ketoacidosis*, a dangerous condition associated with type 1 diabetes.[6] Ketosis is perfectly safe. Babies are in ketosis much of the time, as are metabolically healthy adults during sleep.[7] Ketones have been used as fuel throughout much of human history. If you consider that the human liver can store only around 100 grams of glucose at any given time, early man would have been unable to survive without this protective built-in physiological adaptation to break down stored fat to use for energy during times when food was scarce.[8] Only in modern times have people been able to keep their glycogen stores full by eating three meals a day, plus snacks, while becoming increasingly sedentary. Our hunter-gatherer ancestors lived—in fact those living in non-Westernized parts of the world still live—a ketogenic lifestyle. They are active throughout the day, often performing physically demanding labour. They eat much less often, partaking of traditionally prepared wholefoods that they hunt and gather themselves.[9]

Overconsumption of highly refined foods has led to an unnatural transition towards burning glucose as fuel exclusively, which has in turn led to an explosion of insulin resistance in the United States and worldwide.[10] Imagine that you have a child who is constantly playing very loud music and beating drums, so you take to wearing earplugs. Now your spouse puts on Brahms's lullaby and you don't even hear it—that's what insulin resistance is like. For so many of us with this common condition (and most of us don't know we have it until we

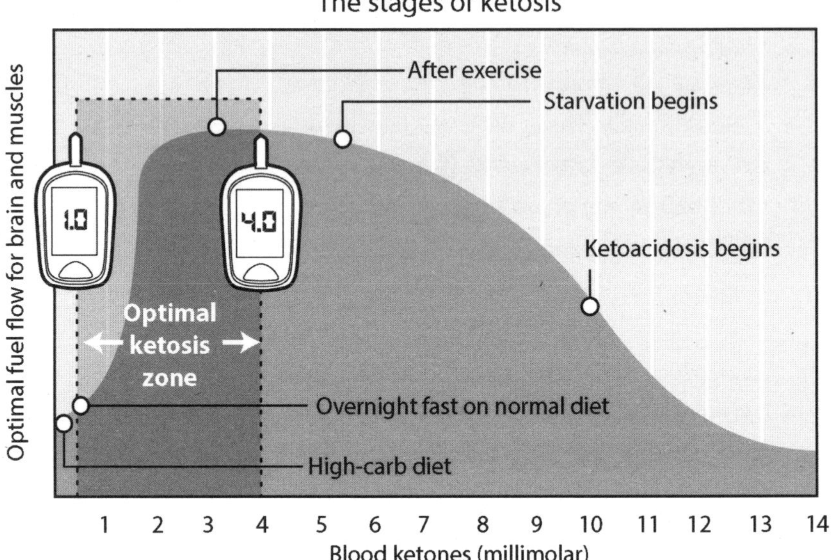

Mild ketosis is the target for KetoFLEX 12/3: beta-hydroxybutyrate (the key ketone) of 1.0–4.0 mmol/L.

develop cognitive decline or diabetes or vascular disease), the years of sugar and high insulin have caused our cells to "turn down the volume" in response to insulin. This is especially bad for your brain, because insulin functions as a trophic factor, meaning that it turns on the very biochemical pathways needed for brain cells and their connections to survive. So it's easy to see why turning down the response to insulin is such an important contributor to Alzheimer's disease—indeed, why some have even called Alzheimer's "type 3 diabetes."[11]

As bad as all of this may sound, the problems with resistance to insulin don't end there! High levels of insulin also block the mobilization of fat into usable energy, causing obesity.[12] Not everyone who's obese is insulin resistant, however; conversely, some people have insulin resistance without being obese (but nevertheless have fat stored around their internal organs), and are called TOFI (thin outside, fat inside).[13]

Symptoms and markers of insulin resistance can include:

- Abdominal fat (visceral)
- An inability to fast
- Hypoglycaemic episodes (low blood sugar)
- BMI >25 (body mass index)
- Fasting glucose >114
- Fasting insulin >5.5
- Haemoglobin A1c > 5.7% (a test that measures the glucose average over two to three months)
- HOMA-IR >1.4 (https://www.mdcalc.com/homa-ir-homeostatic-model-assessment-insulin-resistance)

The likelihood of insulin resistance *in the body* tends to increase with age, although more and more young people are also exhibiting this metabolic condition.[14] As glucose markers increase and a loss of sensitivity to insulin develops, the brain's ability to access the glucose it needs is diminished.[15]

Indeed, insulin resistance *in the brain* also increases as we get older, leading to a fuel deficiency in the brain.[16] Because the likelihood of both insulin resistance and fuel deficiency increases with age, it's hard to separate the two risk factors. Earlier work hypothesized that the decreased usage of neuronal fuel seen in this population is a *consequence* of Alzheimer's disease, as opposed to a risk factor. That position asserts that the brain atrophy accompanying this disease simply necessitates less fuel.[17] This theory falls apart, however, when we consider those at the highest genetic risk.

Carriers of the ApoE4 gene allele, which is the most common genetic risk factor for Alzheimer's disease, exhibit a reduction in cerebral glucose utilization as early as their third decade in similar regions of the brain as Alzheimer's patients.[18] These young ε4+ subjects show no symptoms of cognitive decline despite PET-FDG measurements demonstrating a 5 to 10 per cent reduction in the brain regions associated with memory processing and learning. Brain glucose hypometabolism precedes cognitive decline decades before the first symptoms appear. While we lack definitive proof that this energy deficit *causes* Alzheimer's, this chronic, progressive, brain fuel starvation contributes significantly to the onset of Alzheimer's and offers an opportunity for intervention.

Even when our brains can no longer use glucose effectively, they are able to use ketone bodies to address this deficit. Dr Stephen Cunnane demonstrated that ketones can effectively make up for this neuronal fuel deficit. Additionally, the brain *preferentially* uses these ketone bodies. They enter the brain in direct proportion to their concentration in plasma, irrespective of glucose availability.[19] Thus even a relatively low level of ketones (0.4–0.5 mM BHB, which is beta-hydroxybutyrate) offsets the 5 to 10 per cent neuronal fuel shortage faced by young ApoE4 carriers.[20] Blood measurements (obtained from finger sticks) of BHB are often used to indicate the degree of ketosis. We'll provide instructions for how to track your own levels. We've found that higher amounts (0.5–4.0 mM, and best at 1.0–4.0 mM) are helpful when addressing greater deficits. Through testing and recording, you'll learn where you feel and perform best.

Ketones can fuel the brain very effectively—up to about 75 per cent of its energy needs—but the brain still does need a small amount of glucose. However, this does not mean you need to eat sugar! Even in the absence of sugar consumption, the small amount of glucose needed for the final 25 per cent of brain support may be supplied by the production of glucose by your liver, by a process called gluconeogenesis. The plant-rich diet we recommend, which includes complex carbohydrates but minimizes simple carbohydrates, provides many critical metabolic and cognitive advantages, from fibre to prebiotics to anti-inflammatories to flavanols and many other phytonutrients.

We have strong hints from published research that using ketosis can improve cognition even in those formally diagnosed with Alzheimer's. One of the most well-known case studies, described by Dr Mary Newport, involves the careful documentation of her ApoE4-positive husband's improvement using this approach.[21] As you can see from the drawings opposite by adding coconut oil (which

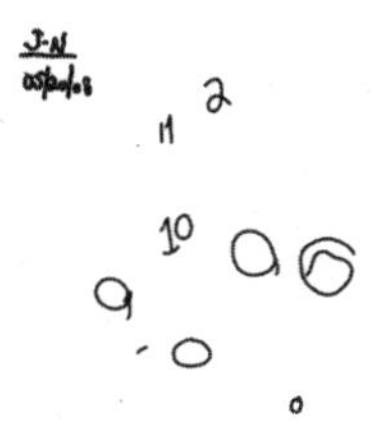

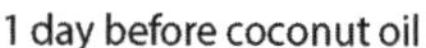

1 day before coconut oil

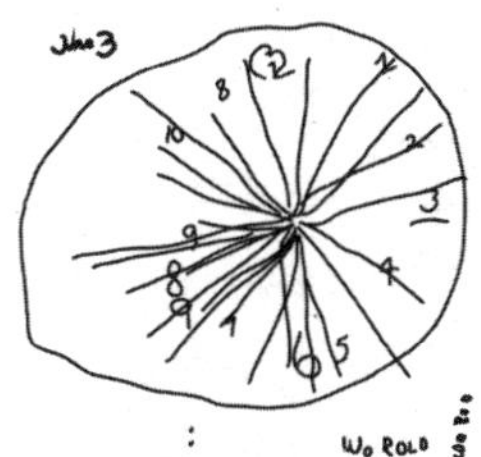

14 days after starting coconut oil

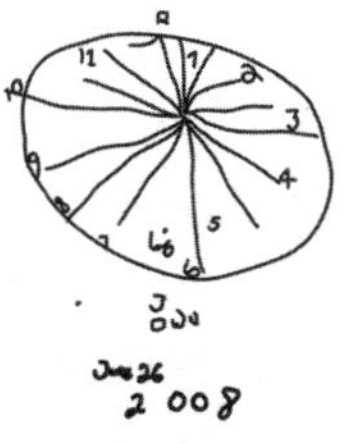

37 days after starting coconut oil

increases ketones) to his diet, Steve Newport experienced a dramatic improvement in cognitive function. Furthermore, his improvement remained stable for two years.

A randomized clinical trial, using only a ketone-supplemented drink, demonstrated modest cognitive improvements in non-ApoE4 carriers. It's worth noting that this trial didn't implement any other strategies, such as a change in diet, and participants reached only very low levels of BHB, 0.4mM, after ninety days.[22] The lack of success in the more disadvantaged ApoE4 carriers begs the question of whether this group needs higher BHB levels and/or additional strategies to benefit.

Impressive results were obtained in a clinical trial in which patients with mild cognitive impairment (MCI, which is the precursor to Alzheimer's) ate either a high-carbohydrate diet (50 per cent of calories) or a low-carbohydrate diet (5 to 10 per cent of calories), and after only six weeks, cognition improved in the low-carb group only, in direct proportion to the degree of ketosis. Not only did cognition improve in the low-carb group, but weight dropped, waist measurements shrank, and fasting glucose and insulin declined—pretty impressive results for only six weeks!

Several recently published case studies with two ApoE4 patients combined additional strategies by using a low-carb diet, fasting, and exercise for even more impressive results. Both were diagnosed with Alzheimer's and experienced reversal of cognitive decline. One also reversed his type 2 diabetes. These examples are illustrative of what we regularly see in patients following the KetoFLEX 12/3 approach.[23]

As you can see from these examples, synergistically combining a low-carb diet with fasting and exercise—KetoFLEX 12/3—is key for sustained improvement as it heals the underlying insulin resistance.

These examples show how powerful insulin sensitivity and ketosis are for cognition. The good news is that the basics—diet, exercise, fasting, with restorative sleep: KetoFLEX 12/3—all support these critical processes and thus enhance cognition. They also provide a strong foundation for all of the other parts of the protocol.

If ketosis is a natural built-in adaptive response to a reduction in glucose levels, why do we have to intervene with a special diet or lifestyle modifications? Over time, those with insulin resistance are no longer able to switch automatically from burning glucose to using their own body fat for fuel.[24] This leads to double jeopardy for the brain, which is deprived of *both* of its fuel sources. The initial goal of the KetoFLEX 12/3 approach is to *shift* from burning glucose (primarily) to burning fat (and the ketones derived from the fat), in order to provide sustainable fuel to the brain. This can be achieved by applying three strategies concurrently: exercise, fasting, and the KetoFLEX 12/3 dietary pattern on a framework of quality sleep. Our approach is a *lifestyle* as opposed to a *diet*; ideally, you'll want to implement all three changes at once. We realize this won't be possible for everyone, so we'll offer some helpful strategies as we go.

ACTION PLAN

- If you are experiencing symptoms of cognitive decline or at risk for cognitive decline, consider adopting the KetoFLEX 12/3 approach as a means of promoting metabolic flexibility, improving cognition, and protecting against cognitive decline.
- The initial goal is to shift from burning glucose primarily to burning fat to achieve a mild level of ketosis.
- The ultimate goal is to heal insulin resistance, create metabolic flexibility, and restore or support healthy cognition.

CHAPTER 5

Put Out the Fire

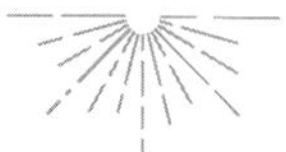

I've been putting out the fire with gasoline.
—DAVID BOWIE

TELLING YOU WHAT YOU *can't* eat may seem like a strange way to introduce a diet, but in this case it's really important. If you continue to eat the "no" foods while incorporating some of our recommended foods, you could create a highly inflammatory environment in your body, *the exact opposite of what we're trying to do.* Putting out the fire is the first step in healing.

JUST SAY *NO*

Simple Carbohydrates

In a misguided effort to reduce the risk of heart disease, the United States formally adopted low-fat dietary recommendations with instructions to increase carbohydrate intake in 1976. By the early 1980s, food manufacturers had figured out a way to profit from these new food guidelines by creating low-fat versions of almost every food imaginable. Consumers were thrilled to have "healthy" versions of their forbidden foods. The resulting food products were highly

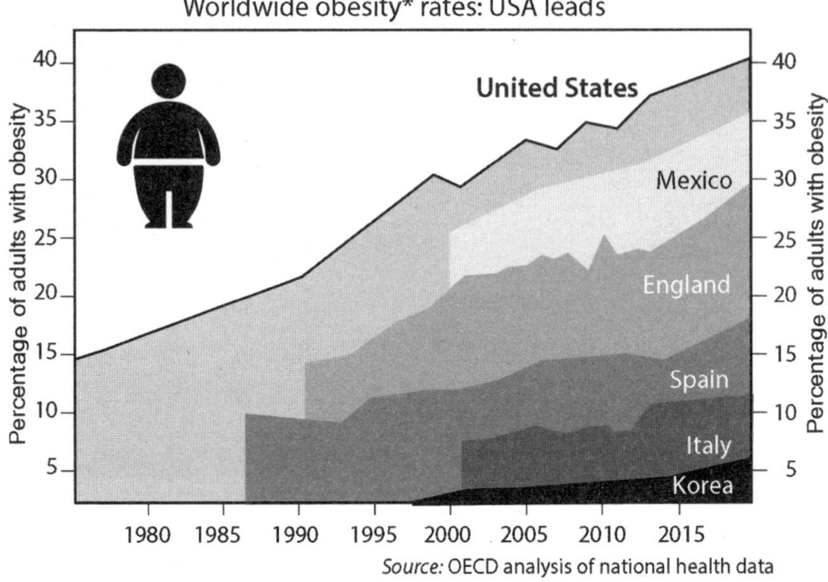

Obesity rates have skyrocketed since the adoption of the low-fat dietary guidelines in the late 1970s.

processed and often loaded with sugar.[1] The rate of obesity in the United States has more than *quadrupled* since the adoption of the low-fat dietary guidelines.[2] More than a third of all American adults (80 million) are now obese. Another third are overweight according to government statistics. Even worse, the rate of severe obesity (usually more than 45 kg overweight) has also quadrupled in this same time period.[3] Sadly, one in five school-age children (6 to 19 years) is now also obese.[4] In the UK, according to NHS, the majority of adults, 63 per cent, are overweight or obese, and 28 per cent of these are obese.*

All of us who are obese have a higher risk for diabetes. Simple carbohydrates, such as sugar, starch, and processed foods, demand high insulin production—more than our bodies are designed to

*National Health Service (2020) 'Statistics on Obesity, Physical Activity and Diet, England 2020'. *Statistics on Obesity, Phyisical Activity and Diet*. Available at: https://digital.nhs.uk/data-and-information/publications/statistical/statistics-on-obesity-physical-activity-and-diet/england-2020/part-3-adult-obesity-copy

produce. Having such chronically high insulin levels causes our cells to scream, "Enough, turn down the volume!" eventually creating resistance to the effects of insulin. This means that not only will your cells not handle sugar as well (and reduced use of glucose in parts of the brain is characteristic of Alzheimer's), they also won't have the survival effect of insulin in the brain—yes, insulin is a wonderful trophic factor for your brain cells, meaning that it keeps them alive. So it's little wonder that turning down the response to insulin is an important contributor to the very neurodegenerative process that occurs in Alzheimer's—in fact, brain insulin resistance is present in almost all cases of Alzheimer's.

The bottom line is simple: we humans are not constructed to eat the amount of sugar and starch that we currently consume, any more than we are built to flap our arms and fly—so we crash when we try either one of those (the crash just takes longer with sugar and starch, and includes hypertension, high cholesterol, diabetes, heart disease, strokes, advanced ageing, arthritis, and dementia).

Fortunately, you can see this whole process creeping up on you by measuring your fasting insulin and your haemoglobin A1c, which is simply your haemoglobin (which carries oxygen to your tissues) with a sugar molecule stuck to it, like a remora stuck on a shark. If your haemoglobin A1c is up to 5.7 per cent or more, then you are already pre-diabetic. A normal A1c falls between 4.0 and 5.6, but we recommend keeping it at 5.3 or lower for best results. Pre-diabetes ranges between 5.7 and 6.4, and full-blown diabetes begins at 6.5, with successively higher levels indicating more poorly controlled diabetes. Even before the haemoglobin A1c creeps up, your fasting insulin may rise, and when it exceeds 5 (measured in mIU/L), that means the islet cells of your pancreas are already working overtime to keep your glucose in check. It's important for you to track your numbers so you can understand where you stand on this spectrum. The good news is that there is a lot you can do about it, and regaining insulin sensitivity will help you not only with your cognition but also with your fat, and it may even help slow your ageing.

Not so long ago—back in 1976—only 5 million Americans were

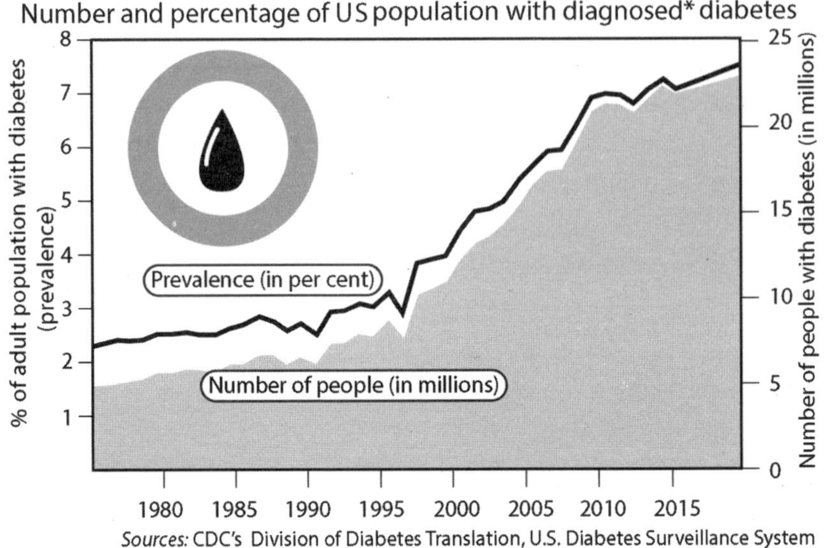

Diabetes rates have increased markedly since 1976.

diabetic. Today, there are more than 100 million of us with diabetes or pre-diabetes![5] As of 2019, Diabetes UK reports that 3.9 million people suffer from diabetes. This dramatic increase reveals why so many more are at high risk for Alzheimer's today. With our diabetes comes inflammation—the sugar binds not only to your haemoglobin but also to many other proteins (the sugar molecules actually *become* part of the proteins), altering both their form and their function. Consequently, your immune system, ever alert for proteins that don't look right, produces an inflammatory response, adding further to your Alzheimer's risk.

The good news is we can fix this, and the sooner the better: decreasing insulin resistance and returning insulin sensitivity can be achieved by replacing simple carbohydrates, sugar, and processed foods with nutrient- and fibre-rich vegetables and healthy fats (while concurrently fasting and exercising) to allow your body to create an even more efficient and effective brain fuel.

Here's what you do. Eliminate simple carbohydrates—sugar,

sweets, biscuits, muffins, cakes, breads, pasta, crackers, white potatoes, grains, soft drinks (both regular and diet, since artificial sweeteners disrupt your gut health), fruit juices, alcohol, processed foods, and anything with high-fructose corn syrup. As you limit your intake of simple carbohydrates, you'll be surprised to find that you fairly quickly lose your desire for sweet-tasting food.

Against the Grain

The KetoFLEX 12/3 approach includes the elimination of all grains (with a few exceptions that we'll discuss in chapter 9). Because of the known inflammatory properties of grains, we recommend that everyone focused on optimizing their cognitive health should avoid them.[6]

Let's start with *gluten* (which can be further broken down into glutenin and gliadin), which is the main glue-like protein in many grains, including wheat, rye, and barley. Over the centuries, the ongoing hybridization of wheat has caused the gluten to become increasingly damaging to human health while higher amounts of gluten have been added in an effort to improve texture and the ability to rise.[7] While gluten often bears much of the blame, *gliadin*, a smaller protein within gluten, is an even bigger culprit. There are now more than 200 gliadin varieties, with glia-α9 being the most potent trigger for the intestinal destruction that occurs with coeliac disease. This gliadin protein used to be quite rare but is now present in most wheat varieties.[8] Additionally, modern wheat has been engineered for increased amounts of a naturally occurring lectin (a lectin is a protein that binds carbohydrates and unfortunately can cause inflammation) called *wheat germ agglutinin* (WGA) to help fend off insects and create a more hardy and sustainable crop.[9] As with WGA, our current wheat crop has been bred to have higher levels of inflammatory *phytates*, also known to help fend off insects and increase fibre content. Phytates are often referred to as "anti-nutrients" because they impair the body's ability to absorb minerals.[10]

Agribusiness has successfully created a hardier, more profitable wheat crop, with little regard for the impact of this on human health. Because this hybridization occurred before the advent of modern genetically modified organisms (GMOs), much of the wheat crop has been able to avoid the negative label despite very similar tampering.[11] These combined changes have led to a dramatic increase in coeliac disease and in non-coeliac sensitivity.[12] The pathological effects of gluten are well established in those suffering from coeliac disease, so most of us who do not suffer from coeliac disease assume that we can eat gluten with impunity (and what tastes better than warm bread?). However, unfortunately, non-coeliac gluten sensitivity (NCGS) affects many of us and can cause similar widespread inflammation.[13] Symptoms include GI issues (bloating, abdominal pain, diarrhoea, etc.), fatigue, bone and joint pain, arthritis, osteoporosis, liver and biliary tract disorders, anaemia, anxiety, depression, peripheral neuropathy, migraine, seizures, infertility, cold sores, and skin rash.[14]

In susceptible people (which may turn out to be everyone!), gliadin can inflame the gut and make it permeable, allowing toxins, food fragments, and fragments of bacteria and other microbes into the bloodstream.[15] Eating gluten increases the expression of *zonulin*, a protein that modulates the permeability of tight junctions (which work like Velcro between the cells in your gut) in the GI tract, with increased leakiness leading to a host of chronic diseases.[16] Those with the ApoE4 gene have increased blood-brain barrier permeability, which may render them more susceptible to the exposure of gluten.[17]

The health implications from gluten go beyond wheat to many other grains and even dairy. Some of these foods are contaminated by gluten, contain gliadin proteins, demonstrate cross-reactivity, or closely mimic gliadin proteins. For those who exhibit any symptoms of NCGS, the foods to avoid include rice, corn, oats, millet, amaranth, bulgur, buckwheat, quinoa, and dairy.[18] Be aware that many non-wheat grains have also been genetically modified, changing the way that pesticides are used. Some grains have been engineered to withstand more herbicides (so nearby weeds can be more liberally sprayed with toxic glyphosate), while others produce their own pesticides, conferring a hardier crop with harmful health implications that we're just beginning to understand fully.[19] Even worse, glyphosate is also used as a desiccant to dry crops for easier harvesting. Think about the implications of this. A chemical designated as a probable human carcinogen by the World Health Organization, which has been indicted multiple times in the US court system with awards in excess of $2 billion, is being sprayed not once, but *twice*, doubling our exposure. Furthermore, non-wheat grains often contain toxins, including arsenic. They are also well known to be high in inflammatory *lectins*, another antinutrient.

Grains can also have a strong effect on blood glucose. Traditionally, farmers have fed grains to their livestock to fatten them up before going to market. The same thing happens to humans, as suggested by the increase in prevalence of obesity and diabetes since the government food pyramid guideline encouraged the heavy consumption of grains. These guidelines just happened to coincide with excess grain production and stores due to government subsidies given to farmers.[20]

You might consider a three-week empirical trial by completely eliminating grains from your diet. Be aware of possible withdrawal side effects that may occur during this period due to the opioid-like characteristics of gluten. They can involve a worsening of GI symptoms and an increase in pain. Symptoms typically last about a week, followed by a dramatic improvement with continued abstinence from gluten, all grains, and dairy.[21] Many patients report marked symptom improvement in that short period of time and choose not to reintroduce inflammatory grains.

If you'd like further corroboration, you can consider blood testing through Cyrex Laboratories. First, we recommend that you use Array 2, which tests for intestinal permeability. If that's positive, you may want to test for gluten sensitivity with Array 3X. If you're experiencing symptoms of cognitive decline, you may want to use the Alzheimer's LINX test, which is designed specifically for the contributors to cognitive decline, such as beta-amyloid and other cross-reactive substances, or Array 20, which tests for blood-brain barrier permeability.[22] In the US, any licensed healthcare practitioner can set up an account to order a Cyrex Laboratories test. In the UK these tests would have to be undertaken through private medical clinics. (Regenerus Labs is the sole provider of Cyrex testing in the UK and Ireland. These advanced tests can only be ordered via a healthcare professional registered in the UK or Ireland, who must be pre-registered with Cyrex.)

Given the KetoFLEX 12/3 wholefood approach, "gluten-free" *processed* foods are not a good idea. Why? Because they are full of chemicals and often little better than the foods they were meant to replace. Instead of gluten-free processed food, experiment with grain-free versions of your favourites using ingredients introduced in the Brain Food Pyramid, chapter 6.

Eliminating grains may be a stumbling block for many people because the science appears to be mixed. On one hand, we have epidemiological evidence that a Mediterranean eating pattern, which includes wholegrains, is healthful.[23] On the other hand, you'll recall that the Mediterranean diet has never been trialled against a non-grain version of itself, so the effect of grains on this diet is unknown. The various diets from Blue Zones, places where people are particularly long-lived and healthy, also include some wholegrains, further contributing to the notion that they have a positive effect.[24] It's worth noting, however, that the wholegrains used in these regions are very different from what passes for "wholegrains" in the United States and many other Western countries. They are typically non-engineered (non-GMO) heritage grains that are free from glyphosate (the toxicant in Roundup). The varieties of wheat are much lower in gluten, lower on the glycaemic index, and prepared in ways that render them safer to eat.[25] The Blue Zone Okinawan diet uses much less rice than many other Asian countries, substituting sweet potatoes instead. Additionally, the Okinawan tradition of *hara hachi bu* means that you stop eating when you are 80 per cent full, leading to an overall lower caloric intake, which further protects against insulin resistance.[26]

Dairy

We also recommend abstaining from conventional dairy for many reasons, which we'll cover in greater depth in chapter 11. As mentioned above, this is especially important for those who have a sensitivity to gluten. Often the damage to the gut from gluten (and other grains) can compromise the ability to digest lactose from dairy. Additionally, the immune system often cross-reacts to the casein proteins in dairy because they are so similar to the gliadin proteins in gluten. This concept is sometimes referred to as molecular mimicry and leads to the same inflammatory response.[27]

We understand that everyone moves at a different pace. Some people may not be ready to completely embrace the KetoFLEX 12/3 nutrition plan. They prefer to ease into the programme by cutting out foods in stages: first sugar, then simple carbohydrates (processed foods), then grains, then dairy. There's no right or wrong way, but those who fully embrace the diet do have the opportunity to heal more quickly. *Warning:* If you continue to splurge on foods in this category, please do not begin incorporating higher amounts of dietary fats, since this combination may create dangerous inflammation and impede healing.

ACTION PLAN

- Eliminate all sugar and simple carbohydrates.
- Eliminate all grains (with exceptions noted in chapter 9).
- Eliminate all conventional dairy.

CAUTIONS

GLUTEN WITHDRAWAL (See page 83.)

CHAPTER 6

Feed Your Head: The Brain Food Pyramid

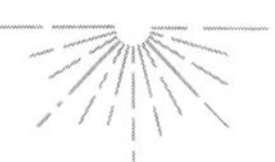

Remember what the dormouse said.

Feed your head, feed your head.

—GRACE SLICK, "WHITE RABBIT"

THE HUMAN BRAIN IS an evolutionary marvel, tripling in size since our first hominid ancestors appeared more than 5 million years ago, with the majority of its expansion having occurred in the last two million years. For much of history, our ancestors' brains were about the size of modern chimpanzees' brains, as evidenced by the finding of "Lucy," a member of an extinct hominid species (*Australopithecus afarensis*) who lived between 3 and 4 million years ago.[1] From that period forward, the human brain evolved in size from 450 cc to 1500 cc, as displayed by a Cro-Magnon man from the *Homo sapiens* species who lived 30,000 years ago.

Our evolved brains are enormous in comparison to our body size. About 500 trillion (500,000,000,000,000) synapses in our brains act as neuron cell connectors, mediating communication. This non-stop activity demands a constant and steady fuel source. While our brains comprise only 2 per cent of our total body mass, they use around 20 per cent of the total energy supply needed for the entire human body.[2] It's vital to ensure that we provide a steady energy supply with high-quality nutrition that optimizes metabolic flexibility.

Interestingly, modern-day human brains are about 10 per cent *smaller* than human brains were at their evolutionary peak, averaging around 1,350 cc. Anthropologists have dated the shrinkage to around 10,000 years ago, when our ancestors transitioned from a hunter-gatherer way of life to an agricultural lifestyle. It has been hypothesized that the reliance upon heavily agricultural sustenance has led to a lack of food diversity, resulting in nutritional deficiencies that continue today.[3]

With the extraordinary abundance of healthful, edible plants available, how did we become so dependent upon agriculturally produced grains? Government-based guidelines, using a food pyramid, focused on pushing inexpensive "nutritious" vitamin-fortified foods to promote health.

The idea of a food pyramid was introduced in 1974 in Sweden, and the first US food pyramid appeared in 1992 and appeared in the UK in 1994 as a pie chart with similar advice to the US pyramid. The food pyramid is a helpful concept, since it guides us to eat more of the healthier foods, depicted at the bottom of the pyramid, and warns us not to eat too many of the less healthy foods at the top of the pyramid.

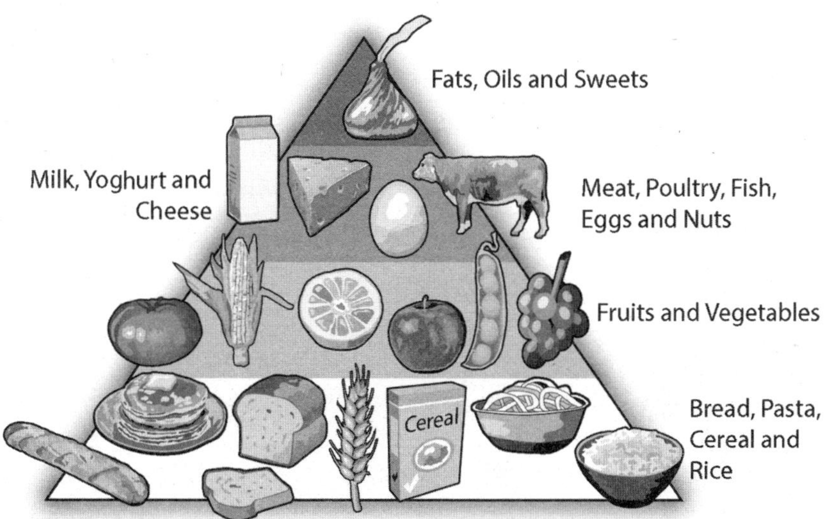

The original food pyramid recommended bread, pasta, cereal, and rice as the major foods to consume—the pyramid's base.

Now that we understand much more about what actually drives cognitive decline than we did back in the twentieth century, we can construct the Brain Food Pyramid, a pyramid optimized for brain function and prevention of cognitive decline. Let's start by examining the original pyramid, which recommended that the foundation of the pyramid—the largest part of our diet—should be from "bread, cereal, rice, and pasta"—"6 to 11 servings per day." In contrast, the fats and oils were at the top—"use sparingly." It has turned out that this is a good recipe for giving ourselves obesity, insulin resistance, diabetes, hypertension, and cognitive decline—exactly what so many of us now suffer from.

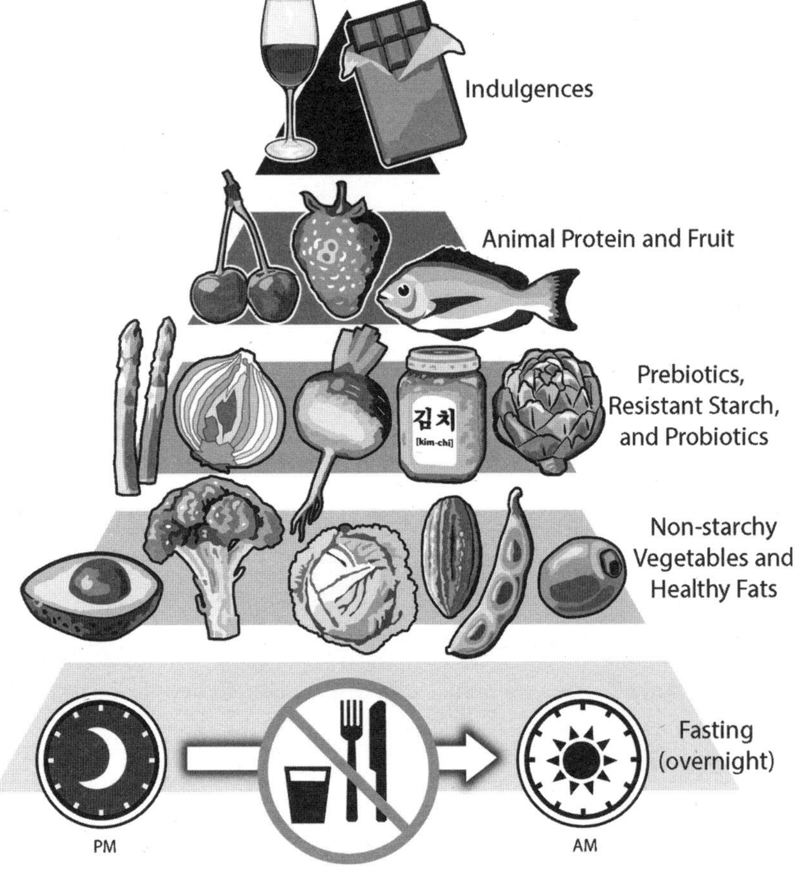

The Brain Food Pyramid puts cognition-enhancing foods and practices such as fasting, healthy fats, and non-starchy vegetables at the base.

Let's look at why a new pyramid is so helpful for cognition, and what the Brain Food Pyramid looks like.

In an effort to meet the nutritional needs of our metabolically demanding brains, the Brain Food Pyramid actually must turn the traditional US Department of Agriculture food pyramid upside down. That's because it focuses on optimizing cognitive and overall health as opposed to encouraging the use of foods that benefit government policy and economics.[4] The advice given to Westerners, and indeed much of the world for too long, has been based on political and financial considerations. Even the American Heart Association has traditionally put its "heart-check" logo on highly processed foods with added sugar because manufacturers paid for the certification and their food products met the criteria for being low in dietary fat.[5] Low-fat Pop-Tarts were touted as "heart healthy" while fresh fruits and vegetables were initially excluded, leading consumers to believe processed foods were the healthier choice.[6] Because of incontrovertible nutritional science and greater public scrutiny, the guidelines of the American Heart Association have evolved and now include some fresh produce and even recognize some healthy fats, such as nuts and avocados.[7]

Another aspect to consider is the fact that wholegrains have been available for only the last 10,000 years. Our human ancestors, all ApoE4 carriers, ate non-grain plants for millions of years before that.[8] It's important to grasp the enormous divide between our modern lifestyle and our still primitive genome. Human genetic evolution occurs very slowly despite the extreme conditions foisted upon our primal biology by our current environment. For example, the ApoE4 gene first came on the scene around 7 million years ago, and approximately 25 per cent of the population still carries this gene. The ApoE3 allele (variant), which is now the most common, did not appear until much more recently—220,000 years ago—while the ApoE2 gene showed up only 80,000 years ago. Evolutionists are unsure exactly what precipitated this evolutionary appearance of ApoE3 and ApoE2, but some have proposed the advent of fire and the ability to eat meat as contributing factors.[9]

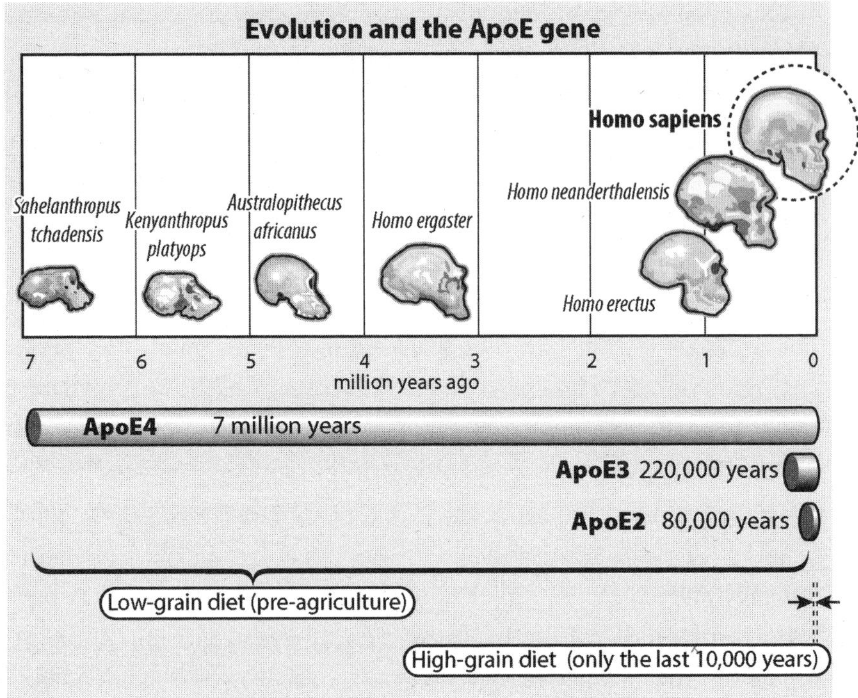

ApoE4 was the original ApoE allele for hominids. ApoE3 and ApoE2 appeared only much more recently in evolution.

As hunter-gatherers, our ancestors likely foraged wild plants (in between the occasional hunt), and thus had a diet extraordinarily rich in fibre. When this fibre is broken down, it ferments in the gut, creating the ketone BHB (beta-hydroxybutyrate), which may have contributed fuel for their brains.[10] The combination of food scarcity and an active lifestyle combined with an extraordinarily high-fibre diet and occasional fatty animal protein likely led to a natural state of ketosis much of the time. The ApoE4 gene is rare in populations with exposure to agriculture, suggesting that the consumption of a diet high in grain may have selected against this genotype.[11] A return to a pre-agricultural diet, *heavy in non-grain plants*, may provide an alternative dietary path for avoiding disease, and also represents a strategy to heal the growing schism between our ancestral genes and our modern world.

Our relatively primitive biology is now exposed to an environment that is very different from the world in which it evolved. In just the last fifty to a hundred years, we have seen an exponential escalation of the toxic effects of our modern environment. We consume an excess of hyper-palatable fake food comprised of simple carbohydrates and engineered grains and oils, laden with edible chemicals. Even the "healthy" produce we eat has been hybridized to have the highest sugar content possible and is often doused in toxic pesticides. The animals we eat have been fed unnatural inflammatory foods, given hormones to promote rapid growth, and raised in toxic living conditions that require high doses of antibiotics. We're too often sedentary, sitting in our cars, at our desks, on our sofas. We endure constant exposure to electromagnetic fields (EMF), Wi-Fi, and artificial blue light that encourages us to disregard our natural *circadian rhythms* (internal clocks directing our sleep/wake cycles). We breathe toxic air that results from industry and transportation. Our lawns are full of hazardous chemicals. We spray our skin with harmful insect repellent. We apply sunscreen with toxic chemicals to protect against the vitamin D our bodies need. The water we drink is full of the residue from all of the chemicals we use in our daily lives. Even our bedding is covered in toxic flame retardant. We no longer interact with a healthy soil that could enhance our microbiome. Instead, we frequently use chemical hand sanitizers to protect ourselves. The list of assaults on our ancient genome is endless and growing. Many of the strategies we recommend are attempts to heal and correct the damage caused by the world we've created rather than an attempt to mimic early man.

We thus offer the Brain Food Pyramid as a guide. We acknowledge the many controversies and unknowns and remain open to continued refinement as new science emerges. We encourage you to use this information to learn about food, not only as "medicine" but also as a delicious opportunity to explore, experiment, and nurture! Simple adjustments in our food choices can provide profound healing. As with all food pyramids, we encourage you to partake generously from the bottom of the food pyramid and more sparingly as you move towards the top. We'll slowly move up the pyramid to discuss each level.

The pace at which these changes are adopted depends upon many individual factors, such as your metabolic state (especially your insulin sensitivity); your ability to move and deal with stress; your sleep habits; and your support systems to help you initiate and maintain change. Modifications can be implemented slowly over weeks, months, or all at once. Those making the transition quickly have the opportunity to promote healing more rapidly, but should also be aware of the possible, usually mild and transitory, side effects that can result, which we'll discuss in chapter 7 with simple work-arounds to help you reach success.

CHAPTER 7

Pyramid Level 1: Clean House

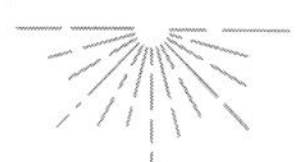

Fasting is the greatest remedy—the physician within.
—PARACELSUS

If you're not supposed to eat at night, why is there a light in the fridge?
—WOODROW PAIGE

WE'RE GOING TO DISCUSS fasting before we begin recommending specific foods. *It's that important.* The 12/3 part of the KetoFLEX 12/3 lifestyle refers to *how many hours* you should be fasting (at least twelve) and *when* you should be fasting (at least three hours before bed). Not only has fasting been a historical part of the evolution of mankind, as an adaptation to food scarcity, it's also been incorporated into all of the major religions since their inception, both for the clarity of mind and the many health benefits.

The health benefits of fasting are numerous through a variety of healing mechanisms. Most important for the purposes of our approach, fasting promotes the restoration of insulin sensitivity, which leads to an improvement in cognition. In our modern era, non-stop access to refined, sugary, processed, chemical-laden food leads to insulin resistance and metabolic inflexibility, whereby the source of fuel is limited to glucose, without the ability to utilize fats or their derivative ketones. Insulin resistance is central to the epidemic of chronic disease, including Alzheimer's. Fasting offers a venue to help restore insulin sensitivity. Insulin sensitivity helps end the cycle of food craving and allows our bodies to burn fat for fuel. Achieving the ability to burn fat, becoming insulin sensitive, and having the metabolic flexibility to use either glucose or ketones as a fuel are key to multiple healing elements. Fasting also leads to a decrease in inflammation and enhances mitochondrial function, boosting longevity. Additionally, fasting reduces the risk of heart disease, cancer, and autoimmune conditions.[1]

Fasting, especially for twelve hours or more, engenders *autophagy*, an evolutionary healing process by which your cells "clean house" and recycle components such as amino acids and mitochondria. Damaged and worn-out cellular constituents such as mitochondria are gobbled up, stripped for parts, and used to make new cellular components.[2] Autophagy also enhances the energy production of our mitochondria, the battery organelles of our cells. Healthy mitochondria are of key importance in preventing and healing neurodegeneration.[3] Other means of promoting autophagy include nutritional ketosis, exercise, protein restriction, and restorative sleep. Even after you've broken your fast with nutritional ketosis, autophagy continues on a neuronal level.[4]

We use the period of sleep to optimize a natural time of fasting every night. Since we need the least amount of energy at night and sleep is the time for detoxification and repair, not digestion, it is best to avoid food for at least three hours before bed. It takes at least twelve hours to deplete glycogen stores (stored glucose), after which you begin to burn fat. Some claim that it takes much longer for glycogen stores to empty (which may be true), but in the context of having achieved the KetoFLEX 12/3 goals, we believe that we are encouraging autophagy through multiple mechanisms that converge to offer benefits *sooner* on a nightly basis. This can be achieved in different ways. Some have early dinners, light dinners, or skip dinner. Alternatively, skipping breakfast is easier for others. Your home, work, and social demands along with your unique circadian rhythm can help guide the best fasting period for you.

The Fasting Goals of KetoFLEX 12/3

- **Fast for at least three to four hours prior to going to bed.** Sleep is an important time for detoxification and repair. As the day winds down, the body needs less food for energy and should be entering a fat-burning state. Sleep, especially that which honours your unique circadian rhythm, is also an opportunity to add hours to a total fasting time.
- **Fast for at least twelve hours between the end of dinner and the beginning of breakfast.** ApoE4 carriers may want to work towards extending the fast to sixteen hours or more. During this period, you may enjoy green tea or black coffee, since they do not break the fast. Those with insulin resistance, who are working to extend their fast, may want to add MCT initially or coconut oil to your morning tea or coffee. These fats provide energy, therefore technically breaking the fast and thus potentially impeding autophagy, but they help you to achieve nutritional ketosis, which can ultimately heal the underlying metabolic issues, enabling you to fast for the prescribed time period.
- **It is best to break the fast with a detoxifying beverage** such as room-temperature water with fresh-squeezed lemon juice or slices of ginger, or a tea such as milk thistle, lemongrass, ginger, or dandelion.
- **As we've described previously, fasting is especially difficult to initiate for those with insulin resistance.** You'll recall that when your body is used to burning glucose steadily as fuel, it has trouble shifting to burning fat. When "fat-adapted," you will be able to go for longer periods without hunger.

Depending upon the severity of your insulin resistance, the transition to the KetoFLEX 12/3 fasting goals may take weeks or even months. By following our guidelines, you should be able to extend the length of your fast a little more each day until you've reached your target. Many patients have found that as they've adopted the KetoFLEX 12/3 lifestyle, they naturally gravitate towards eating only one or two meals per day. This is a mark of success as long as you're maintaining a healthy weight and feeling strong. Indeed, once you are insulin sensitive, a long daily fast soon becomes a way of life and provides an enormous amount of freedom from frequent food shopping, cooking, eating, and cleaning up. Most who've reached this stage report a markedly improved sense of energy and cognitive clarity as well.

Tips for Transitioning to a Longer Fast

- **Distinguish between hunger and true hypoglycaemia (low blood sugar), the latter of which can be dangerous.** Hypoglycaemia leads to symptoms of light-headedness, confusion, slurred speech, blurred vision, hunger, irritability, shaking, anxiety, and sweating, and it may wake you in the middle of the night.[5] If you're uncertain which you're experiencing (assuming the symptoms are mild), test your blood sugar with instructions provided in chapter 18, page 258. In true diabetes, a measurement below 70 mg/dL is considered hypoglycaemic. It's worth noting that those who are insulin sensitive can experience much lower blood glucose levels *without* symptoms.
- **If your blood glucose is below 70 mg/dL and the symptoms are severe, immediately consume some fast-acting source of sugar such as fruit juice.** This may feel counterproductive to the end goal, but it is necessary to address the immediate hypoglycaemia. As you adopt the KetoFLEX 12/3 nutrition recommendations, replacing sugars and refined carbohydrates with fibre-rich, non-starchy vegetables and healthy fats, hypoglycaemic episodes will no longer occur. *Note:* Diabetics must consult with their doctors before beginning this programme so that they can be instructed on how to reduce medication(s) as they heal, to avoid a hypoglycaemic episode.

- **If your blood glucose is within normal range and you are simply hungry, try eating a healthy fat such as nuts, seeds, or avocado slices to encourage ketosis.** Try to extend your fast for five to fifteen minutes longer each day until you reach the recommended goal.
- **Consider using a ketone supplement such as medium-chain triglycerides (MCT oil or coconut oil) or exogenous (*exo* meaning from outside the body) source of ketones such as ketone salts or esters to accelerate ketosis.** (Find other possibilities in chapter 21.) Once insulin sensitivity is restored and you've successfully adopted the KetoFLEX 12/3 lifestyle, you'll be naturally producing ketone bodies endogenously (*endo* meaning from inside the body) by burning your own stored body fat and, over time, will likely not have a need for exogenous ketones. Ideally, supplementation is transitional and short term.

Those who don't break their fast until later in the day often struggle with when to take their morning supplements so as not to interfere with autophagy. The very small number of calories in supplements is of little concern and has minimal effect on autophagy. Some, like resveratrol and curcumin, will even enhance it.[6] Be sure to take fat-soluble supplements (such as vitamins D, E, and K, and curcumin) with fish oil or cod liver oil if you need it for vitamin A due to genetically poor beta-carotene conversion to retinol.

EXCESSIVE WEIGHT LOSS

We've found that some patients have difficulty maintaining their weight, which can become counterproductive. While body mass index is a rough measure, taking into account only height and weight, there is a lot of room for personalization based upon your body frame and muscle composition. We recommend maintaining a minimum BMI of 18.5 for women and 19.0 for men if under age 65 and higher for those over age 65. If your weight drops beyond that, you are at increased risk of sarcopenia (the loss of lean muscle mass) and osteopenia (the loss of bone), both of which accompany ageing and *are correlated with an INCREASED risk of cognitive decline.* (We'll talk more about this in chapter 13.) For now, understand that you must adjust your strategies if your weight drops too low. Here are some helpful tips.

Strategies for Gaining Weight

- **Consider shortening your fast.** Still try to stop eating several hours before bed, but feel free to eat in the morning following the KetoFLEX 12/3 food pyramid.
- **Use more healthy fat!**
    - Add an extra tablespoon or two of high polyphenol extra virgin olive oil (EVOO) to your salads and veggies. This is an easy way to add extra calories.
    - Enjoy an extra handful (or two) of nuts. Nuts are extraordinarily healthful and delicious. Freely enjoy. Macadamias and pecans are especially helpful for weight gain.
    - Add ghee, coconut oil, or MCT to your coffee. This is a simple way to increase calories and induce ketosis. The exogenous ketones from coconut and MCT oil may be especially helpful for those trying to gain weight, as low body fat may prohibit the creation of endogenous ketones.
    - If you develop GI symptoms, consider the use of digestive enzymes. But see the cautions about this in chapter 8.
- **Ensure that you're getting enough protein in your diet** (review the suggestions in chapter 10). Your body cannot synthesize or store the protein it needs for essential body functions. You should include it in your diet, or your body may cannibalize your muscles—not good! While you are

healing your digestive system and recovering from toxic exposures, you may have additional protein requirements. Equally important is adequate stomach acid to ensure proper digestion of protein.

- **Be strong.** Be sure to concentrate on building strong muscles and bones. Devote a part of your exercise programme to strength training and weight-bearing exercise.
- **Don't forget resistant starches.** Add a small amount of cooked and cooled legumes, root vegetables, or tubers at each meal. By using EVOO or ghee as a delicious topping, you'll both blunt any glycaemic response and add extra calories. You can also cycle out of ketosis once or twice per week, with sweet potatoes, for example, to avoid further weight loss.
- **Get involved in meal planning and preparation.** Scour recipes to find innovative ways to make your favourite foods to stimulate your appetite. If you're cooking for someone affected with Alzheimer's, involve him or her in the meal planning and preparation. Seeing, touching, and smelling the food promotes the secretion of our digestive enzymes and prepares our bodies to eat.
- **Relax while eating.** Turn off your TV and your phone. Put away your work. Make mealtime a nurturing and relaxing ritual. Slowly enjoy your food. Linger over a second helping. You're worth it.

ACTION PLAN

- Fast for at least three hours before bed for a total of a minimum of twelve hours.
- ApoE4 carriers may want to try to extend their fast to sixteen-plus hours.

CAUTIONS

- Hypoglycaemia
- Hypotension
- Excessive weight loss
- Keto flu. As you extend your fast and decrease simple carbohydrates, you're likely to begin creating ketone bodies. Congratulations! This is one of the goals of the KetoFLEX 12/3 approach. But some patients report symptoms, dubbed the keto flu, which are transient. Not everyone is affected, and the severity of the symptoms varies from person to person. Dehydration (and the subsequent mineral loss) lies behind most of these transitional side effects. As you extend your fast, your body is burning up the extra glycogen (stored glucose) in your liver and muscles. Breaking down glycogen releases a lot of water. As your carb intake and glycogen stores drop, your kidneys will start dumping this excess water through urination, leading to dehydration.[7] If you're concurrently cutting out processed food, you've dramatically decreased your salt intake. It's especially important while transitioning, and throughout the period of time that you're practising the KetoFLEX 12/3 lifestyle, to stay hydrated and to supplement with sea salt* to replenish lost minerals. This transition leads to lower blood pressure for most people even with the addition of sea salt. A small subset may be susceptible to higher blood pressure with added salt. Be sure to monitor your blood pressure to see how you respond.

Possible Symptoms of the Keto Flu

- Headaches
- Difficulty focusing—"brain fog"
- Fatigue

---

*If you choose a non-iodized salt, be sure to get adequate iodine through your diet from sources such as fish or sea vegetables.

- Nausea
- Bad breath
- Leg cramps
- Faster heart rate
- Light-headedness (hypotension)
- Reduced physical performance

TOXINS IN FAT Some toxins, including persistent organic pollutants, are stored in the fat of animals, including humans. When we begin burning our own fat, we transiently re-expose ourselves to our own stored toxins, which may lead to symptoms that overlap with the keto flu. Because the KetoFLEX 12/3 lifestyle promotes fat burning, it's very important to further support detoxification pathways, especially during the initial period of keto adaptation and while you are losing any excess weight. To promote glutathione production, which aids in detoxification, prioritize cruciferous vegetables, alliums, mushrooms, spinach, asparagus, avocados, okra, and liver. Curcumin, N-acetylcysteine, alpha-lipoic acid, selenium, zinc, and milk thistle supplements can also aid in detoxification.[8] Staying well hydrated with clean water and eating plentiful amounts of plant fibre also promote detoxification.[9] Sweating through exercise or sauna use may also be helpful during this period.[10]

CHAPTER 8

Pyramid Level 2: Indulge Freely

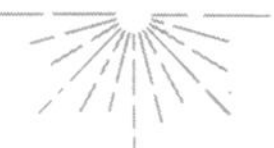

Too much of a good thing can be wonderful.
—MAE WEST

VEGETABLES

Go crazy in the produce aisle or preferably in your garden or local farmers' market. Non-starchy vegetables are among the foods that are essentially unlimited on this KetoFLEX 12/3 eating plan. Freely indulge in vegetables from every colour of the rainbow. Find the most deeply pigmented and vibrant plants that you can source. Look for wild, novel varieties of greens and fragrant herbs. Forget about pale green iceberg lettuce and look for red, burgundy, and bronze-coloured leaves from varieties such as Rossa di Treviso, a radicchio that is an antioxidant superstar, and Outredgeous, a deeply pigmented romaine rich in anthocyanins, a type of neuroprotective flavonoid.[1] Experiment! Challenge yourself to try a new vegetable each time you gather your produce. Become familiar with kohlrabi, artichokes, celeriac, okra, and Mexican yam! Try to source organic, local, and seasonal when possible. At every meal your plate should mostly be covered with a wide variety of raw and lightly cooked vegetables (cooking increases the bioavailability of some nutrients), heavily drizzled with extra virgin olive oil to increase the bioavailability of the phytonutrients and antioxidants.[2]

Choose primarily non-starchy vegetables. Glycaemic index is a scale that provides a relative ranking based on effect on blood glucose levels. These non-starchy vegetables will have a ranking below 35 (plain sugar is the standard at 100). Another helpful term is net carbs, which gives the carbohydrates minus the fibre, in grams. In general, foods with a low glycaemic index or net carbs have less impact on blood glucose.[3] Combining any vegetable with healthy fat, such as high polyphenol extra virgin olive oil, also reduces glycaemic impact. To help you choose the vegetables least likely to affect your glycaemic control, please see the chart below.

VEGETABLES

VEGETABLES	LEAFY (L)	CRUCIFEROUS (C)	FRUITS, LEGUMES, AND FUNGI	HERBS AND SPICES
Artichokes*	Beet greens*	Broccoli*	Acorn squash*** x	Basil*
Asparagus**	Chicories*: endive, escarole, frisée, radicchio	Brussels sprouts*	Aubergine* x	Bay leaves*
Bamboo shoots*	Dandelion greens (C)*	Cabbages (L)*: pak choi, Chinese, savoy, red, green	Avocado*	Black pepper*
Beetroot*** ♦ (cooked)	Kale (C)* ♦	Cauliflower*	Courgettes* ♦ x	Chives*
Beetroot** ♦ (raw)	Lettuces*: leaf (red, green, oak), butter, mesclun (young blend), Romaine (red, green)	Dandelion greens (L)*	Cucumber* x	Coriander*
Carrots*** (cooked)	Purslane*	Horseradish*	Green beans* x	Cinnamon*
Carrots** (raw)	Rocket (C)*	Kale (L)* ♦	Mushrooms*: button, chanterelle, cremini, oyster, porcini, portobello, reishi, shiitake	Coriander (seeds)*

(Table continues)

VEGETABLES	LEAFY (L)	CRUCIFEROUS (C)	FRUITS, LEGUMES, AND FUNGI	HERBS AND SPICES
Celery* ♦	Spinach* ♦	Kohlrabi*	Okra*	Cumin*
Celeriac**	Spring greens (C)*	Radicchio (L)*	Olives*	Dill seed/ weed*
Fennel*	Spring greens (C)*	Radish*	Peas*x: green, snap, snow	Ginger*
Garlic*	Swiss chard (C)*	Rapini*	Pumpkin*** x	Lavender*
Heart of palm*	Turnip greens (C)*	Rocket (L)*	Spaghetti squash* x	Lemongrass*
Jerusalem artichokes*	Watercress (C)	Spring greens (L)*	Sweet peppers* x	Maca (Peruvian ginseng)*
Leeks*		Spring greens (L)*	Tomato* ♦ x	Marjoram*
Mexican yam*		Swiss chard (L)*	Tomatillo* x	Mint*
Onions*		Tenderstem broccoli*	Yellow squash* x	Oregano*
Sea vegetables*		Turnip greens (L)*		Parsley*
Shallots*		Watercress (L)*		Rosemary*
Spring onions*				Saffron*
				Sage*
				Tarragon*
				Thyme*
				Turmeric*
				Wasabi*

KEY
Leafy (L)
Cruciferous (C)
Glycaemic Index: Low* Intermediate High*****
Organic ♦
High in Lectins x

COLOURED VEGETABLES are rich in carotenoids (beta-carotene, lycopene, lutein, and zeaxanthin) and flavonoids, both of which are powerfully anti-inflammatory and neuroprotective.[4] Search for the rainbow. In general, the more deeply pigmented, the greater the health benefits. Dark leafy greens, red cabbage, red onions, carrots (best eaten raw since cooking increases the glycaemic effect), aubergines, tomatoes (especially cooked, which increases lycopene content), and sweet red, yellow, and orange peppers are just a few examples.

LEAFY GREENS engage multiple neuroprotective mechanisms. Healthy seniors who enjoy daily helpings of leafy green vegetables have a slower rate of cognitive decline, compared to those who eat few or no greens.[5] Leafy greens are high in folate, which comes from the term *foliage*. When combined with B_{12} and B_6, folate reduces homocysteine (a protein by-product) in the blood, which, when elevated, contributes to inflammation. Elevated homocysteine corresponds with cognitive decline, white matter damage, brain atrophy, neurofibrillary tangles, and dementia.[6]

DARK LEAFY GREENS including rocket, coriander, butter leaf lettuce, mesclun greens, basil, beetroot greens, oak leaf lettuce, and Swiss chard, as well as rhubarb and beetroot, are the highest sources of dietary nitrates.[7] Yes, rocket is the new Viagra! (Did we get your attention?) Plant-based nitrates convert into nitric oxide, a potent vasodilator, thereby promoting vascular health, naturally relaxing blood vessels, decreasing blood pressure, and increasing blood flow throughout the body, particularly benefiting your heart and brain.[8] Other leafy greens include kale, spinach, spring greens, red romaine, dandelion greens, watercress, rapini, endive, and fennel. Use any and every meal as an opportunity to include fresh or lightly stir-fried nutrient-rich greens.

CRUCIFEROUS VEGETABLES are some of the most powerful and nutrient-dense vegetables. The sulphur component of cruciferous vegetables gives some bitter taste but is responsible for many of the health merits. Sulphur is required for the synthesis of glutathione, the master antioxidant, for detoxification in the liver, and for the production of several amino acids that provide the structural component of many tissues and hormones.[9] Cruciferous vegetables are enormously helpful for their detoxifying effect. The alliums (onions, shallots, garlic, leeks) and the brassicas (cabbage, broccoli, cauliflower, Brussels sprouts, pak choi) aid in detoxification, protect from oxidative damage, and improve glucose metabolism.[10] When cruciferous vegetables are chopped and chewed, their unique sulphur compounds are converted and released. If you are heating them, wait after chopping them for 10 to 45 minutes to allow a heat-sensitive enzyme, myrosinase, in cruciferous vegetables to be released for the conversion into the healthful sulphur compounds.[11] Cruciferous vegetables are best consumed blanched, lightly steamed, or stir-fried at a medium heat to preserve a bit of crunch.[12] Adding mustard seed or other raw cruciferous products, such as broccoli sprouts, can achieve the same benefits, without the wait.[13]

One crucifer, broccoli, activates the Nrf2 pathway.[14] Nrf2 is a powerful protein in each cell that serves as a "master regulator" of the body's detoxicant and antioxidant response. Nrf2 is like a thermostat within our cells that senses the level of oxidative stress and other stressors and activates protective mechanisms. Nrf2 activation is a potent strategy to combat toxins and *oxidative damage* associated with Alzheimer's disease.[15] (Oxidative damage refers to the effects of free radicals and related damaging chemicals.) By consuming broccoli sprouts (3- to 4-day-old broccoli plants), you can access the most potent form of the vegetable activator. You can grow them at home. (Be sure to buy organic, certified pathogen-free seeds, as all sprouts are susceptible to contamination.) Alternatively, you can take sulforaphane as a supplement.

AVOCADOS, OLIVES, AND TOMATOES are the delicious Mediterranean gems of any salad. They're technically fruits, but we've very purposefully included them in the *vegetable* section of our food pyramid to encourage generous consumption. There's a sizable overlap between the categorization of fruits and vegetables when you consider that vegetables are basically any part of a plant that is edible: leaves, stems, roots, tubers, nuts, seeds, or flowers with the seed. Avocados, olives, and tomatoes are flowers with seeds, botanically referred to as fruit. From a culinary perspective, however, they're often used as vegetables due to their savoury taste.

Avocados are one of the healthiest foods you can consume. This fruit has one of the highest beneficial fats (monounsaturated) and almost no sugar. Avocados will not induce glucose spikes and can help you achieve a ketotic state. They are rich in potassium, magnesium, vitamins C and E, and their fat helps you to absorb fat-soluble vitamins (vitamins A, D, E, and K).[16] Avocados are also rich in soluble fibre and support metabolic health as well as small dense LDL and LDL particle number.[17] They can easily be added to every meal and needn't be organic due to their thick, protective skin.

Olives are low in carbohydrates and high in beneficial (monounsaturated) fats, with a rich phytonutrient profile, and thus are a healthy addition to any salad or may be eaten alone.[18] Olives have antioxidant, anti-inflammatory, antiatherogenic, anti-cancer, antimicrobial, and antiviral activities, along with a glucose and lipid-lowering effect.[19] Because olives are naturally bitter, they are cured in brine, contributing to their salty taste. Prior to this step, olives must first be fermented. The fermentation process leads them to be naturally rich in *Lactobacillus*, a gut-friendly bacteria, further contributing to their healthful profile.[20]

Tomatoes are an integral part of the Mediterranean diet, well known for their healthful properties.[21] They're rich in *carotenoids* (plant pigments responsible for bright red, yellow, and orange hues in many fruits and vegetables), specifically lycopene, which protect against cancer, heart disease, oxidative stress, and eye disease.[22] Older adults, with a diet rich in carotenoids combined with omega-3s, displayed improved cognitive performance and greater network efficiency in the brain.[23] Because carotenoids are fat-soluble, ensuring that you're consuming them with dietary fat can greatly improve the amount of neuroprotective polyphenols and carotenoids.[24] Integrating sofrito into your diet may be a simple and delicious way to do just that! This is a finely chopped component of most Mediterranean sauces typically consisting of tomatoes, garlic, onions, and peppers cooked in olive oil. A recent study demonstrated that a single dose of sofrito powerfully downregulated inflammatory markers.[25] It's worth noting that tomatoes in the Mediterranean region are typically peeled and seeded before cooking, reducing their lectin content. All tinned tomatoes are pressure cooked, also reducing lectins. Look for Soil Association (UK) organic, preferably peeled and seeded.

HERBS AND SPICES are integral to cooking wholefoods. These often contain far more of the disease-fighting antioxidants and *polyphenols* than traditional vegetables.[26] (Polyphenols are compounds found in plants that protect against cellular damage.) Herbs and spices also have recognized antiviral and antimicrobial properties.[27] Herbs and spices such as parsley, basil, oriander, rosemary, sage, thyme, oregano, fennel, coriander, cumin, and mint can easily be worked into every meal, even into marinades and oils, to amplify both the flavour and healthful benefits. Many common herbs and spices, such as saffron, turmeric, cinnamon, ginger, ginseng, sage, garlic, black pepper, and paprika have been found to exert neuroprotective qualities that may help prevent and even treat Alzheimer's disease.[28]

- ***TURMERIC*** is a luminary in the spice aisle. It's a major ingredient in curry powder and has been used as a flavour enhancer and medicine in India for thousands of years. Both ground turmeric and shaved turmeric root can be used in cooking to add a pungent, gingery taste, with a tinge of mustard or horseradish (beware that some turmeric is tainted with lead, so it is best to purchase it from a trusted source). Curcumin is the active ingredient in turmeric, and it has both anti-inflammatory effects and beta-amyloid-binding effects. Although the absorption of curcumin is poor, combining curcumin with black pepper increases the bioavailability by 2000 per cent.[29] Additionally, the Indian dish curry contains elements that also increase the bioavailability of curcumin: the fat in coconut milk (turmeric is fat-soluble), quercetin-containing foods (such as onions), and the application of heat. There have been many studies demonstrating the efficacy of curcumin in treating dementia through multiple mechanisms, but one of the most exciting was a small randomized double-blind placebo-controlled trial done at UCLA. Participants between the ages of 50 and 90, with mild memory problems but not diagnosed with Alzheimer's, were randomized to take 90 mg of curcumin or a placebo for eighteen months. The memory function of those who received the curcumin rose by 28 per cent over the course of the study. Their depressive symptoms lessened, as did the level of beta-amyloid and tau in their brains.[30]

- ***SAFFRON***, by far the most precious spice found in most supermarkets and shops selling Asian and Middle Eastern foods and produce, can easily be identified by its long crimson strands, although it's sometimes ground into a powder. Saffron imparts both an earthiness and a sweetness, not unlike honey, when used in cooking and imbues the food with a rich golden colour.[31] Saffron was recently tested on Alzheimer's patients in a small clinical trial with impressive results.[32]
- ***TEAS*** are often comprised of dried herbs, some of which have been found to protect against Alzheimer's. Epigallocatechin-3-gallate (EGCG), a flavonoid found in green tea, penetrates the blood-brain barrier and is the principal anti-inflammatory in green tea. Be sure to keep your water temperature below 76°C to preserve the health benefits. Cold brewing is fine but should be performed for at least two hours. When possible, buy loose-leaf teas (to be used with an infuser), as some companies are now adding plastic to tea bags, which when combined with hot water leaches plastic particles into the tea. Matcha tea has the highest concentration of EGCG, 137 per cent more than green tea. Be sure to source organic matcha tea from Japan (not China) to avoid heavy metal contamination. In the preparation of matcha tea, warm or cold water is fine, as brewing isn't necessary.

ACTION PLAN

- Eat at *least* 6 to 9 servings of deeply pigmented, organic, seasonal, local non-starchy vegetables per day, gradually increasing the amount.

- Include leafy greens, especially those that produce nitric oxide.
- Include cruciferous vegetables, paying attention to preparation to maximize health benefits.
- Challenge yourself to bring home one novel vegetable (or new variety of a familiar vegetable) each time you shop to expand your repertoire.
- Include fresh herbs, spices, and teas.

CAUTIONS

INTERFERENCE WITH WARFARIN If you are taking warfarin, your GP should approve and monitor any change in intake of foods rich in vitamin K, such as leafy greens and other vegetables (and some fruits). Warfarin works as an anticoagulant by interfering with vitamin K, and therefore increases of vitamin K may lessen its efficacy.

PESTICIDES/HERBICIDES Glyphosate and other pervasive herbicides and pesticides are covered in chapter 19. Additionally, other pesticides known to be harmful to human health that have been banned in other countries including the UK and the EU, but are still used in the US include paraquat (linked to Parkinson's disease and kidney and lung problems), 1-3-dichloropropene (classified as a probable human carcinogen by the Environmental Protection Agency), and atrazine (a hormone disrupter, immune system deregulator, possible carcinogen, with effects on reproduction and development).[33] After leaving the EU, the UK may once again allow these chemicals to be used in agriculture

The US Environmental Working Group's annual list of the Dirty Dozen and Clean Fifteen can help you prioritize permitted fruits and vegetables to buy organic. Selecting organic produce may be especially important for ApoE4 carriers. Research shows this group has a significantly increased risk of cognitive impairment with high blood levels of toxic pesticides.[34] Although DDT and DDE have been banned for years in many countries, some legacy contamination still remains today. Evidence shows that soil can remain toxic for up to fifteen years, while aquatic environments show contamination for up to a hundred and fifty years.[35]

Levels can be much higher from produce from other countries where it is still in use today or has more recently been banned. These toxic pesticides accumulate in the body's fat, and 80 per cent of healthy Americans still show demonstrable blood levels.[36] In the UK, buying Soil Association approved organic is the safest way to ensure that you're getting the lowest possible exposure.

GMOS Genetically modified organisms (GMOs) have infiltrated our food supply. The rationale behind them was to breed plants that could tolerate more herbicides and could produce their own pesticides. Engineering these traits has provided economic benefits, but also has led to an increased exposure to the herbicide glyphosate (commercially known as Roundup), and a host of ill health effects.[37] Avoid any GMO food (and the animals that eat them), which includes most soy, corn, rapeseed oil, dairy, sugar, wheat, and courgettes. The UK government (along with 63 other nations around the world) insists on labelling of any GMO content in products. The US does not require this. The label *Certified USDA Organic* means the produce should not be GMO (the same pertains in the UK with Soil Association approval). *Non-GMO Project Verified* is a label that provides testing of residue to 0.9 per cent at multiple levels of production.

BPA/BPS Bisphenol A and bisphenol S are chemical cousins commonly found in plastics, food, beverage tin linings, thermal receipts, and other consumer products. BPA is known to cause harm to the brain, and both chemicals are hormone disrupters. Look for the BPA-free label on plastic or tinned products. If that isn't present, turn it upside down to look for the recycle number. Avoid #7. Be aware that BPA-free may still contain BPS. To avoid both, look for Tetra Pak containers (made from 75 per cent paper board). They are labelled with an FSC designation, from the Forest Stewardship Council. This is especially important for tinned tomatoes, as their acid may cause additional leaching of these toxic chemicals. This is another reason to avoid packaged food altogether and cook from scratch when possible.

HEAVY METALS Heavy metals are a concern in any vegetables coming from developing countries and those from industrialized countries that are known to be highly polluted, such as China and India. Very often waste water as irrigation or by-products from mining or smelting contribute to soil contaminated with heavy metals in these regions.[38] Given that a third of all vegetables and half of all fruits are imported, we have no way of knowing if imported organic produce is safe.[39] It is subject to "spot inspections" and "on-site testing," but we have no way of knowing how often this is occurring.[40] For this reason, we recommend buying only organic.

LECTINS Lectins are proteins that bind to sugars, and may cause inflammation in the digestive system by compromising the gut integrity (leaky gut) and may lead to mild (aches and pains) or widespread systemic autoimmune conditions. Foods high in lectins include grains, pseudograins, legumes, some vegetables (especially nightshades such as tomatoes, potatoes, aubergines, goji berries, and sweet and chilli peppers), nuts (in particular cashews), and seeds. Soaking and pressure-cooking legumes, soaking and/or sprouting nuts or seeds, or peeling the skin and removing the seeds of high-lectin vegetables, especially nightshades, reduce lectins. However, these methods may not be enough for those who are very susceptible to their inflammatory effects. Those individuals may need a programme to help identify and eliminate the cause of their inflammation and subsequent healing of their gut prior to reintroduction (see chapter 9). *The Plant Paradox*, written by Steven Gundry, MD, may be helpful for those who wish to further explore this topic.

FODMAPS Especially when increasing alliums (especially onions and garlic), other cruciferous vegetables, or legumes, everyone is vulnerable to bloating and gas. See the FODMAP section in chapter 9 for more information on how to address this issue. Often, simply reducing the quantity of these foods until the gut has an opportunity to optimize may be all the intervention that's required.

GOITROGENS Historically, goitres (an enlarged thyroid) occurred in response to a lack of iodine in the soil (prior to the introduction of iodized salt). Large amounts of raw cruciferous vegetables (as well as many other foods, medications, and chemicals) inhibit the uptake of iodine by the thyroid gland, reducing the production of thyroid hormone. Cruciferous vegetables should be eaten at least minimally cooked, since cooking reduces the goitrogenic effect. Hashimoto's thyroiditis is most commonly caused by an autoimmune response. But if iodine deficiency is an issue, then you should consider food sources for iodine replacement (sea salt, seaweed and other sea vegetables, fish and eggs) and avoid large amounts (more than 500 grams) of raw crucifers until your iodine levels are adequate. Paradoxically, iodine excess can also be a cause of Hashimoto's thyroiditis, which may be an issue especially if consuming processed and/or restaurant food, which have copious amounts of iodized salt.

OXALATES Foods high in *oxalates*, which are compounds promoting kidney stones and inflammation when eaten in large quantities by those who are genetically susceptible (and anyone with impaired gut health), include pecans, almonds, spinach, rhubarb, beetroot, beetroot greens, and chocolate. Because leafy greens cook down so dramatically, it's very easy to overconsume them. Be on the lookout for smelly urine, frequent bladder infections, kidney stones, even fibromyalgia-like pain and neurologic symptoms. Your doctor can check your urinary oxalate levels to confirm. Reducing high-oxalate foods usually rectifies the problem. Cooking, fermenting, and sprouting reduce oxalates. As your gut heals, you may find that you can slowly increase your intake.

HISTAMINE INTOLERANCE Some people, especially those with leaky gut or those on certain medications (e.g. Metformin), are sensitive to histamine, a neurotransmitter that normally protects our immune, digestive, and nervous systems. If you are intolerant to histamine, you may develop allergy-like symptoms or migraine headaches after ingesting foods high in histamine, such as spinach, avocado, nightshades, fermented foods, bone broth, or tea. See chapter 9 for more information.

HEALTHY FATS

You can liberally enjoy healthy fats within the context of the Keto-FLEX 12/3 lifestyle. Fat is so satiating and calorically dense that it's hard to overindulge. We understand that increasing fat is initially frightening for many people, given the decades of low-fat recommendations still made by many in the medical profession and through our government food guidelines. That thinking is slowly turning around based upon a re-examination of the evidence that led to the ill-founded recommendations.[41]

Most important, healthy fats help to promote the creation of ketone bodies to offset the neural fuel deficit that precedes and accompanies Alzheimer's. By combining healthy fats with an antioxidant-rich plant-based low-carbohydrate diet together with fasting and exercise, you can create ketones more easily than with diet alone.

A diet high in healthy fats optimizes glucose markers more effectively than a diet high in carbohydrates. A recent meta-analysis (a review of multiple studies) of more than 100 papers found that replacing carbohydrates with unsaturated fat improved glucose markers significantly. Reducing carbohydrates and saturated fat alone wasn't enough. Only when both were replaced with foods high in unsaturated fat—healthy vegetable oils such as olive oil, avocados, fatty fish, nuts, and seeds—was significant glucose improvement demonstrated. For each 5 per cent energy increase in monounsaturated fat or polyunsaturated fat, A1c improved by 0.1 per cent. That might not seem like a lot, but the authors estimate that 0.1 per cent reduction in A1c could reduce the incidence of type 2 diabetes by 22 per cent and cardiovascular disease by almost 7 per cent.[42]

Several studies have demonstrated that fats are the component in a Mediterranean diet responsible for its improvement of cognition, even in ApoE4 carriers. A study of the Mediterranean diet that compared a high-fat (olive oil and nuts) version against a low-fat version found better cognition with the higher fat.[43] This trend even held true for ApoE4 carriers.[44] In another recent study, 180 older people participated in a trial where everyone consumed a Mediterranean diet for one year. Half also received supplementation of 30 grams (2 tablespoons) of extra virgin olive oil (EVOO). The group that received the higher dietary fat demonstrated a significant improvement in cognition.[45]

The brain is about 60 to 70 per cent fat. The fat serves to support neurons, mitochondrial membranes, myelin sheaths (insulation for nerve conduction), and other structures. The quality of the fat we consume contributes to the functionality of these structures.[46]

There are four main types of fat. (Most foods contain a mixture but one fat typically predominates.)

1. Monounsaturated fatty acids (MUFAs): avocados, olives, olive oil, nuts, and seeds
2. Polyunsaturated fatty acids (PUFAs)
    - Omega-3:
        - Eicosapentaenoic acid (EPA) and docosahexaenoic acid (DHA): algae, krill, and cold-water fatty fish
        - Alpha-linolenic acid (ALA): walnuts, flaxseed, chia seeds, perilla oil, hempseed, and soybeans
    - Omega-6: nuts, seeds, and the oils that come from nuts and seeds
3. Saturated fatty acids (SFA): animal fats, including meat and dairy; coconuts; and MCT oil
4. Trans fats*: margarine, shortening, other shelf-stable products (biscuits, cakes, crackers, crisps, microwave popcorn, non-dairy coffee whiteners), and fried foods (French fries, doughnuts, and most restaurant deep-fried foods).

Trans fats and industrialized hydrogenated vegetable and seed oils are the only clear-cut demons here. Try to prioritize the use of plant-based monounsaturated, omega-3, and saturated fats. These fats, under the right circumstances (depending on processing methods,

*Food manufacturers in the US can claim 0 trans fats on the label even though they may include up to 0.5 grams per serving. Multiple servings can add up! However, food labelling in the UK and the EU is much more stringent. Read the labels carefully.

sourcing, the presence of low-carbohydrate, high-fibre intake, and a good ratio of omega-6 to omega-3), can make up a substantial portion (calorically) of your diet, leading to a healthy metabolic profile.

The more saturated the fat, the more stable and the less prone to oxidation and rancidity. However, we suggest a limited amount of animal fat, in part because toxins are stored and accumulated in fat.[47] For this reason, wild-caught or grass-fed is *always* preferable for animal products.[48] Beef and lamb in the UK tends to be grass-fed. ApoE4 carriers tend to hyper-absorb dietary fat, leading to elevated cholesterol. Out of an abundance of caution, we recommend limiting saturated fatty acids and prioritizing MUFAs and PUFAs such as olive oil, nuts, seeds, avocados, and fatty fish. (See more on this topic in chapter 8.)

Omega-3 and omega-6 are essential PUFAs, meaning that we must obtain them through our diet, since we cannot synthesize them in our bodies. Because they are polyunsaturated, they are more prone to oxidation and rancidity, which promote inflammation, especially in structures with high fat, like our brains.[49] Omega-3 is anti-inflammatory and omega-6 pro-inflammatory. Our industrialized diet with unhealthy vegetable oils, grains, and grain-fed animals has skewed our intake towards omega-6s. Our ancestral ratio of omega-6s to omega-3s was closer to 1:1, whereas those eating the standard American diet (SAD) today often have an elevated ratio of 25:1.[50] The average Western diet is generally as unhealthy. Achieving a 1:1 ancestral ratio is almost impossible in our modern era, and you needn't become overly concerned with trying to achieve this when eating a wholefoods diet. We suggest a goal of 4:1 or lower, not dropping below 0.5:1, since such low ratios are associated with bleeding due to excessive blood thinning. If you have a bleeding tendency or family history of stroke (especially ApoE4 homozygous men), please see the warning on page 187 in chapter 12.

To encourage a more anti-inflammatory profile, we suggest eliminating all unhealthy omega-6 vegetable oils and increasing healthy omega-3 fats.

Avoid fats that are processed with heat or through chemical extraction. Always look for cold-pressed oils. Buy fats stored in glass jars, since oil can cause plastic to leach, leading to toxic exposure that is cumulative.[51] For any unsaturated oil such as extra virgin olive oil, algal oil, or avocado oil, dark glass is preferable.

HEALTHY FATS

Extra virgin olive oil (high polyphenol, known harvest date, cold-pressed)	Coconut and coconut oil ♦♥ (unrefined, cold-pressed, virgin or extra virgin, no chemical processing)
Avocados and avocado oil	MCT oil ♥
Nuts	Red palm oil ♥ (unrefined, virgin, certified sustainable)
Seeds	Cacao butter
Walnut oil	Fatty fish ♥
Macadamia oil	Egg yolk ♥ (from free-range hens)
Sesame oil	Ghee ♥ (from grass-fed dairy)
Perilla oil	Butter (D) ♥ (from grass-fed dairy)
Algae or algal oil	Lard ♥ (from grass-fed animals)

KEY
Organic ♦
Inflammatory Dairy (D)
High in SFA (saturated fatty acids) ♥

Extra Virgin Olive Oil (EVOO)—a Top Pick for Brain Health

When making dietary fat choices, prioritize fresh, high polyphenol EVOO. Polyphenols are believed to be a key component of EVOO that contributes to its cardio- and neuroprotective properties. There are multiple mechanisms by which EVOO confers health benefits: the promotion of autophagy, improvement in metabolic markers, reduction in neuroinflammation, improvement in synaptic integrity, reduction in beta-amyloid and tau, and increase in BDNF.[52] EVOO also improves lipid profiles by promoting cholesterol efflux (removal), improving the functionality of HDL ("good" cholesterol), and reducing LDL ("bad" cholesterol) oxidation. Our goal is to promote both brain and heart health.[53]

You want the freshest EVOO with the highest polyphenol count that you can tolerate. Higher polyphenols confer a bitterness that is an acquired taste, but one well worth the acquisition. The Ultra Premium Extra Virgin Olive Oil site can help you source the freshest, highest-quality EVOO, with a known harvest date and detailed chemistry, often for the same price as supermarket varieties, the latter of which are frequently mixed with cheaper oils.[54] EVOO should be used primarily as a finishing oil (served at room temperature). It is wonderful to pair with low-glycaemic vinegars or citrus to make a salad dressing. It can also be seasoned with fresh herbs and spices to create a topping or dip for your vegetables. Cooking with EVOO will cause some degradation of the polyphenols and vitamin E content.[55] If you choose to do so, be sure to use a higher polyphenol variety and keep temperatures low to minimize the harmful effects of the heat.

Cooking with Fats

For cooking oils, choose oils with high smoke points, which means they do not produce smoke (associated with damaging the oils) at higher temperatures. The temperature for stovetop cooking at medium heat is around 176°C. Good choices for cooking include avocado oil (271°C smoke point), ghee (251°C), sesame oil (210°C), coconut oil (176°C), and butter (176°C). The smoke point for EVOO is 160–210°C, with the higher number reflecting higher polyphenol content. You can improve the oil's healthful qualities by adding a herb such as rosemary.[56]

Nuts and Seeds: Powerhouses of Nutrition

People who eat nuts live longer.[57] Nuts are both cardio- and neuroprotective, support ketosis, and are an excellent source of healthy fat, protein, vitamins, minerals, and fibre.[58] Nuts and seeds are best fresh, organic, and raw, soaked and sprouted when possible, as these methods reduce lectins, phytates, and enzyme inhibitors, all of which impair digestion and nutrient absorption.[59] Nuts and seeds can be enjoyed raw, as a dairy substitute, lightly sautéed, or roasted. If you prefer the taste of roasted nuts and seeds, it's best to dehydrate or roast them at low temperatures, 76–105°C, with the type of nut or seed dictating the temperature and timing. When roasting nuts and seeds in the oven, be sure to turn them periodically to ensure even cooking. All nuts and seeds have varying ratios of the different types of fats: MUFAs (monounsaturated fatty acids), PUFAs (polyunsaturated fatty acids), and SFAs (saturated fatty acids). PUFAs are particularly susceptible to oxidation and rancidity when exposed to higher roasting temperatures. You can experiment with tossing your nuts and seeds with various spices—paprika, cumin, curry powder, and sea salt are good—prior to roasting. You can also sauté slivered almonds over low heat with sea salt, garlic, and rosemary as a crunchy accompaniment to a salad, or toss raw walnuts with a small amount of stevia and cinnamon for a sweet treat on yoghurt or kefir. (Nut milks are an excellent substitute for dairy products—see chapter 11.)

When you can't prepare your own nuts and seeds, choose dry roasted (with no added oils) as the next best option (although they are cooked at very high temperatures, which will degrade some—not all—of the healthful properties).[60] Nuts roasted with unhealthy oils (listed on page 122) are not recommended. Storing larger quantities of nuts and seeds in the freezer and smaller quantities in the refrigerator helps preserve freshness.

Walnuts, macadamia nuts, pistachios, pecans, chestnuts, almonds, hazelnuts, pine nuts, and sesame or black sesame seeds, black cumin seeds, flaxseed, or hempseed are all excellent options. Cashews, pumpkin seeds, sunflower seeds, and chia seeds, while good choices, may be problematic for people sensitive to lectins. (Soaking and sprouting can be helpful.) Brazil nuts, an excellent source of selenium, should be limited to several a day since the selenium content is 68–91 mcg per nut; just by consuming five, you can exceed the upper limits of recommended levels for adults (400 mcg) and develop toxic side effects.[61]

- Walnuts have been associated with brain health and cognition because of their high omega-3 fatty acid content but should be consumed raw and protected from heat, since PUFAs oxidize easily.[62]

- Hazelnuts have been found to exert a neuroprotective effect, and are especially helpful in protecting against brain atrophy.[63] Additionally, because of their rich MUFA composition, they have been found to reduce LDL and total cholesterol.[64] They have a high phytate (anti-nutrient) content and therefore should be limited in quantity.
- Macadamias have a positive effect on lipid profiles. They have the highest MUFA content of any nut, along with a low carbohydrate and lectin content.[65]
- Pecans, excellent for their high ratio of healthy fat to carbohydrate and protein, improve HOMA-IR (homeostatic model assessment for insulin resistance, a measure of insulin resistance), and reduce risk for cardiometabolic disease.[66]
- Almonds—high in protein, MUFAs, and antioxidants—have been shown to be neuroprotective, improve glycaemic control and lipid profiles, and reduce oxidative stress.[67] The antioxidants are highest in the brown skin, which is also high in lectins.[68] (Those who are sensitive may need to source blanched almonds.) Almonds in the United States are pasteurized by law, even when labelled raw. In the UK, almonds are largely imported from the US. Vendors who sell small quantities may provide true raw almonds.
- Flaxseed, also high in omega-3 fatty acids, benefits heart and overall health.[69] Flaxseed's omega-3 is plant-based and called alpha-linolenic acid (ALA). Flaxseed is the richest source of lignans, a type of polyphenol that helps to balance hormones. It is also an excellent source of antioxidants and fibre. Flaxseed should be eaten raw and either freshly ground or soaked overnight or sprouted to make its nutrient-rich contents more bioavailable and digestible.[70] Flaxseed goes rancid easily, so grind small amounts at a time and store in the refrigerator, with the rest of the whole seeds in the freezer.

Nuts and seeds provide a healthful way of increasing dietary fat and promoting ketosis. They are calorically dense, which can be helpful if you're trying to gain weight. Likewise, if you find that you're gaining weight with the KetoFLEX 12/3, you can reduce intake.

COFFEE LOVERS, REJOICE!

The coffee bean is actually the seed of a coffee berry, which provides a dark aromatic robust beverage that originated in Ethiopia and has been enjoyed since the fifteenth century. Multiple studies have found that our beloved morning java is strongly associated with good health and longevity.[71] Coffee has also been found to provide neuroprotective benefits and is associated with a reduced risk of cognitive decline. Its stimulant effect increases alertness and cognitive performance and slows memory decline in the ageing brain and in Alzheimer's.[72] The polyphenols and bioactive compounds in coffee exert these health effects, with nearly any method of preparation providing benefit, even when decaffeinated. The beneficial effects of coffee include its ability to increase cyclic AMP (a cell messenger critical for memory), create insulin sensitivity, and stimulate an antioxidant response. Coffee upregulates the Nrf2 system, activating protective mechanisms within each cell.[73] The bioactive compounds in coffee exert an anti-inflammatory and antibacterial effect while providing protection against diabetes and some cancers.[74] Phenylindanes, compounds that form during the brewing process, have also been found to inhibit beta-amyloid and tau tangles.[75]

For those concerned that your morning cup of joe will interfere with ketosis, worry no more! Research has found that drinking coffee actually increases plasma ketones.[76] While fasting, enjoy black coffee with approved sweeteners in small amounts as needed. Those who are insulin resistant and are having difficulty with fasting

(continued)

may want to consider adding a small amount of MCT to their coffee until they can heal and begin to create their own endogenous ketones. Also, it's best to source an organic mould-free coffee, particularly if you are dealing with type 3 (toxic) Alzheimer's.

While coffee has many health benefits, we do need to exert some caution. Drinking more than 1 litre (slightly more than four 240 ml cups) per day has been demonstrated to elevate homocysteine levels by 20 per cent.[77] Elevated homocysteine is associated with brain atrophy and diminished cognition.[78] Keep your intake moderate and don't consume after noon, especially if you are a slow metabolizer of caffeine. Excess coffee or coffee consumed later in the day can affect circadian rhythms and sleep quality. Be aware that the acidity in coffee can exacerbate heartburn (gastroesophageal reflux disease, or GERD). Additionally, anyone dealing with chronic stress, accompanied by elevated cortisol, may need to avoid caffeine until the underlying causes can be addressed.

Examples of Unhealthy Fats

- Soybean oil
- Corn oil
- Rapeseed oil
- Peanut oil
- Sunflower oil
- Safflower oil
- Cottonseed oil
- Palm kernel oil
- Trans fats

This list is not exhaustive. In general, avoid seed, grain, bean, or any vegetable oils that are polyunsaturated, omega-6, heat or chemically extracted, GMO, and refined oils.

ACTION PLAN

- Increase healthy fats (with increased plant intake) to heal insulin resistance while creating ketones to fuel your brain.
- Prioritize high polyphenol EVOO, avocados, nuts, and seeds.
- Remember not to combine high-glycaemic and inflammatory foods with dietary fat.
- Be aware that as you heal, your need for dietary fat may decrease over time.

CAUTIONS

GASTROINTESTINAL DISTRESS It may be helpful to adjust your fat intake or, in the case of nuts and seeds, your fat and lectin intake, by increasing slowly. The adjustment may be most difficult for those with compromised gallbladder function. If increasing dietary fat causes you pain in the right upper abdomen, see your GP to rule out gallbladder disease. The gallbladder is the storage facility for bile, which breaks down fat. Those without a gallbladder typically tolerate a higher-fat diet without problems, but some may still need to increase slowly. Those who develop GI issues (including diarrhoea) may consider the use of digestive enzymes with lipase, ox bile, or bitter herbs. See chapter 9 for more.

WEIGHT LOSS Many people who increase dietary fat will experience weight loss because it's so satiating that they inadvertently consume too few calories. (See the caution in chapter 7.)

WEIGHT GAIN Some people will gain weight when they increase dietary fat. They may need to extend their fasting period and increase exercise. They may be consuming more carbohydrates than they think, contributing to persistent insulin resistance. Using a food tracker app like Cronometer can reveal hidden sources of energy such as sugars and grains. Undiagnosed food sensitivities can also

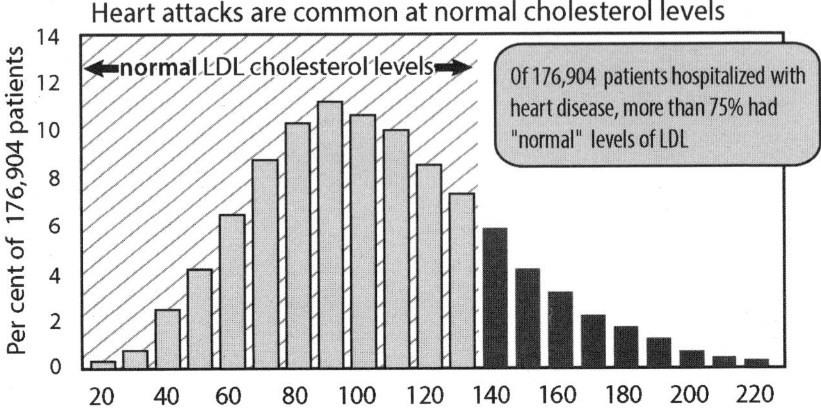

Most myocardial infarctions (heart attacks) occur despite normal levels of LDL cholesterol. A better predictor is the ratio of triglycerides to HDL cholesterol (TG/HDL).

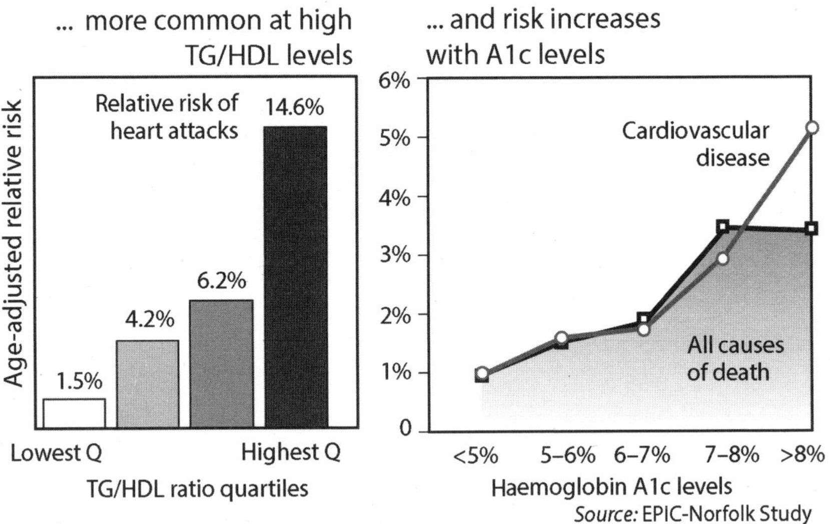

As your haemoglobin A1c rises, so does your risk for cardiovascular disease.

contribute to weight gain through inflammation. (See chapter 9 for how to conduct an elimination diet.)

MOULD IN NUTS AND SEEDS It is important to make sure that any nut or seed does not have a rancid or mouldy smell. Brazil nuts, high in selenium, often contain mould.[79] Avoid peanuts (and especially peanut butter), which are legumes and are associated with mould contamination and the resulting inflammation.[80]

ELEVATED LIPIDS Some who increase their dietary fat (especially saturated fat) may see higher total cholesterol and low-density lipoprotein cholesterol (LDL-C) on their lipid panels. This is especially true for ApoE4 carriers, who are well documented to hyper-absorb dietary fat.[81] Should this be reason for concern? It depends on many other corroborating factors that we'll examine. Our dietary recommendations also lead to favourable changes such as decreased glucose markers including fasting insulin and haemoglobin A1c (HgbA1c), increased high-density lipoprotein cholesterol (HDL-C), and decreased triglycerides (TGs), all of which contribute to an overall decreased risk for heart disease.

The lipid hypothesis—the notion that reducing one's level of cholesterol will lead to a reduction in the risk of suffering a new event of coronary artery disease—has undergone a re-examination over the past several years and remains unproven despite being a guiding force in government food guidelines.[82] Indeed, when you examine the cholesterol of those hospitalized with coronary artery disease, you'll see that most have normal levels of cholesterol.[83]

Examining cholesterol alone is decidedly unhelpful, but looking at the ratios that make up total cholesterol provides much more information and helps us determine actual risk.[84] Total cholesterol is derived by adding LDL-C, HDL-C, and 20 per cent of triglycerides (TG). When you consider the ratio of TGs to HDL-C, the risk pattern becomes much clearer.[85] You want no more than a 2:1 ratio of TGs to HDL-C. Less than 1.1 is ideal.

When you examine glucose markers using haemoglobin A1c levels, you'll see that as A1c rises, the likelihood of a coronary event also rises in a linear relationship.[86] Haemoglobin A1c is short for glycated (containing an added sugar molecule) haemoglobin, and it reflects your fasting blood sugar over approximately three months. Those with the lowest A1c levels are at the lowest risk for heart disease.

Understanding elevated "cholesterol" within this broader context can help you better monitor your risk for heart disease.

There are additional markers that you can follow to track your risk even more accurately. They include oxidized LDL (Ox-LDL, goal <60 U/L) and other advanced lipid particle size tests such as LDL particle size (LDL-P, goal <1200 nmol/L) and small dense LDL (sdLDL, goal <28 mg/dL), all of which closely correlate with haemoglobin A1c. Additionally, if you have a strong family history or other risk factors, you may want to consider a low radiation CT heart scan, which is a coronary artery calcification (CAC) scan; in the UK, you may need to seek out a private practioner to undergo these tests, which will incur a fee. Men over 40 and women over 50 may consider a baseline scan. If you learn that you do have active coronary artery disease, try to find a cardiologist or lipidologist who uses a low-carbohydrate approach to support your desire to protect your brain.

When total cholesterol rises above 200 mg/dL, many doctors are quick to prescribe statins without gathering this additional information to help assess actual risk. Statins can increase the likelihood of cognitive decline.[87] For that reason, when statins are necessary, such as in the case of familial hypercholesteremia, it's important to work with your cardiologist. One approach may be to identify the lowest dose of a hydrophilic (as opposed to lipophilic) statin, combined with ezetimibe to reach your LDL-P goal while still protecting cholesterol synthesis in the brain. If you do experience cognitive decline with a statin, you can track a sterol biomarker called desmosterol. A low level is indicative of a depletion of cholesterol in the brain, and is correlated with cognitive decline.[88]

Let's talk about saturated fat (SFA), since it is on our list of healthy fats. The consumption of SFA is controversial and likely falsely maligned as a risk factor for heart disease, since the milieu in which SFA is consumed is rarely taken into account. A particularly damaging triad of food—the "Berfooda Triangle"—includes saturated fat, simple carbohydrates, and a lack of fibre, as pointed out by Dr Mark Hyman in *Eat Fat, Get Thin*. However, eating a hamburger, fries, and a

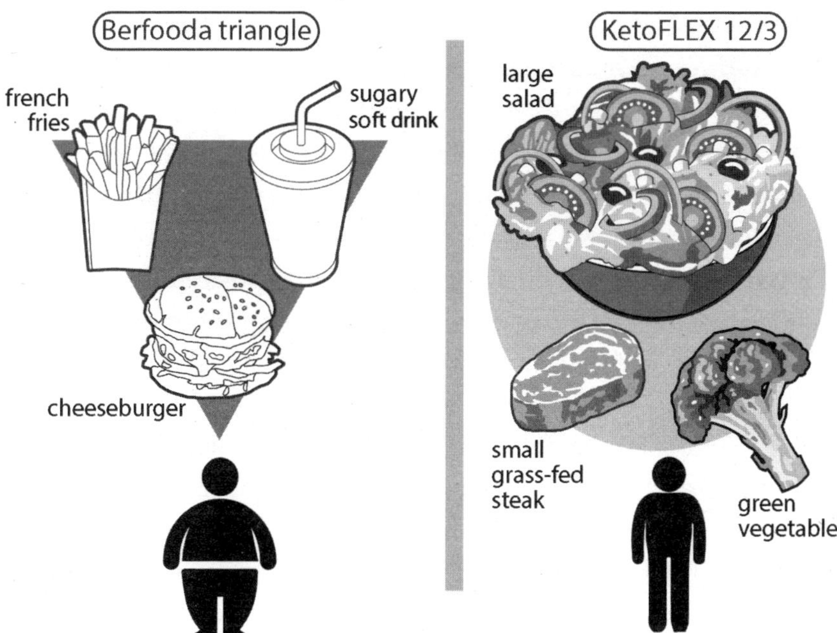

The "Berfooda Triangle." The combination of saturated fat, simple carbohydrates, and lack of fibre is a dangerous one.

soft drink is very different from consuming a small piece of grass-fed beef with a large salad loaded with a variety of nutrient-dense vegetables. The vast majority of studies that have implicated SFA in both heart disease and Alzheimer's failed to take into account the quality of the SFA and the context in which it's consumed.

That said, SFA incontrovertibly raises cholesterol in some people, including ApoE4 carriers.[89] Out of an abundance of caution, therefore, we encourage this population to minimize SFA and prioritize MUFAs and PUFAs—high polyphenol EVOO, avocados, fatty fish, nuts, and seeds—all of which have been demonstrated to *reduce* heart disease.

The role of cholesterol in Alzheimer's disease is still poorly understood. There is mixed evidence demonstrating that high cholesterol (without examination of ratios) at midlife may be associated with

Alzheimer's, but higher amounts seem to be neuroprotective as we age.[90] We recommend emphasizing reduction of inflammatory and glycaemic markers while maintaining a healthy lipid profile.

VASCULAR DEMENTIA OR HEART DISEASE Patients with vascular dementia or known heart disease should prioritize healing their underlying insulin resistance before considering nutritional ketosis. They may want to consider the use of ketone salts or esters during this period to help fuel their brains. *It is very important to eliminate sugars and refined carbohydrates while increasing healthy fats, primarily high polyphenol EVOO, avocados, fatty fish, nuts, and seeds.* People in this group should definitely proceed with the help of a doctor, preferably a cardiologist, who specializes in using a low-carbohydrate approach.

Additionally, you may want to consider using the iHeart fingertip device to measure arterial stiffness as a means of reassurance that your vascular health is improving while adopting the KetoFLEX 12/3 lifestyle. Results from iHeart correlate closely with the SphygmoCor system, the gold standard for measuring pulse wave velocity (PWV). Poor PWV is a significant risk factor for future cardiovascular disease and dementia.[91] (See also chapter 18.)

CHAPTER 9

Pyramid Level 3: Upgrade Your Gut

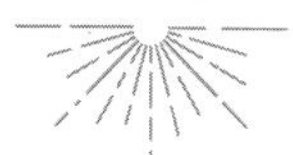

Gut feelings often come from universal knowledge.
—DEBASISH MRIDHA

GUT HEALTH IS THE foundation of any health programme, and it represents an important opportunity for therapeutic intervention in cognitive decline. The brain and the gut are intricately and bidirectionally connected. There's an explosion of scientific literature exploring the manipulation of the gut microbiome for neuroprotection.[1] The gut microbiome provides the basis for healthy function of our nutritional, immune, hormonal, and neurological systems. As we have noted repeatedly, the mismatch between the limits of our genetic design and modern world stressors is emerging as a critical driver of many of our chronic illnesses. Stressful, sedentary, oversanitized lives and diets rampant with sugar but devoid of nutrients or fibre, along with antibiotic, herbicide, pesticide, and other chemical exposures, have been devastating to the integrity of the gut and its microbiome. The explosion of chronic diseases such as obesity, diabetes, and autoimmune and neurological diseases may have roots in common with the dysfunction of the gut microbiome.[2]

If you have any underlying issues such as a leaky gut (an overly permeable gut wall), dysbiosis (a microbial imbalance inside the GI tract), a small intestinal bacterial overgrowth (SIBO, a condition that occurs when bacteria that normally grow in other parts of the gut begin growing in the small intestine), irritable bowel syndrome (or IBS, which manifests as belly pain accompanied by either diarrhoea, constipation, or both), or H. *pylori* (a common infection associated with peptic ulcers), you may need additional interventions to help optimize your health and nutritional programme. We can't overstate how common these GI disorders are and how many people remain undiagnosed and untreated.

The good news is that we hold the power to heal our GI health by paying attention to the symptoms we develop as a result of what and how we eat. By paying close attention to early symptoms, we have the ability to make corrections and heal our guts. In fact, optimizing digestion may allow you to completely avoid (and heal) food allergies and sensitivities. For many, exploring the root cause of underlying GI issues is critical. Here are some points to consider:

Food Allergies or Sensitivities (Intolerances)

- Any true food allergy should be revealed by formal testing with an allergist. Food allergies can be severe and life-threatening, and usually occur closer to the time of ingestion. Symptoms can include tingling or itching in the mouth; itching of the skin, with hives or eczema; swelling of the lips, face, tongue, or throat, or trouble breathing; abdominal pain, nausea, diarrhoea, or vomiting; dizziness, light-headedness, or fainting.
- Food sensitivities are usually timed further from ingestion, are less severe, and often limited to GI symptoms such as wind, bloating, and constipation and/or diarrhoea, but can include rashes, acne, arthritis, widespread body pain, headaches, fatigue, mood swings, irritability, and "brain fog."
- Common food allergies and sensitivities besides grains (especially wheat) and dairy are egg (typically the egg white, not the yolk), peanuts, soy, tree nuts, shellfish, nightshades (such as aubergines, tomatoes, hot and sweet peppers, and potatoes),

and multiple ingredients and chemicals used in processed foods.

- The best way to identify a food sensitivity is to conduct an elimination trial. Eliminate the most common triggers: all grains (especially wheat), dairy, corn, soy, egg, nightshades, and sugar and all processed food for three weeks. Sugar is included in this list, as it is often a culprit for inflammation. If you feel better after the elimination trial, reintroduce one food at a time, starting with egg; approved nightshades; organic, preferably fermented soy; and small amounts of A2 dairy (optional) only. Eat that food twice a day for 2 days, then avoid that food on day 3. On day 4, reintroduce the next food. Keep a journal of your responses. Identifying a food sensitivity can be so rewarding as healing occurs. After an individual's gut heals, some people find that they can even tolerate small doses of the culprit food occasionally. (For some, food sensitivity testing such as Cyrex, Zoomer, Alletess, Meridian Valley Lab, MRT, Alcat, and many others may help illuminate allergens.)

COMMON (OFTEN CUMULATIVE) ROOT CAUSES OF GI DYSFUNCTION

In addition to identifying food allergies and sensitivities and eliminating them, there are many other factors that can impact GI health and cause inflammation to the gut lining, GI imbalances, and delays in gastric emptying. These include:

- Antibiotics
- Anti-inflammatories: aspirin, ibuprofen (e.g. Nurofen), naproxen sodium (e.g. Feminax Ultra)
- Proton-pump inhibitors, or PPIs (e.g. Prilosec, Prevacid)
- H2 receptor antagonists (e.g. Zantac, Pepcid)
- Aluminium hydroxide in antacids (e.g. Tums, Rolaids)

- Anticholinergic drugs: antihistamines (e.g. Benadryl, Zyrtec), tricyclic antidepressants (e.g. amitriptyline, doxepin), barbiturates, and benzodiazepines (e.g. diazepam, Valium)
- Alcohol
- Excessive sugar, especially high-fructose corn syrup such as that used in soft drinks and speciality coffees
- Artificial sweeteners
- Glyphosate
- Stress
- Inadequate stomach acid

A major contributing factor to many GI issues is the lack of adequate stomach acid. Most adults experience a decrease in hydrochloric acid as they age, and others may develop this with chronic stress or hypothyroidism. Exacerbating this is the common use of PPIs and other antacids to deal with heartburn or gastroesophageal reflux disease (GERD), a condition in which acid from the stomach refluxes into the oesophagus. Paradoxically, too little stomach acid can contribute to GERD, as insufficient amounts are available to digest food. The dietary and lifestyle strategies encompassed in the KetoFLEX 12/3 lifestyle can ultimately help to treat GERD, although you may want to consider the additional measures described below.

Lifestyle Strategies to Address GERD

- Reduce belly fat and avoid tight clothing around the waist.
- Avoid triggers such as caffeine, alcohol, nicotine, chocolate, citrus, tomato-based foods, spicy foods, fried foods, gluten, dairy, and processed foods.
- Eat smaller and more frequent meals during this healing period.
- Ensure that you have adequate stomach acid to help digest your food.
- Avoid stress while eating.

- Chew food well and slowly.
- Don't eat within three hours of bedtime.
- Elevate the top of your bed by 15–20 cm.

Weaning Off Heartburn Medicine (PPIs)

It is important to note that long-term use of PPIs is associated with an increased risk of dementia, depression, colorectal cancer, pneumonia, and hip fractures; deficiencies of B_{12}, vitamin C, iron, calcium, magnesium, and zinc; and imbalances in the gut microbiome.[3] Proper acid production in the stomach is important to the work of many essential digestive enzymes, especially pepsin, for the digestion of proteins. Stomach acid is also important for killing bacteria, viruses, parasites, and yeast that we are exposed to in our diets.

Weaning off a PPI is often difficult. Some measures that patients have used successfully include: lowering the dosage slowly while temporarily increasing the use of Pepcid; digestive enzymes, sugar-free DGL (from licorice), aloe, L-glutamine, zinc carnosine, magnesium, and probiotics are also helpful. The supervision of a functional medicine practitioner may be helpful, especially if treatment of H. *pylori* or bacterial or yeast overgrowth is contributing to your GERD.

Strategies for Optimizing Digestion

There are specific strategies you can use to aid digestion while transitioning to your new diet with increased vegetables, fats, resistant starches, prebiotic fibre, and foods rich in probiotics.

- Digestion begins with meal preparation. Try to involve everyone who will be eating in the cooking process. Smelling the food as you cook actually releases pancreatic enzymes that aid in digestion.[4]
- In human history, eating has always been associated with social connection. When you eat a meal with those whom

you care about, your parasympathetic nervous system is triggered to relax, allowing your body to digest food optimally and maximize nutrition.[5] If you are eating alone, consider turning off the TV or your computer and putting down your work. This is a sacred time to relax and nourish yourself.

- Take time to chew. The first step of digestion is proper chewing, which releases several enzymes, including amylase for breaking down carbohydrates and lipase for fats.[6] Try to minimize excessive fluids with your meal so as not to dilute your natural digestive enzymes. Avoid iced beverages so as to maintain your natural body temperature to optimize digestion.
- Consider acid replacement to aid in digestion (unless you suffer from ulcers or oesophagitis). A trial of 1 tablespoon of organic apple cider vinegar in a small glass of water before or after a meal, or supplementing with betaine HCl with pepsin, are methods that have been helpful. (For betaine HCl, start at 500 to 650 mg with a meal that includes 15 to 20 g of protein, then increase by one pill every two days until you feel discomfort. Use the maximum number of pills that does not cause discomfort, but no more than five.) If acid replacement worsens symptoms, consider a trial of ½ teaspoon of bicarbonate of soda in a small glass of water.
- You can enhance digestion by adding bitter herbs (chamomile, milk thistle, dandelion, goldenseal, burdock, gentian), bitter vegetables, or spices (ginger, cinnamon, cardamom), or by using fruits that have natural digestive enzymes such as lemons, avocados, green papayas, green mangoes, or underripened kiwi. Bone broth, resistant starches, and prebiotic and probiotic foods added to your diet will all improve GI health and absorption, and will favourably balance the microbiome. Specific supplements such as bromelain (made from pineapple), papain (made from papaya), or sugar-free DGL (from licorice) may help.
- Elimination, or "pooing," may be the most important aspect of proper digestion. Increasing the intake of food that your

gut loves makes your stools bigger, promoting the ease of elimination and the removal of toxins. Elimination supports your microbiome, improves your glucose control (with fibre) and your lipid profile, reduces your risk of colorectal cancer, helps lower your oestrogen levels so as to avoid uterine and breast cancer, and generally improves your sense of well-being.[7]

- You are constipated if you have fewer than three bowel movements per week or difficulty passing stools. It is optimal to have a large bowel movement at least once a day. A diet high in processed foods, sugar, gluten, dairy, and meat can cause constipation. Exercise, hydration, and an increase in vegetables (especially prebiotic fibre and resistant starches) will help. You may want to consider supplements: organic psyllium fibre, ground flaxseed, acacia fibre, konjac root powder, probiotics, or magnesium citrate.

BONE BROTH TO HELP HEAL LEAKY GUT

Bone broth is an ancestral food that contains *glutamine*, an amino acid that can help to seal a leaky gut or increased intestinal permeability. Glutamine, one of several amino acids in bone broth, and the most abundant in the body, is the preferred fuel of the cells found in the lining of your digestive system. These cells, called enterocytes, form a one-cell-thick barrier and are dynamic players actively involved in shaping the intestine through immune system modulation. Many factors including food antigens, stress, and toxins can affect the integrity of this critical barrier. The glutamine in bone broth nurtures these enterocytes and supports the tight junctions between them, decreasing intestinal permeability.[8]

Despite bone broth's healthful qualities, we recommend minimizing bone broth's use to several servings per week, for multiple reasons. First, especially if the animal grazed in an area with

(continued)

industrial pollutants, the bones may leach heavy metals into the broth. Second, bone broth is a protein and subject to the animal protein restrictions discussed in chapter 10. Additionally, some have expressed concern that the glutamine from bone broth will escape the intestinal barrier and breach a compromised blood-brain barrier, thus negatively affecting neurotransmitters in the brain. This is much more likely to occur from an excess of glutamine found in processed foods such as MSG, and could present a cumulative burden.

Indeed, glutamine is the building block for both glutamate, which has an excitatory role in the brain, and for GABA, which plays a calming role. In a healthy brain, these two neurotransmitters work in a homeostatic manner, balancing each other. However, an imbalance, such as excess glutamate, can conceivably occur. Symptoms could include anxiety, depression, restlessness, an inability to concentrate, headaches, insomnia, fatigue, and an increased sensitivity to pain. If you experience any one of these after using bone broth, discontinue its use and focus on the other ways of healing your gut discussed in this section. Most important, reduce processed foods high in glutamate, including soy sauce, soy protein, fish sauce, wine, beer, cured meats, and any foods with MSG. Dairy and wheat, the use of which is avoided or minimized in our Brain Food Pyramid, are also high in glutamine. Retry bone broth only after significant healing has occurred.

Another potential issue with bone broth involves its histamine content. Histamine is a neurotransmitter that protects our immune, digestive, and nervous systems by alerting our body's response to potential threats. Symptoms of a histamine reaction include headaches, itching, swelling, anxiety, GI upset, and rashes. Histamine intolerance most often occurs with leaky gut, creating a catch-22 with this strategy.[9] Work to identify and eliminate other foods high in histamine while simultaneously using the strategies outlined in this section to heal your gut. Foods high in histamines (often due to food ageing) include smoked meats and fish, fermented foods, vinegar, alcohol, soured foods, dried fruits, and leftovers. Spinach, avocado, citrus, nightshades, nuts, chocolate, black tea, and green tea are also naturally high in histamines. Retry a small amount of bone broth after significant healing has occurred. Some find supplementing with DAO, an enzyme naturally present in the gut that metabolizes histamine, to be helpful.

It's simple to make this gut-nourishing broth. Collect 1.5–2 kg of bones from 100 per cent grass-fed, organically reared animals. Bones from leftover meals are fine or you can purchase them. Cover with 4 litres of water in a pot, slow cooker, or pressure cooker. Ensure that the bones are covered with water. Add 2 tablespoons of vinegar, salt to taste, onions, parsley, and garlic, and bring to a boil, then lower the heat and simmer all day on the hob or in a slow cooker, or about 90 minutes in a pressure cooker. Keep the heat on low so as not to let the broth get to a boil during the simmering period, which could break down the collagen and denature (alter the structure of) the protein. A good broth will jell when cold, rich in collagen and protein. Those concerned about SFA can remove the fatty top layer. Otherwise, strain and enjoy. Bone broth can be frozen to use as the base for other soups or stews, to season vegetables, or to be enjoyed by itself.

If you have any underlying GI issues, proceed slowly with the protocol, prioritizing gut healing. You may need to utilize the help of a functional medicine practitioner to identify and help you address underlying GI issues (see chapter 18). Many patients with chronic GI dysfunction find themselves in endless loops of testing and prescriptions without ever addressing root causes.

As your GI health improves, there will be an improved response to the meaningful changes you are implementing. The healthy bacteria in your microbiome will celebrate with improved digestion, nutrient absorption, and detoxification, which will lead to improved immune and neurological systems. Those wishing to further explore the role of gut health on cognition may want to read *Brain Maker: The Power of Gut Microbes to Heal and Protect Your Brain for Life* by David Perlmutter, MD.

FOODS THAT SUPPORT THE GUT

A combination of *prebiotic fibres*, some eaten as resistant starch, combined with *probiotic foods* provides the ancestral formula necessary for optimal GI digestion. A wide variety of fibre-rich plant-based foods, especially when varied with the seasons, supplies the basic components for this winning formula. Plant carbohydrates are a combination of starch, sugar, and fibre, which vary in type and content in the skin, flesh, and seeds of each plant. Humans do not have the enzymes to digest fibre. Fibre is called prebiotic when it is digested (fermented) by the gut microbiome. There are many types of prebiotic fibre, including a type of starch called resistant starch. Resistant starch resists digestion and acts more like a fibre. Some fibre is not digested by humans or by the gut microbes, but supports the gut by easing elimination, enhancing detoxification, reducing glucose, improving lipid profile, and providing bulk to our bowel movements.

Prebiotics

Prebiotics are vital for gut health. They provide nutritional support for the healthy gut bacteria that we want to cultivate. Humans cannot digest prebiotic fibre. It is instead digested in the colon by beneficial bacteria to support their growth. In turn, their by-products support the health of the intestine. Prebiotic fibre is not fully broken down and absorbed in the small intestine, but rather turned into short-chain fatty acids, like butyrate, by bacteria in the large intestine. These resulting fatty acids may contribute to ketone production to address neuronal fuel deficits and support the creation of a healthy gut wall and microbiome.[10]

Foods rich in prebiotic fibre include fibrous plants, roots, and tubers, many of which are also resistant starches. While cooking renders some of these foods more palatable, it also destroys some of the prebiotic fibres, so cook these minimally for the most impact. Almost all of the foods high in prebiotic fibre, listed below, have low glycaemic impact.

PREBIOTIC FIBRE

Artichoke hearts*	Jerusalem artichokes*
Asparagus*	Mexican yam*
Burdock root*	Konjac root* (elephant yam)
Chicory root*	Leeks*
Dandelion greens*	Mushrooms*
Flaxseed*	Onions*
Garlic*	Persimmons***
Green banana*	Seaweed*

KEY
Glycaemic index: Low* Intermediate** High***

MUSHROOMS are among the prebiotic foods that stand out for brain health. A recent study has shown that eating more than two portions (300 g) of cooked mushrooms per week could lead to a 50 per cent lower risk of mild cognitive decline (MCI), the typical predecessor to Alzheimer's.[11] These humble fungi contain glutathione and another powerful antioxidant called ergothioneine. The porcini mushroom, found in most food shops, has the greatest amounts of these compounds.[12] Mushrooms are also rich in vitamin B and beta-D-glucan. Beta-D-glucan is important to the innate immune system (the ancient part of our immune systems, which functions as a first responder), thought to play a role in the reversal of cognitive decline.[13] Immune-enhancing effects are present in nearly all mushrooms, including white button, cremini, portobello, shiitake, reishi, chanterelle, oyster, and many others. Enjoy raw in salads or lightly sautéed. Mushrooms are delicious when cooked with garlic and onions or added to other vegetables.

Mushrooms also contain bioactive compounds that may help protect against Alzheimer's disease. A study of eleven types of mushrooms, some already used for medicinal purposes, found that they increased grey matter by raising production of nerve growth factor (NGF). The mushrooms studied included lion's mane and *Cordyceps*. Depending upon where you live, lion's mane and *Cordyceps* mushrooms may be difficult to find, but both have been blended into decent-tasting coffees made by Four Sigmatic and are also available in supplement form.

ALLIUMS are another important class of prebiotics, which includes onions, garlic and leeks, shallots, chives, and more. Like mushrooms and cruciferous vegetables, these contribute to the upregulation of glutathione, which in addition to its antioxidant properties is sometimes called the master detoxifier of the body.[14]

There are also supplemental forms of prebiotics, which include psyllium husks, acacia fibre, inulin, fructooligosaccharides (FOS), and galactooligosaccharides (GOS). We recommend starting slowly with foods rich in prebiotic fibre to prevent GI distress. This is especially true with the supplemental forms, as they are very concentrated.

Resistant Starch

Ready for a plot twist? After taking away starchy carbs, we're now going to *recommend* a special category of them: resistant starches. These behave differently from other starchy carbohydrates and have many beneficial health properties. Resistant starches resist digestion, thereby acting more like fibre. This delayed digestion also means that you're not fully absorbing the calories as sugar, as you do with many other carbohydrates and grains.[15] As a type of prebiotic fibre, resistant starch also contributes to butyrate production in the large intestine, which may in turn help to support the gut and supply fuel to the brain.[16]

Throughout much of human history, our ancestors ate high amounts of resistant starch because their food wasn't processed by machinery or broken down by heating; instead it was eaten whole.[17] When food is made highly digestible, through processing, this leads to poor glucose control, poor intestinal health, and weight gain. Cultures that still eat wholefoods, rich in resistant starch, stay lean.[18] An excellent example comes from the residents of Kitava, an island off Papua New Guinea, with a high prevalence of ApoE4 carriers. This culture traditionally ate a majority portion of their calories from resistant starch in the form of yams, sweet potatoes, and taro (as well as coconuts and fish), and have been documented to be healthy and free from the chronic diseases that plague Western civilization.[19]

Resistant starch is thought to confer many health benefits.

- Increased satiety[20]
- Improved insulin sensitivity[21]
- Improved lipids[22]
- Enhanced fat burning[23]
- Improved digestion[24]

PROCEED WITH CAUTION

Despite claims to the contrary, resistant starches may still have a negative effect on your blood glucose levels. Start with small amounts and perform postprandial checks at one and two hours to see the effect they have for you. (See page 258 in chapter 18.) Be aware that the glycaemic effect is highly individualized and may even change from day to day based upon your stress level, sleep, hormonal milieu, gut health, and many more factors. Be careful not to sabotage your ability to heal from insulin resistance, restore metabolic flexibility, and create ketones . . . *all for a sweet potato.* Balance is key with resistant starches. You want enough for the health benefits, but not so much as to impair metabolic healing.

Those who are dealing with type 3 (toxic) Alzheimer's caused by exposure to mycotoxins (mould) or other toxins may need to avoid resistant starch until they've achieved a certain level of healing. Low-amylose diets are very effective for these conditions, which require a strict avoidance of all root vegetables, legumes, grains, and pseudograins.

As always, pay attention to your gut. Those with underlying GI issues may not be able to tolerate resistant starches initially (or prebiotic and probiotic foods), especially those high in lectins. They are best eaten as wholefoods with other vegetable

(continued)

carbohydrates, proteins, and fats. This is another reason to start slowly, experiment with different types, and be prepared to delay this step until further gut healing has occurred.

We've coded the various resistant starches to alert you to the fact that resistant starch, despite claims to the contrary, may still have a negative effect on your blood glucose levels. We recommend increasing the resistant starch content and decreasing the effect on blood glucose by cooking resistant starches that are meant to be cooked (potatoes, other root vegetables, legumes, and rice) and then cooling them before eating. Be aware that some people still can't tolerate these higher glycaemic foods even if they've been previously cooked and cooled. You can easily test your postprandial blood glucose to see the effect a particular food has for you. (See page 258 in chapter 18.) Also be aware that high lectin levels may be an issue with some of these resistant starches, including legumes, nuts (especially cashews), and seeds.

RESISTANT STARCH

Legumes (beans and lentils)**	**Yams***
Chestnuts	**Sweet potatoes***
Pistachios*	**Potatoes*** x (coloured)**
Cashews* x	**Green bananas* (uncooked)**
Cassava root (tapioca)**	**Green plantains* (uncooked)**
Taro root*	**Green mangoes** (uncooked)**
Turnips	**Green papayas**
Parsnips*	**Persimmons***
Swede*	**Teff*** x**
Mexican yam*	**Buckwheat** x**
Yucca	**Sorghum***
Tiger nut	**Millet**

KEY
Glycaemic Index: Low* Intermediate High*****
High in Lectins x

LEGUMES Legumes, although not an ancestral food, are excellent sources of resistant starch, and are especially helpful for vegetarians and vegans to meet their protein and mineral needs. Furthermore, since their fibre and resistant starch content is higher than most grains, they do not contribute as much to elevated glucose levels.

Legumes, however, can be problematic because they contain lectins, phytates, and enzyme inhibitors, which may contribute to inflammation, and impair digestion and nutrient absorption. Here are preparation and cooking methods to *reduce* these effects:

- Soak dry beans overnight (48 hours is better).
- Add ⅙ teaspoon of bicarbonate of soda per litre of water during soaking.
- Change the water up to three times per day while soaking. (Be sure to replace the bicarb with each change.)
- Rinse thoroughly before cooking.
- Cook low and slow (all day is best).
- Remove the foam during cooking.
- Pressure-cooking with a modern pressure cooker (such as an Instant Pot) is fine.
- During cooking, add a 10 cm strip of kombu, a type of seaweed.
- Add spices during cooking such as fennel, garlic, cumin, turmeric, ginger, cloves, and cinnamon.

All of these techniques will render the beans more digestible and less likely to produce wind, and will help to increase the absorption of the nutrients. If you are short on time, tinned beans are a decent option, as they are already pressure-cooked and lower in lectins. Be sure to find a BPA/BPS-free of organic beans.

TUBERS Potatoes, sweet potatoes, yams, and other tubers are enlarged roots or stems that are mostly starch, some resistant to digestion. Our ancestors have eaten them for millennia, especially after fire helped to make them more digestible. This allowed for the absorption of more nutrients but diminished the amount of resistant starch. Cooling helps to regain that resistant starch partially. Deeply pigmented vegetables such as red, purple, orange, and yellow potatoes, as well as sweet potatoes, yams, and taro, carry advantages in higher nutrient value. For example, sweet potatoes have very high beta-carotene (a precursor to vitamin A) but have four times the sugar content compared with baking potatoes. Adding healthy oils can help to blunt the glycaemic effect.

Those who are sensitive to nightshades may need to avoid potatoes. (Sweet potatoes and yams are not in the nightshade family.) Avoid green skin on any potato. This is a fungus and can be cut off. Those who are sensitive to nightshades would still be better served choosing healthier options from the KetoFLEX 12/3 Brain Food Pyramid, but these can be occasionally considered.

NOT FOR EVERYONE!

These are essentially "cheats" for those who are insulin sensitive, metabolically flexible, and physically active, who need extra calories.

Non-gluten grains and pseudograins include teff, buckwheat, sorghum, and millet and appear on the resistant starch list on page 142. Rice, oats, and popcorn are additional options. The most important consideration is their glycaemic potential and the need to monitor responses to these carbohydrates. In addition, the lectin content may be too high to consider any of these grains, especially if any autoimmune or GI issues are present. Unlike legumes, it is difficult to reduce the lectin level of grains. While not ancestral, these grains do have some modest benefits as resistant starches and nutrients.

- Rice is the staple food of more than half of the world's population, with 90 per cent of its consumption being in Asia. Brown, black, and wild rice have higher nutrient values and more fibre than white rice. White rice, however, has a lower lectin content, as the hull has been removed, but a higher glycaemic effect. Sushi rice is naturally cooked and cooled. Cooking and cooling increases the resistant starch value of rice. You can add healthy oils to help blunt the glycaemic effect. Rice also concentrates inorganic arsenic from soil, but toxicity is only potentially problematic with chronic consumption.

- Oats, which are steel-cut (least processed) or whole, thick rolled and raw, have large amounts of beta-glucans, a type of soluble fibre and resistant starch. Oats have unique anti-inflammatory compounds and a high nutrient content. The glycaemic effects of even the least processed of oats can still be too high in net carbs. Steel-cut oats can be soaked, cooked, and even cooled to increase the resistant starch. Organic whole raw or toasted oats, as in muesli, can be used with coconut, berries, cinnamon, and approved milks and sweeteners. Care must be taken to purchase *certified* gluten-free oats to prevent cross-contamination.
- Popcorn is addictive! That may be reason enough to avoid mentioning this snack food, since it is so easy to eat too much! There are some redeeming qualities to this grain, however. There are nutrients, antioxidants, quite a lot of fibre, including resistant starch; 240 g of organic non-GMO gluten-free air-popped popcorn has about 11 grams of fibre (4 grams being resistant starch), providing a net carb of 16 grams. Air-pop, drizzle with olive oil, and add sea salt, rosemary, or other herbs, spices, and nutritional yeast or crumbled seaweed flakes. *Limit* the amount. Cinema popcorn is not a good choice: in the US, a small bag is 420 g, a medium is 960 g, a large is 1200 g, and all of the popcorn in cinemas is full of

(continued)

toxic ingredients. Microwave popcorn is even more toxic. Check your response to the glycaemic effect before making a habit of this. Also, consider that corn is a grain with potential to be as allergenic as wheat, and many should avoid consuming it.

The current intake of resistant starch among those eating a typical modern diet is less than 5 grams a day.[25] The amount of resistant starch we recommend is between 20 and 40 grams a day. We recommend that you slowly increase your intake, paying close attention to the effect on both your digestion and blood glucose control. Be sure to eat resistant starches with other foods as a part of a meal. Adding extra fat (like EVOO) can also help to blunt a blood glucose spike.

Probiotics

Probiotic foods contain beneficial bacteria, which convert carbohydrates into lactic acid (fermentation) and compete with pathogenic bacteria. Before the ability to refrigerate foods, all cultures developed methods to make foods last longer and render them more digestible through fermentation, which creates healthful microbiomes. For millennia, these techniques have been used to make foods more digestible and longer lasting. Locally available foods and unique tastes have led to the creation of a wide variety of probiotic foods and beverages associated with different cultures. Vinegar, heat, and pasteurization all kill bacteria. Avoid any probiotic food with vinegar or added sugar. If choosing foods that have been heated or pasteurized, ensure the label states that live active cultures have been re-added. Here is a list of recommended probiotic foods:

PROBIOTICS

Sauerkraut* **Fermented, finely shredded cabbage**	**Tempeh* ♦** **Fermented soybean patty with Indonesian origins**
Kvass** **Fermented beetroot juice beverage with Eastern European origins (Look for lowest sugar.)**	**Natto** ♦**
Pickles* **Fermented cucumbers**	**Kombucha**** **Fermented tea with Manchurian origins (Look for lowest sugar.)**
Assorted fermented vegetables* **Pickled in brine, pasteurized**	**Non-dairy yoghurt or kefir*** **From coconuts or almonds**
Kimchi* **Spicy fermented cabbage and other vegetables with Korean origins**	**Buttermilk (D)**** **From grass-fed A2 dairy**
Brined olives* **No vinegar**	**Dairy yoghurt or kefir (D)** ♥** **From grass-fed A2 dairy (Look for full fat, no added sugar, with live, active cultures.)**
Miso ♦** **Japanese paste made from fermented soybeans, rice, chickpeas, rye, or barley**	

KEY
Glycaemic Index: Low* Intermediate High*****
Organic ♦
Inflammatory Dairy (D) ***Although the lactose is reduced by fermentation, the protein still may be inflammatory.***
High in SFA (saturated fatty acids) ♥

It's a good idea to incorporate probiotic foods into your daily meals. If you have access to your own organic garden, eat without "triple-washing"! Our ancestors didn't sterilize their food, which likely benefited their guts. Healthy soil is the key to health.

Emerging microbiome research is yielding important data on which strains may relate to specific disease states. Most of these probiotic foods are providing *Lactobacillus* and *Bifidobacteria* strains (except natto, which has *Bacillus subtilis*). Probiotic supplements, on the other hand, may be helpful to repopulate the gut, especially after antibiotic use. However, probiotic supplements appear to influence the gut microbiome in the short term rather than populate it in the long term.

ACTION PLAN

- If you have any chronic GI issues: work to address root causes, incorporate strategies for optimizing digestion, and consider a three-week elimination diet (including FODMAPs if necessary) to identify hidden food sensitivities.
- Slowly incorporate foods with prebiotic fibre into each meal.
- If resistant starch is appropriate for you, look for opportunities to add small amounts into your diet, using healthy fats to reduce the glycaemic effect if necessary.
- Once insulin sensitivity and gut health have been remediated, a long-term goal is the incorporation of more resistant starches.
- Experiment with adding a variety of probiotic foods into your diet.

CAUTIONS

GI DISTRESS Eating too many prebiotic fibres, resistant starch, or probiotic food too quickly can lead to GI distress such as mild abdominal pain, cramps, diarrhoea, wind, and bloating. We recommend starting with small amounts and increasing gradually. Because these side effects are closely related to leaky gut, dysbiosis, SIBO, and IBS, people suffering with these conditions may have a greater propensity for GI side effects.[26]

FODMAPS If you've already conducted a general elimination diet to determine underlying food sensitivities and you still have some lingering GI symptoms, you might want to consider an additional elimination trial of high FODMAP foods. FODMAP is an acronym for a collection of short-chain carbohydrates and sugar alcohols that can be poorly absorbed, resulting in GI distress. FODMAPs are fermentable oligosaccharides, disaccharides, monosaccharides, and polyols. Many high-FODMAP foods are actually very healthy foods that we recommend in our diet. They're just poorly digested by some, and thus eating them in large quantities may cause digestive issues for many people. The goal is to heal our guts to the point where they can digest these foods without problems.

Low-FODMAP diets are used on a temporary basis to treat conditions like IBS, SIBO, and other functional GI disorders such as altered motility. Low-FODMAP diets can also be prescribed to ease symptoms from other conditions, such as Hashimoto's thyroiditis, multiple sclerosis, eczema, rheumatoid arthritis, and fibromyalgia. Additionally, this diet may be helpful for those who have trouble tolerating high-histamine foods, which include fermented foods, bone broth, leftovers, alcohol, and many other foods. Abstain from fermented foods and probiotics during your low-FODMAP trial.

When people with IBS consume FODMAPs, the FODMAPs are rapidly fermented by the bacteria living in the intestines, causing wind to be produced. This results in bloating and impacts the ability of the gut to contract properly, leading to either loose stools or constipation. SIBO occurs when bacteria normally living in the large intestine make their way into the small intestine. The overgrowth of bacteria in the small intestine can lead to intestinal permeability, acid reflux, bloating, and IBS symptoms that often occur immediately after eating fibrous foods (including prebiotics and resistant starch) and fermented foods. Eliminating FODMAPs cuts off the food supply to the pathogenic bacteria in the small intestine. A low-FODMAP diet alone may not be enough to treat SIBO, but it's a good first step. Specialized antibiotics or antimicrobial treatments are sometimes needed. A functional medicine physician can guide you in testing for and treating SIBO.

Symptoms that may indicate you have a sensitivity to FODMAPs include:

- Wind
- Bloating
- Abdominal distention
- Abdominal pain
- Diarrhoea

- Constipation
- A feeling of early satiety

As with any elimination diet, you'll lower your intake of FODMAPs for three to six weeks to see if it helps to improve your symptoms, allowing your gut to heal before slowly reintroducing one food at a time to identify which foods are causing symptoms. Be aware that it's often the *quantity* of FODMAPs that may be causing the problem, and simply reducing the amount at any one meal can sometimes prevent symptoms. We know that elimination diets are difficult, but they offer powerful information that you can use for the rest of your life to personalize a sustainable diet that nourishes your body and optimizes your health.

HISTAMINE INTOLERANCE As noted in the previous chapter, some people, especially those with leaky gut, are sensitive to histamine, a neurotransmitter that normally protects our immune, digestive, and nervous systems. They often present with allergy-like symptoms after ingesting foods high in histamines. Some foods high in histamine include vinegar, fermented foods, and bone broth. See the box on bone broth on page 135 for more information.

REBOUND GERD FROM TRYING TO WEAN OFF PPIS (See page 132.)

ELEVATED GLUCOSE READING (See page 141.)

CHAPTER 10

Pyramid Level 4: Choose Wisely

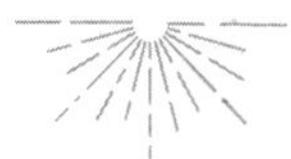

We are our choices.

—JEAN-PAUL SARTRE

ANIMAL PROTEIN

Ancestrally, wild animals grazed the land and ate their natural diets, providing our ancestors with clean, healthy animal protein that was naturally lean, rich in omega-3 fats and conjugated linoleic acid (CLA), which is associated with improved immune function and reduced inflammation. In an effort to increase efficiency and profit, large modern agricultural enterprises, in the United States particularly, employ concentrated animal feeding operations (CAFOs) to provide the meat available in supermarkets today. (In the UK, much of the beef, lamb and pork sold is not so intensively raised; beef and lamb are mostly grass-fed, with limitations imposed on growth promoters and antibiotic use.) These CAFOs facilities house animals in very confined and often unsanitary quarters, administer antibiotics to address disease, and utilize growth hormones to increase their size quickly. These antibiotics and hormones are passed on to us, endangering our health with antibiotic resistance and imbalanced hormone profiles, which lead to earlier puberty and insulin resistance.[1] CAFO animals are also fed very unnatural diets, typically inexpensive grains contaminated with glyphosate, and the resulting inflammation is passed on to us.[2]

Even when we avoid grains for the health benefits, we may still suffer the ill effects from grains simply by eating the grain-fed CAFO animals.

Many traditional long-lived healthy societies, such as the Okinawans, ate limited amounts of wild or pastured animals.[3] Nothing of the animal was wasted. Compare this to our modern-day practice of eating large quantities of primarily muscle meat (such as chicken breast and ground beef), which is rich in the essential amino acid methionine, while glycine, another amino acid found in collagen, bone, skin, and organ meat, is rarely consumed. Methionine restriction is associated with a more favourable metabolic picture (increased insulin sensitivity and fat burning) and longevity, while methionine excess can contribute to homocysteine elevation if not recycled properly.[4] To optimize health, methionine should be balanced with glycine and other amino acids. Adding grass-fed bone broth and organ meats to your diet is a simple way to achieve this balance.[5] Liver in small amounts is extraordinarily healthful, providing high levels of retinol, B_{12}, and choline.

For the purpose of reversal of cognitive decline, we recommend clean animal protein, in adequate amounts as determined by an individual's needs. That means sourcing animals that have lived and eaten as close as possible to what their natural states would dictate.

Calculating Protein Requirements

KetoFLEX 12/3, inherent in its name (FLEX = flexitarian), provides an opportunity to include animal protein or not. If you decide to include animal protein, think of it as a condiment or a side dish, not a main course.

Early humans likely ate whatever was available, which probably included insects, bark, roots, tubers, plants, fish, eggs, and the occasional feast from a successful hunt.[6] Animal protein was likely a rare treat, not the main part of every meal. While we need protein for essential body functions, the average Westerner eats too much. Dr Valter Longo's work reveals that lower protein intake at midlife, with higher amounts as we age, is correlated with longevity.[7] Many healthy people can limit animal protein consumption to 0.8 to 1 gram of protein per kilogram of lean body mass (LBM) per day, with the understanding that actual protein needs for each person are highly individualized. (Detailed instructions for determining your protein needs can be found in chapter 12.) Depending upon your starting place, you may need more protein initially, as you work to heal underlying damage, transitioning to less as you heal. It's important to identify your personalized protein needs by being aware that specific groups of people may need more protein:

- Those with chronic GI issues, including GERD (especially those using PPIs and other antacids), SIBO, IBS, etc.
- Those diagnosed with type 3 ("toxic") Alzheimer's
- Those with underlying illness, active infections, and recovering from surgery
- Those over age 65, especially those with marked muscle loss
- Those with suboptimal BMIs (below 18.5 for women and below 19.0 for men)
- Those who engage in rigorous sports or physically demanding work

Be aware that not everyone who falls into these categories *automatically* needs more dietary protein. This is especially true for those who are healthy, have optimized GI digestion (especially adequate stomach acid), and are actively encouraging muscle growth through daily challenging movement. If you fall into one or more of the bulleted categories above, increase your dietary protein by 10 to 20 per cent beyond our recommendations, to 1.1 to 1.2 grams of protein per kilogram of lean body mass, until you can address the specific root cause of whatever is causing you to have an increased need for or insufficient metabolism of protein, with the ultimate goal of working towards our recommended amount.

To prevent muscle loss while reducing protein, it's vital to incorporate strength training into your lifestyle. Look for opportunities to add weight-bearing movement into your day (see chapter 13). While reducing protein, pay close attention to how you feel in terms of strength. Those who are losing muscle or excessive weight may need to reconsider protein intake or possible GI dysfunction leading to reduced protein absorption.

Those who are otherwise healthy, strong, and thriving on our protein recommendations may want to consider further restricting protein to 15 to 25 grams per day, several times a week, to encourage autophagy, your cellular housekeeping programme, to promote healing. You may even want to consider abstaining from animal protein one or more days per week.

All plants have some protein. There is *no need* to limit your protein from plants when used as a wholefoods. In fact, we recommend using a variety of plants for protein (and more!), as many as possible. Vegetarians and vegans can achieve adequate protein from legumes, nuts, seeds, and vegetables. For instance, the protein in 28 grams of pistachios equals that in one free-range egg; however, plant protein is often incomplete and generally less bioavailable. Those relying solely on plant proteins should therefore consider potential deficiencies in omega-3s, vitamin B_{12}, retinol, vitamin D, zinc, and choline—all vital for brain health. See chapter 12 for more information specifically for vegans and vegetarians.

Seafood and Eggs for Brain Health

You might be wondering which animal foods are most important for optimal cognition. Wild-caught seafood and free-range eggs are the clear winners! Although we discuss seafood and eggs in this section on animal protein, it is mostly their unique fat that makes fatty fish (omega-3 fatty acids, especially DHA) and egg yolks (choline) important. Both are critical for synaptic support.[8]

DHA Our brains are more than 60 per cent fat, and docosahexaenoic acid (DHA) comprises 90 per cent of omega-3 fatty acids in the brain. The brain is unable to manufacture DHA locally and maintains these high DHA levels primarily through the uptake of DHA from lipids in circulating blood that cross the blood-brain barrier.[9] Maintenance of DHA concentration is important throughout the life cycle, starting with pregnancy, lactation, and infancy for proper brain and eye development, with implications later in life. DHA continues to be important for young brains, since they don't complete myelination until the third decade. Myelination is the process of forming a myelin sheath (or insulation) around the brain cell wiring.[10] DHA incorporates into the cell membranes, increasing fluidity, which is important for cell transport and communication. In fact, DHA is one of the most important fats for synaptic structure. DHA also increases BDNF, a growth factor that has an anti-Alzheimer's effect, promoting the survival of new brain cells and protecting existing ones.[11] The role of DHA may be especially critical for ageing brains, since they tend to shrink in size and exhibit increased oxidation and changes in membrane lipid composition.[12] A wealth of evidence suggests that maintaining an adequate level of omega-3 fatty acids (both EPA and DHA) provides powerful neuroprotection when you carefully account for potential confounders, described below.

Maximizing Neuroprotection from Omega-3 Fatty Acids

1. Make sure that you're getting enough. Because of multiple genetic and dietary interactions, the only way to do this is to measure blood levels, through a simple test called the omega-3 index. This test measures the red blood cell level of both EPA and DHA. Non-ApoE4 carriers should aim for a goal of 8 to 10 per cent, while ApoE4 carriers should try to reach ≥10 per cent.[13] Your omega-6 to omega-3 ratio should be in the range of 1:1 to 4:1. If you have a bleeding tendency or family history of haemorrhagic stroke (especially ApoE4 homozygote men), please be aware that ratios <0.5:1 may be associated with a bleeding tendency.
2. Ensure that you've met your homocysteine goal of ≤ 7 μmol/L. New evidence, which partially addresses previous inconsistent research results, suggests that omega-3 fatty acids do not benefit cognition unless elevated homocysteine has been addressed.[14]

CHOLINE Egg yolks, fish, and liver are among the best dietary sources for choline, a micronutrient critical to the brain. Choline stimulates the production of acetylcholine, a neurotransmitter responsible for synaptic connections essential to memory. Phosphatidylcholine, a phospholipid (a class of lipids that represents a major component of all cell membranes) of which choline is one component, is reduced in the brains of Alzheimer's patients. Higher levels are associated with memory performance and resistance to cognitive decline.[15] Choline has also been found to aid in the reduction of homocysteine, implicated in both dementia and cardiovascular disease as mentioned earlier. A recent study demonstrated that choline not only improved spatial memory in pregnant mice, but did so for several generations, without further supplementation, underscoring its neuroprotective importance.[16]

Sourcing Animal Protein

FISH Look for fish that are wild-caught, high in omega-3s, cold-water, and low in mercury. It's helpful to remember the SMASH (salmon, mackerel, anchovies, sardines, and herring) acronym when choosing fish. Fresh or flash-frozen are best. Jarred is preferable to BPA-free tins. The oceans, lakes, and all waterways are dynamic ecosystems continually being exposed to varying degrees of toxins. Seafood that is sourced away from industrialization is typically safer, excluding environmental disasters. Fish high in mercury are typically those with long lives (thus bioaccumulation) and large mouths (eating up the food chain), such as tuna, swordfish, and shark, and should be avoided. In general, fish that are smaller and lower on the food chain are the safest. Also avoid smoked fishes, which contain nitrates and are associated with stomach cancer.

Salmon is high in omega-3 and is less contaminated. The best source is wild-caught from the Pacific, especially from Alaska. Sockeye, king, coho, keta, and pink are good options. Fresh wild-caught salmon is typically available from May through September, but flash-frozen salmon is usually available at many supermarkets year-round. Beware of farmed salmon, which represents the majority of the salmon in the market. Many restaurants even represent farmed salmon as wild-caught. Wild-caught salmon is a much deeper reddish orange hue with a more gamy taste, while farmed salmon is milder in flavour, paler in colour, and riddled with white fatty marbling due to a lack of exercise in captivity. Most farmed salmon is extremely toxic with pesticides, persistent organic pollutants (POPs), polychlorinated biphenyls (PCBs), mercury, cadmium, dioxins, and antibiotics. Due to their crowded, filthy, stressed conditions and unnatural GMO feed, these fish are diseased, often riddled with sea lice and unhealthful to consume. The nutrient quality, including omega-3 fats, is also compromised.[17]

With the exception of salmon, the rest of the fish in the SMASH acronym are always wild-caught. North Atlantic-caught mackerel is a good option, as are herring and mackerel caught in a purse-seine net in the North Atlantic (in the UK look for the Marine Stewardship Council symbol on all fish you buy). Avoid king and Spanish mackerel, which are high in mercury. The soft bones from anchovies and sardines are exceptionally healthful for their calcium, collagen, and other nutrients. Atlantic and Pacific herring are both good options. If you like Scandinavian pickled herring, look for a low-sugar variety or consider pickling them yourself. Other good fish options low in mercury include sustainably caught wild cod, pollack, and sole (or flounder).

SHELLFISH, CRUSTACEANS, AND MOLLUSKS These should be wild-caught when available. Shrimp (and prawns) should always be wild-caught. The majority of shrimp sold in the UK and the US are farmed and imported and should be avoided. Farmed scallops, clams, mussels, and oysters are generally considered safe. Crabs are wild-caught and generally considered to be safe, although some have higher *dioxin* levels. Dioxin is an environmental pollutant that can be harmful to human health. Avoid imitation crabmeat, which has high levels of inflammatory transglutaminase that can penetrate the blood-brain barrier and disrupt neurotransmitters.

Marine Stewardship Council in the UK and globally, offers guidance on how to choose sustainably caught fish. When you choose MSC-labelled fish, you are choosing wild-caught seafood that can be traced to a sustainable source. Additionally, searching for labels such as *Fishwise and Seafood Safe* can also help you source the least toxic and most sustainably harvested fish.

EGGS Not unexpectedly, the healthiest eggs come from the healthiest hens, which are those that have the greatest exposure to non-toxic open pastures. Eggs from free-range hens are also an excellent source of omega-3 fatty acids (up to 13 times more than eggs from standard, non-free-range chickens), B_{12} (70 per cent more), folate (50 per cent more), and the fat-soluble vitamins, especially E, A, and beta-carotene, providing at least double that of conventional eggs.[18] The deeper orange-coloured yolks from free-range hens are a reflection of their ability to consume their natural omnivorous diet, which includes grass, weeds, seeds, insects, and worms. Within the UK, all eggs sold at retail level must follow strict labelling requirements as to whether they are organic, free-range, barn-raised or from caged hens. They must also indicate on the egg this same level of labelling in code, along with the country of original and the production site code. Eggs are also graded and labelled by quality, weight, and a best-before date. In the US, labeling in this area is unregulated, and we still recommend sourcing eggs with a pasture-raised label together with *Animal Welfare Approved* or *Certified Humane*.

GRASS-FED MEAT Your goal is to source 100 per cent grass-fed meat from animals that graze on healthy pastures, without exposure to antibiotics or growth hormones. Grass-fed meat is leaner, with a healthier nutrient profile. Most British beef cattle and lamb are reared outdoors and have access to pasture, but the only way to be sure is to look at the labels or shop at a reputable butcher. Look for organic, grass-fed, or access to pasture on the labels. Grass-fed meat should be cooked low and slow to create a mild exterior sear, allowing the naturally occurring sugars to caramelize on the surface, while protecting muscle fibres from contracting too quickly and becoming tough.

In the US, however, USDA certified organic meat may *not* be your best option, because these animals still receive supplemental grains, albeit *organic* grains. Also, be aware that the rollback of country of origin labelling in the US is making it harder to find 100 per cent grass-fed meat. Look for the American Grassfed Association's *Certified*

Grassfed label or use their site to find a rancher near you. Another helpful tool is the EatWild website. New Zealand lamb, which is widely available, is always grass-fed. In the US, a good online source for grass-fed meat and liver is US Wellness Meats. Because red meat (beef, lamb, bison, pork) contains high amounts of the sugar molecule Neu5Gc (N-glycolylneuraminic acid), we recommend limiting red meat. In the US, we also advise against eating any venison (deer, moose, elk) because of chronic wasting disease, spreading among the North American herds and affecting Norway and South Korea. (See more under Cautions on the next page.)

POULTRY Your goal is to find the almost impossible: a 100 per cent free-range chicken, duck, goose, or turkey. There are many unregulated labels in the US—*cage-free, free-range, free-roaming,* or *pastured*—that may lead you to believe the bird roams freely and hasn't received supplemental grains, but that is rarely the case. While these birds may be afforded the limited opportunity to roam outdoors, they are typically still given supplemental feed comprised of grains, which can be inflammatory for you in the same way as if you had eaten the grains yourself. Those labelled *USDA Organic* are a little better, as they are free from antibiotics and growth hormones. They eat only organic feed, which still includes grains but safer versions, free from pesticides and contamination. The labelling regulations in the UK and throughout the EU are more stringent, with traceability and clarity being particularly important issues.

When possible, talk directly to the farmer and ask what the birds have been fed. You want poultry that have been given the freedom to roam and eat grass, weeds, grubs, and insects on land that is free from pesticides, herbicides, and other contamination. Truly free-range poultry naturally have higher levels of omega-3s. They're much smaller than conventionally raised birds and are generally tougher but can be rendered tender when slow-cooked in liquid. There is some debate about whether or not poultry can receive adequate nutrition from simply foraging, and it's impossible to raise poultry that are 100 per cent free-range in the winter months in northern climates, as the bird's food supply is typically covered in snow. (If you live in a northern climate, we recommend purchasing flash-frozen poultry that has been pastured before winter.) EatWild provides a search engine to help you find poultry that has at least six hours a day of pasture grazing but may still receive some grain or seed depending on the weather conditions.

ACTION PLAN

- Healthy people should limit animal protein consumption to 0.8 to 1 gram per kilogram of lean body mass per day, with some exceptions above.
- Be aware that protein goals may be reduced as healing progresses, to enhance autophagy.
- All plants contain some protein. There is no need to limit your protein from whole plants.
- Prioritize wild-caught seafood and free-range eggs.

CAUTIONS

FARMED SALMON (See page 157.)

FARMED SHRIMP (See page 157.)

ANTIBIOTIC AND HORMONE EXPOSURE Carefully source grass-fed meat that hasn't been exposed to antibiotics and hormones per our instructions above. Organic poultry is always free from antibiotics and hormones but still receives supplemental organic grains.

HEAVY METALS AND OTHER ENVIRONMENTAL CONTAMINATION Because toxins—mercury, lead, cadmium, and countless others—have become so pervasive in the water and land where animals live, *they are impossible to avoid.* Bioaccumulation and the storage of toxins in the fat and bones of animals, including our own, continue to confound our efforts to reduce our toxic burden. In addition to heavy metals, our oceans are becoming filled with thousands of tons of plastic waste elements (microplastics) consumed by even the smallest fish. These toxins accumulate in the fat of animals we consume and in turn are passed on to us. Many of these toxins have cumulative effects on our health. While our guidelines provide instructions on how to source the cleanest animal proteins possible, toxic contamination is another reason to limit animal protein altogether.

GRAIN EXPOSURE (See page 151.)

ELEVATED GLUCOSE MARKERS Many who embark on lowering their carbohydrate consumption consume extra protein, as they are not comfortable with increasing the fat in their diet. Excess protein, like excess carbs, can cause a spike in blood glucose. Limiting your protein, by using fat with non-starchy vegetables, can help to keep you both satiated and in ketosis, thereby keeping blood glucose low.

ELEVATED HOMOCYSTEINE (See pages 152 and 155.)

TMAO (TRIMETHYLAMINE N-OXIDE) Some studies have suggested that eating red meat raises TMAO, which in turn increases the risk for heart disease, cancer, and all-cause mortality. However, the epidemiological evidence is inconsistent and virtually disappears when kidney disease and insulin resistance are considered as contributing factors.[19] Additionally, none of these studies takes into account the health of the microbiome (where TMAO originates) and may underestimate the healthy user bias—the concept that those who eschew red meat may have overall healthier habits. We suspect that the small amount of unprocessed clean animal protein we recommend in the context of a heavily plant-based diet and healthy lifestyle will minimize the potential negative effect of TMAO.

EGGS AND PROSTATE CANCER An inconsistent correlation has been found between egg consumption and prostate cancer that holds true only for North America. In countries where there is high egg consumption and plentiful vegetable intake, this correlation disappears. Newer research suggests that the unhealthy user bias traditionally associated with egg intake may be mediating this risk.[20] We suspect that men who are otherwise following our heavily plant-based, no-sugar guidelines will minimize the potential risk. Men at higher risk due to progressive benign prostate enlargement or who are diagnosed with prostate cancer should be careful to meet but not exceed their choline needs.

IGF-1 ELEVATION Excess protein, especially when combined with a sedentary lifestyle and a Westernized diet, can elevate insulin-like growth factor 1 (IGF-1), a protein that has a similar molecular structure as insulin. Excess levels of IGF-1 are correlated with some cancers, including cancer of the colon, pancreas, endometrium, breast, and prostate.[21]

AGES Advanced glycation end products (AGEs) are harmful compounds that result when proteins and lipids become glycated. They are naturally present in uncooked animal protein and other foods. Cooking animal protein, especially at high heat or with added sugar, dramatically increases AGEs, as exemplified by visible browning and charring. AGEs are also formed endogenously by consuming proteins and lipids when they combine with sugar in the bloodstream. Both endogenous and exogenous AGEs result in premature ageing, and the development and worsening of many chronic degenerative diseases, including Alzheimer's, atherosclerosis, diabetes, and kidney disease.[22] When cooking animal protein, use moist heat (casserole, stew, poach) instead of dry heat (grill, roast, fry). Lower temperatures over a longer cooking period with marinades made from acidic ingredients such as vinegar, citrus, or wine and with rosemary or other herbs help to mitigate the effects. Many find using a slow cooker helpful.[23]

NEU5GC (N-GLYCOLYLNEURAMINIC ACID) Neu5Gc is a sugar molecule found in most mammals but not humans. Preliminary evidence suggests that after humans ingest Neu5Gc (prevalent in red meat), they may not recognize the molecule and create inflammatory antibodies in response. Those with the highest quartile of Neu5Gc antibodies were found to have a three times higher risk of colorectal cancer than those in the lowest quartile.[24]

CHRONIC WASTING DISEASE: This is a fatal prion disease affecting deer, moose, and elk in North America, Norway, and South Korea. The CDC has warned against eating venison from infected animals. Because there is an extended incubation period before symptoms appear, we advise against eating any venison.[25]

FRUITS

Some call fruit "God's sweets." In their ancestral form, fruits were rich in phytonutrients and healthful fibre. Sadly, many modern fruits bear little resemblance to their predecessors. Fruits that are readily available in our shops today have often been selectively bred to be sweeter, larger, easier to eat, and more durable for transport, resulting in unnatural varieties that are low in fibre and high in sugar, harming metabolic health. Ancestrally, fruits were consumed at the end of summer to fatten for the winter. Some describe our current obesity epidemic as stemming from "the winter that never comes." That is beautifully exemplified with the ready availability of every fruit imaginable no matter the season.

Carefully selected, a small serving of fruit, especially combined with nuts, can be a perfect dessert safely enjoyed at the end of a meal.[26] Choose organic, local, and seasonal fruits with a low glycaemic index or net carbs. A perfect example would be a tart wild crab apple combined with a few English walnuts enjoyed in the late summer or early autumn. Below see a complete list of all recommended fruits, with accompanying glycaemic warnings.

FRUITS

Bilberries**	Green mangoes**
Blackberries**	Green papayas**
Black currants*	Green plantains*
Blueberries**	Kiwis* (unripe)
Boysenberries**	Lemons*
Cherries* (tart)	Limes*
Coconuts* ♥	Mulberries**
Crab apples** (wild, in season)	Persimmons***
Cranberries*	Pomegranates***
Grapefruits*	Raspberries**
Green bananas*	Strawberries** ♦

KEY
Glycaemic Index: Low* Intermediate** High***
Organic ♦
High in SFA (saturated fatty acids) ♥

Some fruits, such as wild berries, may be eaten out of season in order to take advantage of their powerful neuroprotective properties. Wild unsweetened berries, including blueberries, strawberries, raspberries, mulberries, bilberries, black currants, blackberries, boysenberries, cranberries, and pomegranates, should be prioritized because their polyphenolic compounds exert a therapeutic effect in both preventing and remediating cognitive decline. Their dark pigments, called anthocyanins, and other flavonols contribute to their neuroprotective properties.[27]

Blueberries have been particularly well studied for memory enhancement. In two separate randomized controlled trials, they improved aspects of cognition including verbal memory, working memory, and task switching, which is an important component of executive function.[28] Additionally, functional MRI tests demonstrate higher levels of blood-oxygen-dependent signals in the brains of those with mild cognitive impairment after consuming blueberries.[29] Tart cherries, which are technically drupes, not berries, have also been shown to improve cardiometabolic health, oxidative stress, and inflammation. A small, randomized controlled trial demonstrated that those who supplemented with cherries showed improvements in verbal fluency and short- and long-term memory.[30] Persimmons, an excellent source of prebiotic fibre, have demonstrated neuroprotective properties but are fairly high on the glycaemic index and thus should be enjoyed cautiously.[31]

Wild unsweetened fresh berries and cherries are preferable, but frozen are fine. (Surprisingly, even dried fruit retains high levels of nutrients, just in condensed packages.) Be careful to source *unsweetened* versions. Always eat the whole fruit as opposed to the juice, to maintain the fibre and reduce the glycaemic index. Some berries, such as cranberries and black currants, are very tart and unpalatable for some. Explore different ways of using small amounts of approved sweeteners to render them more palatable.

Other fruits that can be liberally enjoyed out of season are lemons and limes. They are excellent sources of vitamin C and are naturally low in glucose. These bright citrus powerhouses of flavour add a refreshing flavour punch to salads, animal proteins, desserts, and more. Even zesting their tough outer peel is an easy and nutritious way to put an extra zing of flavour into many foods; choose unwaxed citrus for zesting, preferably organic. (Note: Acidic foods soften your tooth enamel. It is best to wait for a half hour after eating any acidic food before brushing your teeth.)

We caution against eating most ripe tropical fruits, as they tend to be very high on the glycaemic index. Some exceptions are unsweetened coconut (technically a drupe) and all of the resistant starches previously mentioned, including unripened green plantains, bananas, mangoes, and papayas. Be careful not to cook green bananas and plantains, as that degrades the resistant starch. As mentioned earlier, kiwi has natural digestive enzymes and has also been found to improve lipid profiles and reduce lipid oxidation.[32]

BEETROOT If fruits are "God's sweets," then beetroots are his *jewels.* Beetroots, a deep ruby red, *sugary* but non-starchy root vegetable, provide big benefits to both the heart and brain through different mechanisms. Beetroots are well known for being a rich source of nitrates, which are converted into nitric oxide in the vascular endothelium. Nitric oxide acts a vasodilator, which helps to decrease blood pressure and improve blood flow, thereby supporting cerebral and cardiac vascular health, and is particularly appropriate for vascular cognitive decline. Another way that beetroots may benefit the brain is by combining them for their uridine content with omega-3 fatty acids and choline to support synaptic growth.[33] A recent laboratory study demonstrated that betanin, a compound in beetroots that is responsible for their distinctive red colour, may help slow the accumulation of beta-amyloid in the brain.[34] Beetroots also have potent antioxidant and anti-inflammatory detoxification properties.[35] Beetroots and their leafy greens are also rich in carotenoids, which have been shown to aid in eye health.[36]

Raw beetroots, which are delicious in salads, have the lowest glycaemic impact. Cooked beetroots have a distinctive earthy taste, not unlike potatoes. They can be steamed or roasted, maintaining their firmness. It is important not to overcook them, as this will diminish their nutrients and increase their sugar content. Serving them with EVOO or butter can also help to blunt the glycaemic effect. You may keep the skin on, particularly with young beetroot (which are tender and less bitter), if you're roasting them or making kvass, an Eastern European lacto-fermented beetroot juice. The skin is rich with microbes, which confer healthy microbiotica for the kvass. It is best to avoid pickling beetroots with vinegar, as that destroys the healthy gut bacteria. As with all higher glycaemic foods with healthful properties, *balance is key*. Eat small amounts as part of a meal and check your postprandial blood glucose at one and two hours to see the effect on you.

ACTION PLAN

- Eat heirloom fruit seasonally. Depending upon what part of the world you live in, there may be many other options available to you locally. Always balance nutritive value against glycaemic concerns.
- Enjoy small portions of wild berries year-round.
- Unripened tropical fruit (green plantains, bananas, mangoes, papayas, and kiwi) may be eaten in small amounts as resistant starches and for their natural digestive enzymes.
- Lemons and limes are great sources of vitamin C and can be enjoyed liberally.

CAUTIONS

ELEVATED BLOOD GLUCOSE This is discussed above. Be sure to conduct one- and two-hour postprandial blood glucose checks to see the effect a given fruit has for you. See chapter 18, page 259, to find target goals. Combining fruits with nuts can reduce the glycaemic effects, as can eating fruit at the end of a meal.

OXALATES Beetroots and several of the recommended fruits, including raspberries, cranberries, blueberries, papayas, and kiwis, are high in oxalates. Oxalates are plant-based compounds that may promote inflammation or kidney stones when eaten in large quantities by those who are genetically susceptible or who have impaired gut health.

CHAPTER 11

Pyramid Level 5: Risky Business

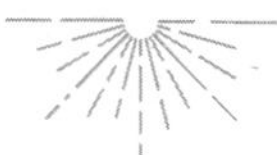

Earth provides enough to satisfy every man's need,

but not every man's greed.

—MAHATMA GANDHI

SWEETENERS

You'll be amazed at how quickly you lose your taste for sweet foods after adopting a low-glycaemic wholefood diet. You may even find yourself eating lemon and lime slices the way you once ate an orange! This retraining of your taste buds is a positive sign that you've weaned yourself off hyper-palatable fake food loaded with added sugar. Savour this sweet victory and don't sabotage your progress with sweeteners. The last thing we want to do is to reacclimate your taste buds to the sweet food we've encouraged you to abandon. Evidence also suggests that the sweetness from even non-caloric sweeteners still tricks our bodies into producing insulin and other hormones involved in glucose regulation, which can be harmful to your metabolic healing.[1] There are several natural sweeteners that may be considered for limited use.

STEVIA Very small amounts of stevia in pure forms are acceptable. The stevia plant is extraordinarily sweet and grown in many parts of the world including Japan, China, Brazil, and Paraguay. It's 200 to 300 times more intense than ordinary table sugar, and thus little is needed. Stevia contains zero calories and is often combined with other sweeteners. You want to avoid blends and find a pure source with as few ingredients as possible. SweetLeaf is an acceptable brand. Some people complain that stevia has an unpleasant aftertaste, while others don't notice it.

MONK FRUIT Small amounts of pure monk fruit sweetener are also acceptable. Monk fruit, or *luo han guo*, is a small round fruit grown in South East Asia. It's said to be named after Buddhist monks who grew it eight centuries ago. Monk fruit is 100 to 250 times sweeter than table sugar but has zero calories. Like stevia, it's often combined with other sweeteners. Avoid blends and find a brand with as few ingredients as possible. Pure Monk is one example of an acceptable brand.

HONEY With our focus on ancestral foods, we'd be remiss not to include honey for its many health benefits. Unfortunately, it also has a very high glycaemic index and is appropriate only in very small amounts for those who are *not* insulin resistant, and with a meal high in fibre and fat to blunt its effect. Local raw (unpasteurized) honey is comprised of organic acids and phenolic compounds that combine to provide powerful antioxidants.[2] Honey is also a prebiotic, with natural digestive enzymes that can help contribute to gut health.[3] Honey has both antimicrobial and antifungal properties, and very preliminary evidence suggests that, if locally sourced, it may help to desensitize against allergies.[4] Be sure to perform postprandial blood glucose checks to test the effect honey has for you. Do not use honey in your coffee while fasting, as it will impede your ability to achieve ketosis. Beekeeper's Naturals, while not local for everyone, is an example of a good product that is also addressing the bee colony collapse issue threatening our global food supply.

SUGAR ALCOHOLS While they can occur naturally from rotting fruit and fermented food, the vast majority of commercially available products (erythritol, sorbitol, and mannitol) are highly engineered and come from the glucose in GMO cornstarch. Xylitol is the exception and comes from the glucose in hardwood. Sugar alcohols are well known to cause GI side effects and sometimes headaches. They can exacerbate underlying IBS or SIBO. Even small amounts can cause a laxative effect.[5] Additionally, sugar alcohols appear to unfavourably alter the gut microbiome by feeding harmful microbial species including *E. coli, Salmonella, Shigella,* and *Streptococcus.*[6]

ACTION PLAN

- If necessary, use limited amounts of approved sweeteners.

CAUTIONS

GLUCOSE ELEVATION Honey can cause glucose elevations and is recommended in only small amounts for those who are metabolically healthy (see above).

ALLERGIES Anyone with bee sting allergies should be cautious with honey.

COCOA FLAVANOLS

Our decadent, beloved chocolate, rich in cocoa flavanols, can still be enjoyed, just in small amounts. While the flavanols derived from the cocoa bean provide significant health benefits, they also come with significant toxicity concerns, landing them in the indulgence category. Cocoa flavanols are a highly unique blend of phytonutrients found only in the cacao bean, not to be confused with the coffee bean. Further confusing the issues, the terms *cacao* (kə-'kaů) and *cocoa* ('kō-kō) are often mistakenly used interchangeably. *Cacao* refers to the raw beans that are found inside of large fruit pods from the cacao tree, whereas *cocoa* refers to the processed product once the beans have been harvested, fermented, dried, and roasted at high temperatures. Cocoa flavanols are commonly enjoyed as cacao nibs, cocoa powder, cacao powder, and chocolate.

A strong body of evidence suggests that cocoa flavanols provide neuroprotection. Several studies have demonstrated that cocoa flavanols not only improve cognitive function but also show improvements in circulation to specific parts of the brain involved with age-related memory decline as measured by imaging.[7] Cocoa flavanols improve blood vessel function, thereby improving the delivery of oxygen and nutrients throughout the body, resulting in improved blood pressure and overall metabolic health.[8]

Unfortunately, we need to weigh the benefits of cocoa flavanols against the potential for toxicity. Cadmium and lead, while naturally present in the Earth's crust, affect many cocoa products primarily through man-made pollution. Both are heavy metals that accumulate in the body and have been implicated as having detrimental effects on human health. Cadmium affects the central nervous system, leading to reduced attention, impaired ability to smell, and memory deficits. Additionally, it has been implicated as a toxin that affects many organs and is classified as a carcinogen.[9] The World Health Organization (WHO) recommends limiting cadmium consumption to no more than a maximum of 0.3 micrograms (mcg) per gram (g) in dried plant materials.[10] The United States hasn't set a national standard, but California requires warning labels on any food containing more than 4.1 mcg of cadmium per daily serving. Lead also affects many body organs and is distributed to the brain, where it can lead to often irreversible brain damage, affecting cognition and intellect. Children and pregnant women are particularly vulnerable.[11] According to the WHO, there is no safe limit for lead in food.[12] The US Food and Drug Administration (FDA) limits the maximum amount allowable in food to 3.0 micrograms per day for children and 12.5 for adults.[13] California limits lead exposure to just 5.0 micrograms a day for everyone, from all sources.[14]

When choosing a dietary source for cocoa flavanols, you must take into account multiple variables. Your goal is to find cacao with:

- High flavanols. In general, the higher the cacao, the higher the level of flavanols.[15]
- Low sugar. The same rule applies. In general, the higher the cacao, the lower the sugar.

- Low cadmium. Using the limits from above, source the lowest cadmium.
- Low lead. Using the limits from above, source the lowest lead.

We've got some tips and resources to help you evaluate all of the moving parts. First, always look for the highest cacao percentage that you can tolerate. One hundred per cent cacao will always have the highest level of flavanols and the lowest level of sugar, but it's pretty bitter and definitely an acquired taste. Always try to find chocolate with 85 per cent cacao or higher. ConsumerLab.com, a subscription resource that evaluates many health and nutrition products, offers an in-depth evaluation of flavanols (and some toxins) for many chocolate, cacao, and cocoa products. To determine the levels of sugar, simply read the nutritional information on the back of the package and always try to choose the option with the least sugar. A free online resource called As You Sow is excellent for evaluating the levels of both cadmium and lead using our limits from above. Their Toxic Chocolate search engine also allows you to filter for your desired level of cacao. (Do not rely on the USDA organic seal to protect against heavy metal contaminants.) The EWG Food Scores search engine may also be helpful, but it provides only a ranking as opposed to listing actual levels of specific toxins and doesn't allow you to filter by cacao percentage. There are a multitude of cocoa flavanol products available. Some are very common, such as chocolate and cocoa, while others are more exotic, such as cacao nibs and cacao powder. Many products make extraordinary health claims without mentioning the inherent toxins.

CACAO NIBS These robust, crunchy darlings of the health food world are the purest form of cocoa beans; lightly roasted and ground-up bits that can be found in both fermented and non-fermented versions. The non-fermented varieties are slightly less bitter. In addition to providing the phytonutrient benefits described above, they're also a decent source of prebiotic fibre. Sadly, they also tend to be very high in cadmium, with only several coming close to or meeting the WHO cutoff of 0.3 mcg per gram. We caution readers to consume no more than an occasional serving of 1 tablespoon with the lowest toxicity you can find.

COCOA POWDER Cocoa powder is used to create cocoa beverages and chocolate. It is roasted at much higher temperatures and more finely ground. In its pure form, it's unsweetened and still retains significant, yet reduced, amounts of the healthful flavanols described above. Cadmium levels and lead are even more concentrated in cocoa powders, with *none* meeting the WHO limitations. For that reason, we recommend *abstaining* from cocoa powder.

CACAO POWDER This is different from cocoa powder. It's made by cold-pressing cacao nibs into a paste and then drying that into a powder. Because this is the most concentrated source of cacao, it also has the highest toxicity for both cadmium and lead. We are unable to recommend any commercially available products.

CHOCOLATE Luckily, cadmium and lead levels are typically the least concentrated in chocolate, but chocolate can come with a whopping amount of sugar and negligible amounts of the healthful flavanols. Your goal is to source the lowest amount of tolerable sugar with the highest flavanol content and lowest toxicity. The percentages of cacao on chocolate bars actually refer to how much of the bar, by weight, is made from pure cacao beans and their by-products. By default, higher percentages of cacao contain less sugar and higher flavanols. A few squares of carefully chosen chocolate per day can be a safe (yet decadently delicious) treat to savour after a healthy meal.

ACTION PLAN

- To derive the health benefits of flavanols, enjoy small amounts of chocolate high in cacao and low in sugar, cadmium, and lead.
- Because of toxicity concerns, limit cacao nibs and avoid cocoa and cacao powder.
- Consider a flavanol supplement.

CAUTIONS

GLUCOSE ELEVATIONS (See page 167.)
HEAVY METAL TOXICITY (See page 170.)

DAIRY

Because dairy products cause inflammation in so many people, and since inflammation is a key driver of Alzheimer's disease, we recommend against the use of dairy. If you're used to pouring a generous dollop of cream in your coffee, this recommendation can hurt. We get it and will suggest some healthful work-arounds.

Dairy is inflammatory for several reasons. Almost 70 per cent of the world's population is lactose intolerant, and many aren't even aware of their own intolerance. Lactose intolerance is defined by a reduced ability to digest lactose after infancy. This is especially true of non-Europeans, with up to 90 per cent of East Asians being affected.[16] Common symptoms of lactose intolerance include stomach pain, bloating, gas, and diarrhoea. Less well-known symptoms include reduced GI motility, nausea, vomiting, constipation, eczema, sinusitis, arthritis, muscle and joint pain, tiredness, heart arrhythmia, short-term memory loss, headache, mouth ulcers, and other symptoms, suggesting widespread inflammation affecting multiple body systems.[17]

Dairy may also be inflammatory to anyone with gluten sensitivity because of molecular mimicry. The casein protein in dairy is similar enough to the gliadin protein in gluten that it confuses the immune system. When we're sensitive to a food, our adaptive immune systems create antibodies to the "bad guy," which in this case is *gluten*. Every time we ingest gluten, the alarm bells are sounded and our antibodies go on attack. However, our immune systems aren't perfect, and proteins that are molecularly similar, like casein is to gliadin, can be mistaken for the original antigen, causing a ratcheting up of inflammatory cytokines and a steady state of chronic inflammation if the offending food(s) aren't eliminated.[18]

Even those who don't have gluten sensitivity or lactose intolerance may still be sensitive to dairy because of the evolving nature of our milk supply. Nature has beautifully supplied all mammals with the perfect food to nurture their offspring—*breast milk*. For millennia, each mammal species used their breast milk exclusively for their own young. Cow's milk is clearly not an ancestral food. Not until the advent of agriculture and the domestication of animals around 10,000 years ago did humans begin to use the milk of ruminants for their own nutrition.[19]

Originally all mammals, including humans, produced a type of milk called A2. Somewhere around 8,000 years ago, a mutation occurred in Europe, leading to a new type of cow's milk called A1. No one knows for sure how or why this occurred. Some theorize that the mutated A1 breeds may have been better milk producers and farmers might have naturally gravitated towards them for breeding to increase production. Over time, the vast majority of cow's milk in the Western world eventually transitioned to a blend, comprised primarily of A1 milk.[20]

Around twenty-five years ago, scientists made an interesting discovery when they found a small molecular variation between the two types of milk. Beta-casein, the most abundant protein in milk, is composed of 209 amino acids. It turns out that at the 67th position, the ancestral A2 milk had the amino acid *proline*, whereas the newer A1 casein had *histidine*. Just a single amino acid out of 209 may not sound like much of a change, but even such a small change may alter the structure (as an example, sickle cell disease is caused by a single amino acid change in haemoglobin), which may be recognized by our immune systems.[21] Indeed, evidence began to accumulate that the newer A1 milk might be linked to many inflammatory diseases, including type 1 diabetes and cardiovascular disease.[22] Further research has revealed that the digestion of A1 milk produces inflammatory compounds in the GI tract that can cause digestive problems and even neurological deficits.[23] Not surprisingly, this hypothesis has received dairy industry pushback from A1 farmers, who question the financial motivation of this research, some of which has been funded by the A2 industry. Independent research, however, suggests that there's enough "smoke" for concern.[24] Given the close relationship between gut and brain health and the inflammatory component of Alzheimer's, we recommend switching from A1 to A2 dairy products if you are planning to include dairy in your diet, and minimizing your total exposure.

MILK It's becoming fairly easy to find A2 milk in most food shops. Of course you want to select grass-fed, A2 whole milk, which might be a bit more difficult. It's important to understand that the fat in whole milk blunts the effects of the natural sugar in the milk. Goat, sheep, buffalo, camel, or yak milk is always grass-fed and naturally A2. Decent substitutes include unsweetened versions of milk from almonds (from blanched almonds if you're sensitive to lectins), coconut, flax, hazelnut, hemp, macadamia, and organic soy milk. (Cashew milk may be too inflammatory, as it's high in lectins. Rice milk is too high in carbohydrates.) Use the Cornucopia Institute's Plant-Based Beverage Report and Scorecard to find the healthiest options. Any of these can be used in your coffee as a substitute for cream. Some people also enjoy a little coconut oil or vanilla-infused ghee in their coffee.

Remember, dairy and dairy substitutes in your coffee will end your fast. If you drink coffee during your fast, take it black with only a tiny bit of approved sweetener. Those who are insulin resistant and working to extend their fast may use a little bit of coconut oil to help promote ketosis. See more in chapter 7, "Tips for Transitioning to a Longer Fast."

YOGHURT You may occasionally enjoy a small amount of yoghurt from the milk of any of the approved animals mentioned above. Try to source organic and grass-fed with live and active cultures. Look for the list of cultures on the packaging of yoghurt in the UK. Always buy unsweetened, organic yoghurt. You can mix with a few nuts and wild berries for sweetness. If needed, feel free to add a small bit of an approved sweetener. You can also try to find unsweetened organic coconut or soy yoghurts. Yoghurts without a lot of added sugars and other ingredients can be hard to locate, leading many people to make their own.

KEFIR Kefir is a fermented drink with a sour taste that's very healthful because of the live active probiotics. Kefir typically has a larger number and a wider variety of healthy bacteria than yoghurt. All of the same caveats for yoghurt apply to kefir.

CHEESE Cheeses from any of the approved animals above are acceptable in small amounts. Goat, sheep, and some water buffalo cheeses are widely available.

ACTION PLAN

- Avoid all conventional animal dairy.
- You may have small amounts of A2 dairy if tolerated and desired.

CAUTIONS

GI DISTRESS (See page 173.)

INFLAMMATION (See page 173.)

ELEVATED LIPIDS Most full-fat dairy products are high in saturated fat and can contribute to higher LDL-C for some people, primarily ApoE4 carriers. This doesn't mean total avoidance, but rather mindful consideration. (See page 113 in chapter 8.)

CANCER POTENTIAL Dairy cows are milked throughout their pregnancies, exposing us to reproductive levels of hormone in their milk. The stimulation of hormone-sensitive cancers, such as those that occur in the breast, uterine, and prostate tumours, might be an issue with the hormones and growth factors in dairy products.[25] (The UK dairy industry, however, faces tough regulations on the use of hormones and growth factors.) The correlation is particularly strong for prostate cancer risk.[26]

ALCOHOL

Cheers . . . to *life*! This one may be tough to hear, but we're going to give it to you straight. It's abundantly clear that heavy alcohol use is associated with a greater risk of developing dementia.[27] The amount of alcohol that constitutes heavy drinking is less clear and further confounds the issue; complete abstinence also appears to increase risk.[28] The quality of evidence, however, is insufficient to suggest that those who currently abstain should begin to drink alcohol. Focused research has shown that ApoE4 carriers do poorly with any amount of alcohol.[29]

Alcohol harms us in many ways. It acts as a neurotoxin that damages multiple structures in the brain, leading to seizures (usually on withdrawal), brain atrophy, memory loss, sleep interference, and cerebellar damage (causing unsteadiness, slurred speech, and inability to walk). It also interferes with ketosis.[30] It burdens our liver's detoxification pathway, critical to overall health.[31] Alcohol blocks our ability to reach REM sleep, thereby fragmenting sleep and disrupting memory formation and overall cognition. (REM, which stands for *rapid eye movement*, is one of several stages of sleep that is repeatedly cycled throughout the night.)[32] Additionally, alcohol is a cause of cancer in the liver, rectum, throat, and the breast for women.[33]

Out of an abundance of caution, we advise against drinking for any high-risk group including anyone currently exhibiting symptoms of cognitive decline, carriers of the ApoE4 gene, and anyone with a past or present history of alcohol abuse. For these groups, *and perhaps others*, any amount of alcohol may increase your risk of developing cognitive decline. Alcohol abuse is detrimental to overall health. Anyone who thinks they may have a problem should seek help. Women who are pregnant or breastfeeding should abstain from all alcohol.

If you choose to indulge occasionally, we suggest only dry red wine in small amounts. Some evidence suggests that red wine confers health benefits not found in other alcoholic beverages.[34] We encourage you to limit your intake to 100 ml. The standard pour for a single serving of red wine is 150 ml, although many restaurants pour substantially more. It's very helpful to use your food scale or a measuring cup with millilitres to get a visual illustration of what constitutes 100 ml.

As many of us know, drinking wine also limits your inhibition and encourages more drinking and unhealthy food bingeing. The sugar content of red wine can also knock you out of ketosis. It's also best to drink wine following a healthful meal. It can be very instructive to do one- and two-hour postprandial blood sugar checks after you've had a glass of wine. A good wine merchant or wine specialist in some supermarkets can advise on sources of organic low-alcohol sugar-free wine, free from mycotoxins and chemical additives and low in sulfites.

There's no better feeling on earth than to wake up refreshed, clearheaded, and excited to take on the day. If you decide to occasionally indulge in alcohol, record the effect it has on your blood sugar, sleep quality, and cognition.

ACTION PLAN

- Alcohol is a neurotoxin, and thus best avoided by anyone suffering from cognitive decline or at risk for cognitive decline.
- If you decide to indulge occasionally, consider small amounts of organic, sugar-free, low-alcohol red wine.

CAUTIONS

(See above.)

CHAPTER 12

Big Little Details

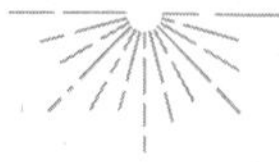

We think in generalities, but we live in detail.
—ALFRED NORTH WHITEHEAD

VEGANS AND VEGETARIANS

Whether you prefer to be a vegetarian, a vegan, or an omnivore, the goal is simply to create the neurochemistry that prevents and reverses cognitive decline. You can do that with or without meat, as long as you are aware of what adjustments to make in each case.

The KetoFLEX 12/3 dietary plan is plant-rich for *everyone*. Animal protein is optional. Vegetarians and vegans can achieve adequate protein from properly prepared nuts, seeds, legumes, and vegetables. Many plant proteins, however, are incomplete because they lack sufficient quantities of some essential amino acids. By consuming a variety and large quantity of plant proteins, however, you can achieve exposure to all nine essential amino acids.

PLANT FOODS HIGH IN PROTEIN

Edamame (CP)* ♦ x (150 g = 22 g protein)	**Chia seeds (CP)* x (28 g = 4.7 g protein)**
Tempeh (CP)* ♦ (100 g = 19 g protein)*	**Walnuts* (28 g = 4.3 g protein)**
Lentils x (75 g = 18 g protein)**	**Wild rice*** x (100 g = 3.5 g protein)**

(Table continues)

Natto (CP)** ♦ (100 g = 18 g protein)	Almond butter* (1 tsp = 3.3 g protein)
Beans** x (average, 60 g = 15 g protein)	Brussels sprouts* x (100 g = 3.3 g protein)
Miso (CP)** ♦ (100 g = 12 g protein)	Asparagus* (125 g = 2.9 g)
Hemp hearts (CP)* (28 g = 10 g protein)	Broccoli* (175 g = 2.6 g protein)
Amaranth*** x (245 g = 9.4 g protein)	Cauliflower* (150 g = 2 g)
Tofu (CP)** ♦ * (100 g = 9.2 protein)	Spring greens* (75 g = 1.5 g protein)
Teff*** x (250 g = 9.1 protein)	Alfalfa sprouts* (18 g = 1.3 g protein)
Green peas* x (150 g = 9 g protein)	Spinach* ♦ (25 g = 1 g protein)
Quinoa (CP)*** x (185 g = 8.1 g protein)	Pak choi* (70 g = 1 g protein)
Almonds* x (28 g = 6 g protein)	Leaf cabbage* (75 g = 0.9 g protein)
Pistachios* (28 g = 6 g protein)	Watercress* (34 g = 0.8 g protein)

KEY
Complete Proteins (CP)
Glycaemic Index: Low* Intermediate High*****
Organic ♦
High in Lectins x

Not all plant proteins are incomplete. Hemp, chia, quinoa, and soy are examples of complete plant proteins. Hemp hearts, the inside of hempseed, are delicious when sprinkled on salads. Unsweetened hemp milk is a great substitute for cow's milk. Chia seeds can be soaked to reduce phytates and easily incorporated into smoothies and puddings. After examining the totality of evidence, we feel that soy within the KetoFLEX 12/3 context can be a healthy option when choosing organic (non-GMO), preferably fermented, and paying attention to the minimal potential for goitrogenic effects. (See page 112 in chapter 8.) Tempeh, miso, and natto are also good options, since their fermentation process destroys some of the anti-nutrients. Organic tofu and edamame are fine but should be limited because of the phytates, which can interfere with nutrient absorption, especially if you are soy intolerant. Quinoa may need to be limited due to the high carbohydrate content. (Let your blood glucose be your guide.) We do not recommend any protein supplements (powders), either animal or plant-based, with the exceptions of spirulina and nutritional yeast.

Cronometer, an online food diary, can help you track the quantity of each amino acid to ensure that you're meeting your goals. (See "Tracking Macronutrient Ratios" on page 190 for details.) Plant proteins are generally less bioavailable than animal proteins, largely due to their anti-nutrients, including lectins, phytates, and oxalates. You'll recall that these plant compounds reduce the absorption of nutrients from the digestive system. Properly preparing plant proteins—using techniques such as soaking, sprouting, fermentation, and cooking—can aid in addressing this issue. Optimizing GI health is also critical to improve nutrient absorption. (See chapter 9 for details.)

Both vegans and vegetarians, using a wholefoods approach, can safely implement this diet by practising some important precautions. Please note that strict veganism can lead to very similar nutritional deficiencies that are observed in Alzheimer's patients: low levels of omega-3 fats, choline, vitamin B_{12}, vitamin D, retinol, and zinc. All of these nutrients are vital for brain health, specifically synaptic formation, maintenance, and support, as well as many other bodily functions. It's also important to ensure adequate vitamin K_2 intake to enable the efficacy of vitamin D and retinol, while protecting your bones and arteries. Your genetics can also contribute to your body's ability to utilize these nutrients, which we'll talk about in the next section. If you are vigilant and carefully choose food sources or use supplements when necessary to overcome these deficits, a diet free from animal products can be very healthful. Omnivores don't get a free pass on this one! *Everyone*, based upon their genetic susceptibilities and unique diet, is vulnerable to a deficiency in any of these nutrients vital for cognitive optimization and overall health.

OMEGA-3 Alpha-linolenic acid (ALA) is a vegan source of omega-3 fat and is found in many healthful foods: chia seeds, Brussels sprouts, hemp seed, walnuts, flaxseed, seaweed, and perilla oil. ALA, however, must be converted to the longer chain, more bioactive EPA (eicosapentaenoic acid) and DHA (docosahexaenoic acid) to provide the benefits necessary for optimal brain health. Unfortunately, the body's ability to convert ALA is limited to 5 per cent for EPA, while less than 0.5 per cent is converted to DHA.[1] This conversion ratio diminishes even further with specific genetics, gender (women of childbearing age convert more effectively), age, and ill health.[2] Increasing food sources of ALA and supplementing with algal oil can be helpful for those who prefer not to eat fish. The goal is to attain an Omega-3 Index (a blood test that accesses the EPA + DHA content of red blood cells) of 8 to 10 per cent for non-ApoE4 carriers and $\geq$10 per cent for ApoE4 carriers, and a ratio of omega-6s to omega-3s of 4:1 or lower, but not below 1:1, to prevent excessive blood thinning.

CHOLINE Choline is an essential nutrient that exerts a powerful neuroprotective effect. It's a major component of membrane phospholipids such as phosphatidylcholine, and a precursor to the neurotransmitter acetylcholine, which is critical for memory. Choline is necessary for the creation and maintenance of neural synapses. Supporting the cholinergic system is vital for preservation of brain health.[3] Many people are deficient in choline, but those who eat an exclusively plant-based diet are especially vulnerable, since high amounts are found in many animal-based foods. Plant sources of choline include broccoli, almonds, walnuts, pinto beans, avocados, Brussels sprouts, Swiss chard, and spring greens, but it's difficult to meet your nutritional needs using only plant sources. Lacto-ovo vegetarians, who avoid all fish, poultry, and meat but do consume eggs and dairy, can also use eggs to help reach their daily goal. Citicoline is a plant-based supplement. Alpha-GPC is another alternative that can be vegan-friendly. The goal for dietary intake is 550 mg/day for men and 425 mg/day for women.

VITAMIN B12 B_{12} is a vital nutrient for brain and overall health. The bottom of the current US reference range (200–900 pg/mL) is set too low, since anaemia and dementia symptoms may be seen below 350 pg/mL, a supposedly "normal" level. B_{12}, in combination with folate and B_6, is necessary for homocysteine optimization. Elevated homocysteine is associated with impaired cognition and increased brain atrophy.[4] The recommended homocysteine goal is 7 µmol/L or lower, which is difficult to achieve with suboptimal B_{12} or folate. (For tips on lowering homocysteine, see "Using Genes to Guide Your Dietary Choices" later in this chapter.)

There are a few select plants that provide B_{12}: specific mushrooms (chanterelle, black trumpet, and shiitake) and an edible alga called green or purple nori. Some fortified options include nutritional yeast (often used by vegans as a substitute for Parmesan cheese) and some versions of unsweetened almond and coconut milk. B_{12} supplements are readily available. Sublingual methylcobalamin is a good source. Vegan True Methylcobalamin contains no animal-derived ingredients. The goal is to attain a level of 500–1500 pg/mL.

VITAMIN D Vitamin D is also known as the sunshine vitamin, but in our modern predominantly sheltered lifestyle, few people get enough sun exposure to achieve optimal levels. Vitamin D binds to the vitamin D receptor, enters the nucleus, and turns on over 900 genes. One of the most important roles of vitamin D is the creation and maintenance of brain synapses. Reduced levels are associated with cognitive decline.[5] The majority of foods high in vitamin D are found in animal sources, but mushrooms and fortified unsweetened almond and coconut milks are decent plant sources. Lacto-ovo vegetarians can get vitamin D through egg yolks, A2 milk, and cheese. Vitamin D_2 is always plant-based. Vitamin D_3 from lichen is also vegan friendly. The goal is to attain a level between 50 and 80 ng/mL (this is routinely measured in the 25-hydroxy vitamin D test). Note that anyone taking more than 1000 IU of vitamin D each day should include vitamin K_2 (at least 100 mcg). See more on vitamin K_2 on the next page.

RETINOL/VITAMIN A Vitamin A is composed of two retinoids: retinol and carotenoids, including beta-carotene. Beta-carotene is abundantly available in many plants including sweet potatoes, carrots, and dark leafy greens. Retinol is found primarily in animal products such as cod liver oil, liver, kidney, eggs, and dairy. Vegans who carry specific polymorphisms that poorly convert beta-carotene to retinol may be deficient in this essential nutrient. Vitamin A is widely associated with eye health and immune function. Even marginally low levels are associated with the development of Alzheimer's disease. A recent study found low levels of retinol associated with increased risk of developing cognitive decline for both ApoE4 and ApoE2 carriers.[6] Eating plenty of foods rich in beta-carotene along with a dietary source of fat (since vitamin A is fat-soluble, it is poorly absorbed in the absence of fat) is often enough. Vegans, especially those genetically at risk, may want to ensure they have adequate levels. The reference range for serum retinol is 38–98 mcg/dL. You want to target the middle of the range, preferably with diet. If supplementation is necessary, use retinyl palmitate.

VITAMIN K_2 The fat-soluble vitamins, particularly vitamin D and vitamin A, rely on adequate levels of vitamin K in order to operate efficiently. Vitamin K is vital for proper blood clotting and bone, heart, and cognitive health.[7] It aids in directing calcium to the bones and away from the arteries where it can do damage. There are two types of vitamin K: K_1 and K_2. Vitamin K_1 is abundant in many leafy greens and vegetables, including kale, spinach, turnip greens, spring greens, Swiss chard, parsley, romaine, green leaf lettuce, Brussels sprouts, broccoli, cauliflower, and cabbage, but it is poorly absorbed by the body. K_2, on the other hand, is mainly found in animals, with the primary exception being natto, which many find difficult to eat because of the strong taste. Vegans can get some K_2 from fermented foods such as sauerkraut, plant-based kefir, unpasteurized kombucha, or vegan kimchi, but amounts are inconsistent. There are vegan K_2 supplements made from natto that can ensure adequate intake.

ZINC Too little zinc and too much copper are associated with dementia. These minerals have an interrelated antagonistic relationship, competing with each other for absorption. Without adequate zinc, copper builds up in the tissues of the body. This accumulation can have detrimental health effects. This is a common problem for strict vegans, since their diets tend to be naturally low in zinc and high in copper. Zinc deficiency is also very common (especially in those taking proton-pump inhibitors), affecting approximately a billion people globally. Zinc plays a vital role in the brain, as well as decreasing inflammation and boosting immune function. While zinc is abundant and highly bioavailable in meat, eggs, and seafood, it's also found in many legumes, including green and black soybeans (tofu and tempeh) chickpeas, lentils, and many nuts and seeds—

walnuts, cashews, almonds, and pecans, and seeds from pumpkin, sunflower, and hemp. Unfortunately these plant sources are also high in anti-nutrients. For this reason, it's very important to prepare them properly. Be aware that many legumes, nuts, and seeds are also high in copper, which must concurrently be reduced to create a healthful balance. For that reason, it might be wise to consider a small amount of supplementation. Fortified nutritional yeast is a good option. Two tablespoons provide 20 per cent of your daily needs. Your goal is to attain a zinc level of 100 mcg/dL with an equal value of copper for a 1:1 ratio. If needed, vegan zinc supplements are widely available, but carefully track and tweak, since a little goes a long way. For those with zinc deficiency, taking 20 to 50 mg of zinc picolinate is helpful; more than 50 mg of zinc per day should not be taken except under a doctor's supervision.

USING GENES TO GUIDE YOUR DIETARY CHOICES

Genetic information can help us to make more informed and effective choices. If you've participated in direct-to-consumer genetic testing through a company like 23andMe, you already have access to parts of your genome. By using the "Browse Raw Data" tool, you can easily access the genes we discuss below; this may aid you in optimizing your nutrition for brain health. Additionally, there are many online services, ranging from very pricey to quite affordable, that offer to interpret genetic information and provide you with a personalized report to optimize health. FoundMyFitness offers a comprehensive genetic report that's regularly updated and available in exchange for a donation of as little as £7.50 ($10).

Before we dive in, if you haven't previously done genetic testing there are some important financial, legal, and even emotional aspects to consider before purchasing the test. Knowledge of ApoE4 status, for instance, can be initially distressing and overwhelming. The ApoE4.Info non-profit has put together a decision guide that may be helpful if you're unsure about checking your status. Many who do learn their ApoE4 status are grateful for the knowledge and have used it to improve their health.[8] Indeed, genetic information can be used to help us make more healthful choices. Knowledge is power!

Each of the trillion cells that comprise the human body has a nucleus that houses its DNA (deoxyribonucleic acid), the genetic blueprint responsible for traits that are passed down from generation to generation. Our DNA is made up of four different types of nucleotides, each with a unique base: cytosine (C), adenine (A), guanine (G), and thymine (T). The specific sequence of these nucleotides codes for your protein sequences, as well as regulatory information. Every person has two copies of each gene: one inherited from each biological parent (except that males, since they have only one X chromosome and one Y chromosome, have only a single copy of most of the genes on the X chromosome). New cells are made when the original cell divides into two. Each resulting cell harbours our entire genetic code in its nucleus. Although our genomes are nearly identical—the genome sequence of each of us is about 99.9 per cent identical to that of every other person—each of us has more than 3,000 differences from any other individual, and this is what makes each of us genetically unique. These more than 3,000 differences are mostly changes of a single "letter" (A, C, G, or T) at a single site, and these are thus called single nucleotide polymorphisms (SNPs), pronounced "snips."

These SNPs generate biological variations between people by causing differences in the recipes for proteins written in genes. Those differences can in turn influence a variety of traits, including how we metabolize our food, our propensity for specific nutrient deficiencies, and our susceptibility to specific diseases. By using the "Browse Raw Data" tool at 23andMe, you can plug these SNPs into the search engine to check your genetic status. This knowledge can serve as a starting point for fine-tuning your dietary choices to complement your genome.

We have listed below some of the important genes that affect our nutrition. Note that these various SNPs throughout your genome are labelled and numbered, using rs followed by the reference number (rs stands for Reference SNP Cluster ID).

Omega-3

- rs1535 (G;G) Poor conversion of ALA to EPA.

Young healthy females convert only 5 per cent of their total ALA intake into EPA. With this polymorphism, the conversion rate is even lower—29 per cent lower relative to the highest converter (A;A). (A;G) is an intermediate converter, with an 18.6 per cent poorer conversion rate.[9] This may be particularly relevant to strict vegans who rely on ALA conversion to meet their EPA and DHA needs.

Omega-3/ApoE4

- rs429358 (C;T) and rs7412 (C;C) One copy of ApoE4.
- rs429358 (C;C) and rs7412 (C;C) Two copies of ApoE4.

ApoE4 carriers were previously thought *not* to derive cognitive benefit from a diet rich in omega-3s, whereas other ApoE genotypes enjoyed a decreased risk of cognitive decline.[10] A recent paper hypothesized that ApoE4 carriers fail to show similar cognitive benefit from omega-3 fats because they may need a different form, phospholipid DHA, found in fish, fish eggs (like salmon roe), and krill oil.[11] Additionally, ApoE4 carriers demonstrate lower levels of omega-3 fatty acids in their blood following both consumption of fish and supplementation.[12] Evidence is mounting that this group may actually need higher amounts of omega-3 fatty acids due to their perturbed metabolism of fatty acids. Indeed, this genotype preferentially metabolizes DHA, while other APOE genotypes conserve it.[13] In a data set comprised of all ApoE4 carriers, those with the highest omega-3 status performed better on cognitive testing and demonstrated larger brain volumes than ApoE4 carriers with lower levels.[14]

Please note that for those with a bleeding tendency, omega-3 fatty acids should be minimized. This is of particular importance for those with cerebral amyloid angiopathy (CAA), which should be suspected especially in men who are ApoE4 homozygotes and have a family history of haemorrhagic stroke. If this condition is suspected, then an MRI with a microhaemorrhage sequence (MP-RAGE) is important to determine whether any indication of early, unrecognized bleeding has occurred.

Choline

- rs174548 (G;G) (C;G)

These polymorphisms are associated with a reduced phosphatidylcholine level. G is the risk allele, with homozygotes showing the lowest levels. Heterozygotes have intermediate levels. Phosphatidylcholine is a class of phospholipids that includes choline, a precursor to the neurotransmitter acetylcholine, which is vital for memory formation and is reduced in the brains of patients with Alzheimer's.

- rs7946 (T;T) (C;T)

These polymorphisms are correlated with lower phosphatidylcholine production in the liver. T is the risk allele, with homozygotes producing the lowest levels. Lower phosphatidylcholine can also lead to a reduced clearance of fat from the liver.[15] Inadequate choline status can also put you at risk for elevated homocysteine.[16] Those at risk of lower levels may want to increase dietary intake and/or supplement.

B12

- rs602662 (A;G) (G;G)
- rs601338 (A;G) (G;G)

These polymorphisms result in B_{12} levels that are lower than normal due to malabsorption. G is the risk allele, with homozygotes being more severely impacted. B_{12} deficiency is a reversible cause of dementia.[17] Sublingual B_{12} is especially effective in overcoming malabsorption. This may be especially relevant to vegans and anyone struggling to reach adequate levels.[18] The (A;A) variant of both polymorphisms is associated with better absorption and higher levels.

MTHFR (methylenetetrahydrofolate reductase)

- rs1801133 (T;T) (C;T) Reduced MTHFR enzyme activity; (T;T) has a 65 per cent decrease and (C;T) has a 35 per cent decrease.
- rs1801131 (C;C) (A;C) Reduced MTHFR efficiency; (C;C) has a 40 per cent decrease and (A;C) has a 17 per cent decrease.

These common alleles, separately and when combined, affect 70 per cent of the population and lead to reduced folate metabolism and overall methylation, which have widespread effects on health. Individuals with these polymorphisms are at risk for higher homocysteine levels, which are strongly correlated with diminished cognition and brain atrophy.[19] Your goal is to achieve a level ≤ 7.0 µmol/L. Those who carry the rs1801133 polymorphisms above may also need to pay particular attention to riboflavin status.[20] Those with reduced methylation, in general, should take methylated forms of vitamin B_{12} and folate along with the active form of B_6, P5P (pyridoxal 5-phosphate). Also, be aware that the B vitamins are not effective in reducing homocysteine without an adequate omega-3 and choline status.[21] Additionally, a revealing new paper suggests that inadequate vitamin B status, leading to elevated homocysteine, actually *prevents* those who are using omega-3 fatty acids from deriving cognitive benefit, which may help explain previous inconsistent reports in the medical literature. It's stunning to see how interconnected each of these nutrients is, and it underscores the importance of knowing and addressing your unique vulnerabilities.

Vitamin D

- rs10741657 (G;G)
- rs12794714 (A;A)
- rs2060793 (A;A)

Above are several variations in the CYP2R1 gene (vitamin D 25-hydroxylase) that can lead to decreased circulating vitamin D levels. Those with vitamin D deficiencies are nearly twice as likely to experience dementia.[22] If you have any of these polymorphisms, supplementing with vitamin D may not be as effective. You should carefully track your serum levels, adjusting your dosage of vitamin D to ensure that you're maintaining an optimal level.

Retinol/Vitamin A

- rs7501331 (C;T) (T;T)
- rs12934922 (A;T) (T;T)

Both of these polymorphisms separately and combined lead to a reduced ability to convert plant beta-carotene into retinol or vitamin A. Animal forms of retinol (cod liver oil or liver) are the most bioavailable and may be helpful in overcoming these polymorphisms. Even a marginal vitamin A deficiency may be associated with impaired cognition and reduced neuroplasticity and neurogenesis.[23] Additionally, there is a synergy between vitamins A, D, K, and others to be optimally effective and to reduce cardiovascular risk.[24]

TRACKING MACRONUTRIENT RATIOS

When you are first learning how to achieve ketosis, it can be very helpful to track macronutrient ratios. Within a few weeks, you'll soon learn which food patterns get you into ketosis, and more important, you'll become familiar with the transformative feeling of ketosis. Before we dive in, we want to emphasize that macronutrient ratios have a lot of wiggle room for personalization. It's important that you check your ketone levels to know whether or not you're succeeding in achieving ketosis. (See instructions in chapter 18, "Tools for Success.") A fasting BHB of >0.5 mM is your morning goal, with your level rising to about 1.5 (and as high as 4.0) during the day. Some people get their highest reading of the day right before breaking their fast. Others get their highest level later after a full day of combining the KetoFLEX 12/3 strategies: fasting plus exercise plus a low-carb diet. Experiment to see when you capture your highest reading. (Be aware that it will typically be lowest in the morning because of the "dawn effect," whereby your liver sends out glucose to help prepare you to meet the demands of the day ahead.) Once you've tracked for several weeks or even months, you'll know what kinds of foods you should be eating to achieve your goal, and you'll instinctively recognize what ketosis *feels* like, so you'll no longer feel the need to track. Many people report a calm, steady feeling of energy, without the blood sugar highs and lows, accompanied by a distinct feeling of cognitive clarity.

Macronutrients are simply foods that your body needs in large quantities to optimally function. You'll recall that they are broken down into three categories: protein, fat, and carbohydrates. Most foods are a combination of several different macronutrients. Each gram of protein or carbohydrate supplies 4 calories, while each gram of fat supplies 9 calories. (This will become important later as we crunch the numbers.)

1. **TDEE** To get started on figuring out the macronutrient ratios that are best for you, you need to determine your total daily energy expenditure (TDEE). TDEE is your basal metabolic rate (BMR) or the rate that you use calories at rest, plus your activity level or caloric use.

TDEE = BMR + Activity Level

To determine your BMR, use this calculator (https://www.calculator.net/bmr-calculator.html): Simply plug in your age, gender, height, and weight and you'll get a variety of results based on your activity level. This is your caloric requirement to maintain your current weight. (In "How to Track" on page 196 we'll talk about how to lose or gain weight.) Let's start by doing an example together. We'll use a 65-year-old, 5-foot-6-inch woman weighing 130 pounds (59 kg) who engages in exercise four to five times per week. When we plug her numbers into the calculator above, we get:

TDEE (1760) = BMR (1201) + Activity Level (559)

Next, let's work on finding ideal macronutrients ratios. We'll start with protein.

2. **Protein** We recommend 0.8 to 1 gram (g) of clean protein for each kilogram (kg) of lean body mass (LBM) per day. Those who are more active should use the top end of that range, whereas those who are less active should stick with the lower amount.

   You can learn your LBM by using a simple online lean body mass calculator. When we plug in our example's gender, height, and weight, we learn she has an LBM of 101. Divide that by 2.2 to get her LBM in kilograms. Next let's take that weight in kilograms and multiply it by 1 gram of protein (due to her high activity level) to calculate her protein requirement for one day.

101 lbs LBM ÷ 2.2 kg/lb = 45.9 (46 kg) LBM
46 kg LBM x 1 g protein/kg LBM = 46 g protein/day

Now that we've determined her ideal number of protein grams, we simply multiply that number by 4 to identify how many protein calories per day she requires (since each gram of protein = 4 calories). To learn what per cent of her calories should be from protein, let's divide that number into her TDEE.

46 g protein/day x 4 calories/g protein = 184 calories of protein
1760 calories TDEE ÷ 184 calories protein/day = 9.57 per cent (10 per cent)

This woman needs 10 per cent of her total calories to come from protein. To help you envision what that would look like, see our list below.

- 2 small free-range eggs (10 g protein)
- 140 g wild-caught salmon (36 g protein)

3. **Fat** Let's move on to fat. When you are initially trying to achieve the ketosis goals to address insulin resistance and/or cognitive decline, we recommend *starting* with 75 per cent of your calories coming from fat. This will vary a bit for everyone. Those who are able to employ a long daily fast and exercise may be able to use considerably less dietary fat, since fasting and exercise also produce ketones. Those who are still working towards achieving those goals may initially need more fat and less carbohydrate. While protein needs will remain fairly steady (but generally decrease over time as healing occurs), fat and carbohydrates can be adjusted on a sliding scale to help you reach ketosis. Only by regularly testing your BHB will you know what amount is right for you.

   That may seem like a lot of fat, but it's really not when you consider that fat is much more calorically dense than protein or carbohydrates. You'll recall that whereas proteins and carbohydrates both contribute 4 calories per gram, fat is more than twice that, at 9 calories per gram. An easy way to include extra fat is to generously finish salads and vegetables with delicious, healthful, high polyphenol extra virgin olive oil (EVOO). It's delicious when paired with an acid, such as your favourite balsamic vinegar or a squeeze of lemon or lime juice. You may want to season your olive oil with your favourite fresh herbs and spices in a small ramekin on your plate so you can dip each bite of vegetables to enhance the taste and bioavailability of nutrients. Avocados, nuts, and seeds can easily be tossed into salads or enjoyed as snacks.

   To determine how many calories from fat our example needs, we just multiply TDEE by 75 per cent. To learn how many grams of fat, we just divide the total fat calories by 9, since each gram of fat provides 9 calories.

1760 calories (TDEE) x 0.75 = 1320 fat/day
1320 calories fat/day ÷ 9 calories/g fat = 146.7g (147g)/day

Our example could easily achieve her 75 per cent goal with the following foods:

- 4 tablespoons high polyphenol EVOO (53.3 g fat)
- 1 small avocado (21 g fat)
- 2 tablespoons sunflower seeds (8 g fat)
- 30 g macadamia nuts (25 g fat)
- 30 g walnuts (19.1 g fat)
- 2 free-range eggs (9.3 g fat)*
- 140 g wild-caught salmon (11.5 g fat)*

*Added earlier. You'll recall that most foods are a combination of several macronutrients, so some fall into more than one category.

Remember, the fat you will need to achieve metabolic flexibility, insulin sensitivity, and cognitive clarity will change over time. Many participants find that they need less fat the longer they practise the protocol because the KetoFLEX 12/3 lifestyle (diet plus fasting plus exercise) naturally leads to ketosis with less dietary fat. Also, once insulin resistance is healed and metabolic flexibility restored, you can experiment with adding more healthful resistant starches while recording the effect on your cognition. Some people find that once they are healthier, they no longer need higher levels of ketosis. Remember, this is a personalized programme. Allow your biomarkers (fasting glucose, insulin, and A1c, as well as cognitive performance) to guide your dietary choices.

4. **Carbohydrates** We'll finish off with carbohydrates. To determine our example's carb ratio, we simply add her protein percentage (10 per cent) plus her fat percentage (75 percent). Then subtract that from 100.

100 per cent - (10 per cent protein + 75 per cent fat) = 15 per cent carbs

The woman in our example can enjoy 15 per cent of her caloric needs from carbs. To determine how many calories from carbs the woman in our example should eat, we multiply TDEE by 15 per cent. To determine how many grams of carbs, we just divide the total by 4, since each gram of carbs is 4 calories.

1760 calories (TDEE) x 0.15 = 264 calories/day
264 calories/day ÷ 4 calories/g carb = 66 g carbs/day

While we've previously referenced "net carbs" (total carbs − total fibre = net carbs) to highlight the importance of fibre, for the sole purpose of our calculations, you need to use total carbs. At first glance, 15 per cent total carbs (or 66 grams) may not seem like a lot, but when you consider that our goal is to prioritize organic, seasonal, local, nutrient-dense, non-starchy vegetables from every colour of the rainbow, you may be surprised at how many you can enjoy! Below is an example of what 66 grams of carbs could look like. (For those used to calculating net carbs, our list below adds up to 39.3 g.)

- 20 g rocket (0.7 g)
- 225 g spinach (1.1 g)
- 75 g red romaine (1.5 g)
- 30 g cooked kale (1.4 g)
- 40 g mushrooms (1.6 g)
- 175 g cooked broccoli (11.2 g)
- 325 g cooked cauliflower (5.1 g)
- 10 medium spears cooked asparagus (6.2 g)
- 65 g Mexican yam (1.6 g)
- 20 g fresh basil (0.3 g)
- 40 g fermented veggies (4 g)

- ¼ medium sweet potato, cooked and cooled as resistant starch (5.9 g)
- 2 free-range eggs (1 g)*
- 1 small avocado (11.8)*
- 30 g walnuts (4 g)*
- 30 g macadamia nuts (4.6 g)*
- 2.5 tablespoons sunflower seeds (3.9 g)*

*Added earlier. You'll recall that most foods are a combination of several macronutrients, so some fall into more than one category.

HOW TO TRACK

Now that you get the maths and can figure out your personalized macronutrient ratios, let's talk about how to track them. Cronometer is a free online resource that can be helpful. It serves as a food diary, allowing you to enter the food you eat in real time while it calculates your macronutrient ratios for you and displays them in a pie chart. To use Cronometer for tracking macronutrient ratios, see instructions below.

1. On your Target page (under Settings) in the "Macronutrients" section, for "Tracking carbohydrates as," be sure to specify "total" carbs as opposed to "net" carbs.
2. Also in the "Macronutrients" section, choose "Macro Ratios" instead of "Fixed Values" or "Ketogenic Calculator." (We don't recommend their calculator, as KetoFLEX 12/3 users typically end up being able to eat more carbohydrates because we combine diet with fasting and exercise.)
3. In the "Macronutrients" section, input your custom "Protein," "Carbohydrate," and "Fat."
4. To see your macronutrient ratios displayed in a pie chart, go to Display (under Settings) and turn on your toggle switch for Show Calories Summary in Diary. Your macronutrient ratios

will show up in a circular graph labelled "Consumed," right beneath the food diary.

Cronometer has many useful features and some limitations. See below for more.

- **Weight** Cronometer is helpful if you have weight to gain or lose. You start by entering your current height and weight on the Profile page (under Settings), then enter your goal weight on the Target page. You can determine the pace at which you want to lose or gain weight. We recommend no more than 0.5 to 1 kg a week for healthful, steady results. Cronometer will automatically calculate your TDEE to help you reach your goal.
- **Saturated Fat** Those who hyper-absorb dietary fat (typically ApoE4 carriers) may want to track SFA. Using the Food Diary option, look below the graphs to "Lipids." There you'll see a breakdown of all of your dietary fats and will be able to track the amount of saturated fat in your diet.
- **Ratio of Omega-3s to Omega-6s** In the Food Diary option, under "Lipids," you can track this ratio and purposefully tweak it towards the anti-inflammatory pattern of our ancestors by eating more foods rich in ALA, EPA, and DHA while concurrently reducing omega-6s, especially from non-wholefoods sources.
- **Complete and Incomplete Protein** Be aware that the Cronometer protein total doesn't distinguish between complete and incomplete protein, which may lead you to think you're exceeding your protein goal with incomplete proteins (like leafy greens) when you're not. For the purpose of tracking, you needn't include incomplete plant proteins in your protein total. The last thing we want to do is limit your plant intake! You can use the "Add Note" option of the Food Diary to separately calculate and track your complete protein.

- **Essential Amino Acids** Vegans and vegetarians can use Cronometer to track intake of all nine essential amino acids (histidine, isoleucine, leucine, lysine, methionine, phenylalanine, threonine, tryptophan, and valine) to ensure that you're achieving your goals. Under "Nutrient Targets," scroll down to "Protein."
- **Micronutrients** Cronometer also tracks micronutrient intake but should be used only as a rough guide. For instance, it doesn't distinguish between beta-carotene and retinol or ALA, EPA, and DHA. Don't assume that you've met various nutrient goals without taking this into account. Similarly, if Cronometer indicates that you've met a specific nutrient goal, don't assume that translates to your blood level. As the "Using Genes to Guide Your Dietary Choices" section indicates, our ability to synthesize various nutrients from food relies on our genetics and our overall state of health.

If you decide to track macronutrient ratios, invest in a good quality food scale. You'll save a lot of time if you use a scale rather than trying to measure food the old-fashioned way. (See more in chapter 18, "Tools for Success.")

We've put together a few examples of the types of delicious meals you can enjoy. Please remember that these are just suggestions. Everything can be tailored to your preferences, allergies, and sensitivities. The sky is the limit. Be creative. This first meal is an example of a KetoFLEX 12/3 "breakfast" despite the fact that it would typically be eaten early in the afternoon after a twelve-to-sixteen-hour fast.

This meal features two free-range eggs, steamed broccoli with red pepper, and stir-fried spinach with sweet onion. For gut health, some cooked and cooled sweet potato wedges (as a resistant starch) and fermented sauerkraut (as a probiotic) are included with 240 ml of bone broth. Include a ramekin of high polyphenol EVOO, so each bite of vegetable can be dipped into the oil.

A second example is of another typical meal eaten later in the day, featuring wild-caught Alaskan salmon, steamed asparagus, red cabbage, spinach, celery, cherry tomatoes, Kalamata olives, slivered almonds, avocado slices, and high polyphenol extra virgin olive oil with lemon.

These are just two of many examples of delicious meals that support insulin sensitivity and mild ketosis and provide nutrients that support cognition.

CHAPTER 13

Exercise: Whatever Moves You

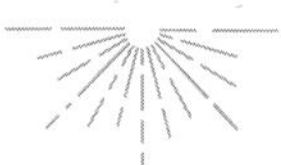

We do not stop exercising because we grow old—

we grow old because we stop exercising.

—KENNETH COOPER

The one thing that can solve most of our problems is dancing.

—JAMES BROWN

THE THIRD COMPONENT OF the KetoFLEX 12/3 lifestyle is exercise. It's simple: your body was designed to move—a lot. When our ancestors began transitioning from a more sedentary existence towards a hunter-gatherer lifestyle, the increase in aerobic activity may very well have contributed to the evolution of greater longevity. As hominids appeared, we came down from the trees onto the savannah and began travelling long distances in our search for food and running to chase our prey. Our longevity increased in direct proportion to our activity level.[1] The same strategy that enabled our ApoE4 predecessors to thrive provides important clues for optimizing our lives today. Evolution suggests that we were born to run. In fact, of all of the strategies we recommend, none has more scientific evidence than exercise.[2] *Being active is the single most important strategy you can employ to prevent and remediate cognitive decline.* But just as for each of the components of the protocol, it alone is rarely sufficient—it exerts its best effects when used in concert with the other features of the protocol. Indeed, a recent paper examined 41 previous studies and found that including cognitive challenges with physical exercise enhanced cognitive gains.[3]

Exercise protects us at a cellular level. It upregulates Nrf2, which protects our cells by conferring epigenetic protection for greater resilience to environmental stressors and by increasing the cells' capacity to prevent and resist disease.[4] Exercise is also an important strategy to heal the damaged mitochondria that accompany insulin resistance. While fasting combined with our dietary recommendations can aid in recovery, combining those strategies *with* exercise is vital.[5] Mitochondria are often described as the batteries found in each cell of our body. Exercise upregulates mitochondria and essentially "turns on" metabolic flexibility—the ability to metabolize either fat or glucose as fuel depending upon its availability.[6] A steady energy supply is vital for cognition when you consider that the brain, which comprises only 2 per cent of the body's total weight, greedily requires 20 per cent of the body's overall energy supply.[7]

Exercise is beneficial in many other ways. It can help you maintain a healthy BMI and reduce insulin resistance, blood pressure, and the risk for heart disease and stroke.[8] It also reduces stress and anxiety while improving mood and sleep.[9] The great news is that *any* form of exercise helps by increasing brain volume—everything from walking to gardening to dancing.[10] When starting any exercise programme, be sure to check with your doctor to make sure that you're healthy enough to engage in your preferred activity. It's always tempting to overdo, but you ultimately hurt yourself if you sustain an injury and have to refrain from exercise while you heal.

Everyone wants to know the best form of exercise for brain health. Aerobic exercise has been studied in greater depth than strength training and might take a slight lead, but both have been found to be vitally important as we age. The term *aerobic exercise* is used for any sustained physical activity—examples are walking, jogging, cycling, or rowing—that improves the efficiency of the body's cardiovascular system. A 2018 meta-analysis examining twenty-three previous interventions found that exercise can delay the decline in cognitive function of those diagnosed with or at risk for Alzheimer's, with aerobic exercise having the most favourable effect.[11]

A recent study examined the effectiveness of two different exercise interventions using a group of seventy seniors diagnosed with mild cognitive impairment (MCI). Everyone exercised four days a week for 45 minutes to an hour. One group engaged in a stretching regimen and the other engaged in aerobic activity, primarily using a treadmill. After only six months, the results were startling. Brain imaging showed that those who participated in vigorous aerobic exercise actually had reduced levels of tau, a protein associated with the tangles and neurite retraction of Alzheimer's. Additionally, the aerobic exercisers had better blood flow in the memory and processing centres of their brains as well as measurable improvement in the attention, planning, and organizing abilities referred to as executive function.[12] Older adults with higher cardiorespiratory fitness also have better preservation of overall brain volume, increased cortical thickness, and greater white matter integrity.[13]

Aerobic exercise is thought to be helpful in several ways. Most important, it provides a more constant and sustained level of cerebral blood flow.[14] Increasing blood flow to the brain is vitally important, as a deficit in this is one of the first measurable manifestations of the Alzheimer's disease process.[15] Aerobic exercise also upregulates brain-derived neurotrophic factor (BDNF), an important protein that stimulates the production of new brain cells (neural precursors) and supports existing synaptic connections. Decreased BDNF levels constitute a lack of trophic support and contribute to cognitive impairment.[16]

A newfound mechanism by which exercise benefits the brain was recently discovered with the revelation of a novel role for glial cells in the brain. These cells form a waste disposal system for the brain labelled the *glymphatic system*; it behaves in a fashion similar to the lymphatic system in the body. Beta-amyloid and other extracellular proteins are cleared from the brain through this newly discovered pathway.[17] Exercise powerfully stimulates glymphatic flow, with a more than twofold increase found in mice that had exercised for five weeks.[18] (Sleep is another powerful and independent driver of the glymphatic system that we'll discuss in chapter 14.)

Strength training as it relates to cognitive health hasn't been as well studied, but being strong is an important part of general health. A recent meta-analysis examined twenty-four studies and found that strength training yielded strong positive improvements in scores used for Alzheimer's screening, with the greatest improvement in the area of executive functioning.[19] Strength training prevents sarcopenia, the natural loss of lean muscle mass that occurs with ageing.[20] Sarcopenia is correlated with cognitive decline.[21] Strength training also prevents the loss of bone, which reduces the risk of cognitive decline, slows ageing, and prevents brain atrophy.[22] Adults who strength-train demonstrate cognitive improvement, fewer white matter lesions in the brain, and an enhanced gait, and can more easily perform daily tasks of living.[23]

RETHINK EXERCISE. Rather than viewing your workout as an obligation, make it the highlight of your day. Whether it's a long meditative hike in nature or a social group bike ride, schedule everything else around this sacred time. This is your dedicated time to move your strong body. If you keep the experience joyful and fun, it will soon become a self-perpetuating habit. Intellectually understanding that exercise is a powerful neuroprotective strategy is important, but translating that knowledge into daily practice is what matters.

GET OUTSIDE. Research shows that spending time in nature is good for your health and, not surprisingly, your brain.[24] Spending time outdoors has been proven to reduce stress, boost creativity and problem-solving skills, sharpen mental focus, and minimize rumination.[25] Another important benefit from exercising outdoors, especially in the morning, is the improved sleep that results from exposing your eyes to sunlight, which helps to support a healthy circadian rhythm.[26]

TAKE A WALK. One of the simplest forms of aerobic exercise, which incorporates strength training because it's naturally weight bearing, is walking. Try to incorporate a daily walk into your routine. Walk with purpose, as if you were late for an appointment. Depending on your current fitness level, you may need to start slowly. That's okay.

Just try to increase the length of your walk by a few minutes per day until you reach thirty minutes or more.

We can't overstate the importance of having the correct footwear when engaging in a walking programme for fitness. Many people train in the wrong shoes and end up with debilitating hip, knee, and ankle injuries. If you plan to mix your speed up, *which we highly recommend*, go with a running shoe as opposed to a walking shoe. Running shoes tend to have superior cushioning and are typically lighter in weight than walking shoes. Running in shoes specifically designed for walking can lead to an injury. Find an athletic store that has a trained specialist who can study your gait as you walk (or run) to help you identify the best shoe for your needs. Many people either over- or underpronate, meaning your foot rolls slightly inwards or outwards as you walk. Once you've found your perfect shoe, you'll be amazed at the difference in your performance. Depending upon your mileage, be alert to even a slight persistent pain in your ankle, knee, or hip after six months to a year. This is typically caused by excessive wear and may be a sign that it's time for a new pair of shoes. Below are strategies for getting the most out of your walk.

- **Walk with a friend.** Connecting with others is vital for brain health.[27] Socialize as you exercise.
- **Play with speed.** As you feel stronger on your daily walk, consider increasing your speed and even adding periods of running or sprinting.
- **Add music.** When you are walking alone, listen to your favourite music and even sing along. You could also listen to meditative music to unwind as you walk.
- **Train your brain.** Incorporate cognitive training into your daily walk. While walking, practise saying the alphabet backward. Try to count backwards from one hundred by sixes, sevens, eights, and nines.
- **Learn while you "burn."** Use exercise as a time to learn while you're burning your own body fat, harnessing the power of the mind-body connection. Learn a new language

or listen to educational podcasts or auditory books while exercising. There is something very powerful about "getting in your head" while working out your body. When you are exercising alone, it makes the time go much more quickly and gives you a double sense of accomplishment.

- **Use a weighted vest.** This is especially helpful for those working to increase bone density. Research has shown that this is a safe and effective way of increasing the demand on your body and improving bone density.[28] The vest should be no more than 4 to 10 per cent of your body weight. Start with a low weight and slowly move up. It's great to get a vest that has the option to add weight as you become stronger.
- **Add walking lunges.** Incorporating a few sets of walking lunges adds variety to your walk, while increasing your leg strength.
- **Make nature your gym.** You needn't stop with lunges. Look for opportunities to add other calisthenics on your walk. When you pass a bench or a log, for instance, stop for a set of triceps dips or push-ups. Be creative and have fun.
- **Consider getting a dog.** There are many healthful aspects to pet ownership, but the responsibility of having to walk a dog several times throughout the day may provide the motivation you need for a number of daily walks.[29] Dogs also provide excellent companionship and make us more social.
- **Track your progress.** Use a pedometer to monitor your motion. To reduce your accumulated exposure to radiation, we recommend a basic, inexpensive model rather than newer devices or apps that use Wi-Fi. OneTweak is an example of an acceptable pedometer. Start with a realistic goal based upon your current level of fitness, working towards 10,000 steps a day. Use your journal to track how exercise is affecting your cognition, mood, sleep, and appearance.

MIX IT UP. You needn't stick with walking every day. Keep it fun. Keep it fresh. Cross-training is important. Wake up new muscles by switching activities. Consider joining a local gym, YMCA, or senior or community centre for group strength classes or working with a trainer to specifically develop a programme to meet your goals. It's often more enjoyable to train while benefiting from a supportive relationship or spirited group atmosphere.

Swim a few days a week. Take a boxing class or sharpen your reflexes with Ping-Pong. Try pickleball or Zumba. Joyfully experiment to keep your body strong. Consider cycling. There are now bicycles for every terrain and level of fitness: mountain bikes, road bikes, beach cruisers, and even recumbent bikes. More and more cities are creating dedicated cycling paths that take you out of pollution and traffic and provide an opportunity to spend time in nature. If you live in a northern climate, don't let the cold weather stop you. Snowshoeing is an excellent workout. Cross-country skiing is even better. Both provide an opportunity to enjoy the quiet beauty of freshly fallen snow. If you live near a body of water, you might try kayaking for a terrific upper-body workout. If you already have a sport you like, such as golf, look for ways to make it even more challenging. Ditch the cart, carry your clubs, and walk the course. If you're already playing tennis, take lessons to up your game. Join a competitive league. It's a great opportunity to socialize while increasing your level of exercise.

Don't forget dancing! A recent six-month study compared various forms of exercise to learning complex choreographed dancing with multiple partners, and only the dance intervention demonstrated a significant improvement in brain imaging. Researchers theorize that the combination of physical, cognitive, and social engagement worked synergistically to provide the greatest benefit.[30]

STRIKE UP THE BAND. A great way to develop a strengthening programme without a home gym (or having to join one) is by using resistance bands. Resistance bands are inexpensive, lightweight, and portable, and they can easily be stowed away when not in use. They're perfect for anyone who travels often. These are essentially large rubber bands manufactured with different tensions depending upon your fitness level. They can be used in a wide variety of ways that mimic the use of both machines and free weights.

HARNESS THE MIND-BODY CONNECTION. Yoga and Pilates both offer stress relief and improve flexibility, balance, and overall body strength. Yoga focuses more on flexibility and broad muscle groups and has a spiritual element, while Pilates focuses more on body control, muscle toning, and core strength. Each discipline requires a strong mind-body connection that has been shown to benefit cognition as well as many other health parameters.[31] Qigong and tai chi are other good options that require a strong mind-body connection with a meditative component for stress reduction. (See chapter 15 for more.) Some yoga postures may even promote neuroprotection in surprising ways. Dr Rammohan Rao, a neuroscientist and experienced yoga practitioner, promotes the practice of gentle inversion postures such as downward dog to activate the glymphatic system.

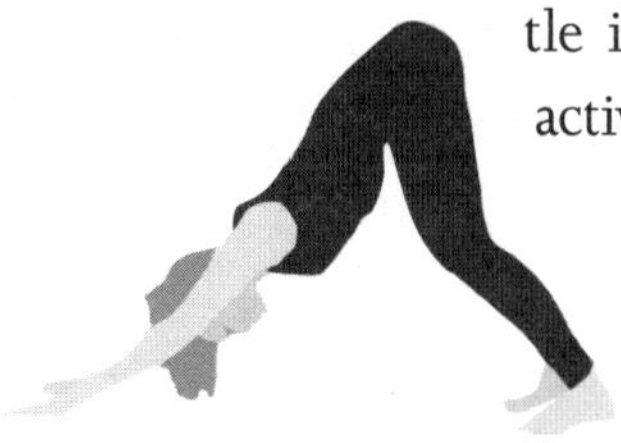

JUMP TO IT. Another fun (and surprisingly efficient) activity to consider is *rebounding*. Rebounding simply involves jumping up and down on a mini trampoline. There are many health benefits, but one of the most important is the activation of lymphatic circulation, prompting the clearance of toxins.[32] The lymphatic system is a network of tissues and organs that help rid the body of toxins, waste, and other unwanted materials. This is especially important for those dealing with type 3 (toxic) Alzheimer's.[33] The primary function of the lymphatic system is to transport lymph, a fluid containing infection-fighting white blood cells, throughout the body. Unlike your circulatory system, which uses the heart as a pump, your lymphatic system is completely dependent upon physical activity or massage to promote activation.

The downward dog yoga pose.

Other benefits of rebounding include:

- An excellent aerobic workout—68 per cent more effective than running, and yet requires less effort[34]
- Improved maximum oxygen uptake (VO_2 max)[35]

- Powerful stimulation of the immune system[36]
- Increase in bone density[37]
- Low impact; gentle on the joints[38]
- Improvement in digestion and stimulation of bowel movements for those who experience constipation[39]
- Improved balance—vital to seniors as they age[40]

If you have concerns about your steadiness on the rebounder, be sure to buy a unit that comes with a balance bar. If you have bladder control issues, empty your bladder before a workout and take frequent breaks if you feel the urge. Start with a health bounce, maintaining connection with the trampoline floor. As you feel ready, begin jumping up, keeping your feet within several centimetres of the surface. At your own pace, work your way up to fifteen minutes of steady jumping. As your proficiency increases, you can add variety with jumping jacks, high knees, waist twists, and running in place.

KICK IT UP. An interesting study demonstrated that leg power reliably predicted both cognitive ageing and global brain structure.[41] Pushing more weight on a leg press predicted better cognitive testing, greater brain volume, and healthier cognitive ageing over the ensuing decade. Given the significance of leg strength, you may want to start including daily squats into your exercise routine. If your leg muscles are weak, you can get started by standing in front of a chair as if you were going to sit down. Move your buttocks towards the seat and hold that position right above the chair for as long as possible. You should feel a burn in your front thigh muscles, the quadriceps. It's okay to fall into the seat if you feel the need. (That's why you're starting in front of a chair.) Try to resume standing and repeat for several repetitions. Over time, your leg muscles will get stronger. Work up to three sets of fifteen repetitions daily.

"HIIT" ME WITH YOUR BEST SHOT. High-intensity interval training (HIIT) is a good alternative for anyone who's already fit and has limited time to work out. HIIT involves short bursts of intensive training intermixed with periods of recovery. The goal is to push your muscles and cardiovascular system to maximum capacity for short periods. A

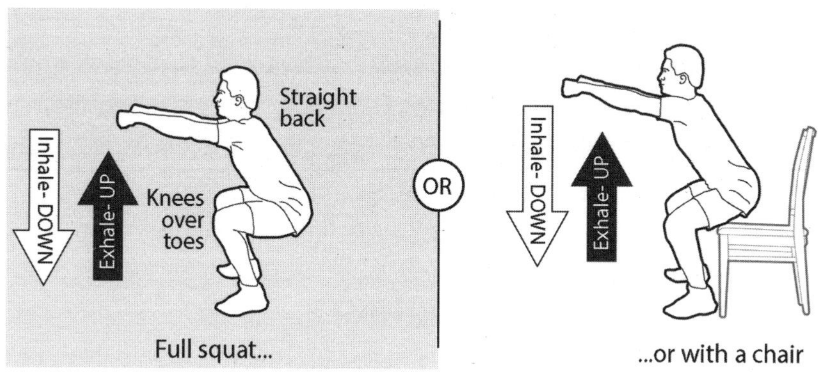

Improving leg muscles with squats.

typical session is quite short, often less than thirty minutes, based upon your current fitness level. HIIT has been shown to provide very similar health benefits as traditional exercise in a shorter amount of time, including lower body fat, heart rate, and blood pressure.[42] Additionally HIIT may be even more helpful than traditional exercise at reducing blood sugar and improving insulin sensitivity.[43] Most important, HIIT has been found to improve cognition function in older adults, with the greatest improvements seen in speed processing, then memory and executive function.[44]

Before trying HIIT, you need to know your maximum heart rate. Subtract your age from 220. For instance, if you're 60, subtract 60 from 220 to get a maximum heart rate of 160. This is the average maximum number of times your heart should beat per minute during exercise. There are endless variations of this strategy involving calisthenics, walking/running, weights, and more. A classic example can be performed on a stationary bike. After a brief warm-up, find a comfortable steady state where you achieve a speed and tension level that expends about 50 per cent of your maximum ability. After pedalling at this rate for 2 to 4 minutes, bring your speed and tension all the way up to 100 per cent capacity for 30 seconds to 1 minute, depending on your fitness level, returning to your steady state for another 2 to 4 minutes. A typical session involves four to six high-intensity periods, always returning to a steady state in between and followed by a cooldown. Those who are fit and looking for a challenge may want to check out Orangetheory Fitness. This is a franchise that offers group classes all over the world and uses HIIT with heart rate monitors to ensure that participants stay within their safe range while still being challenged.

TOO INTENSE?

Steven Gundry, a cardiac surgeon and the author of *The Plant Paradox,* has found that some very intense workouts, like extreme HIIT, engaging in marathons, and other intense activities can temporarily increase troponin, a protein that measures damage to heart muscles. A troponin blood test is traditionally used in the accident and emergency department of a hospital to determine if a patient is suffering a myocardial infarction (heart attack). Dr Gundry uses a highly sensitive (100 times) version of the cardiac troponin test. Interestingly, he's found that ApoE4 carriers appear to experience elevations with extreme workouts. This correlates beautifully with prior work finding the ApoE4 allele to be pro-inflammatory.[45] Does this mean that ApoE4 carriers shouldn't utilize HIIT? On the contrary. This high-risk group may actually need intensive exercise the most. His findings do, however, provide a warning for this group against engaging in *extraordinarily* intense exercise. HIIT can be performed to a less extreme intensity. Evolutionarily, as hunter-gatherers, we know that ApoE4 carriers moved throughout the day, gathering food punctuated by periods of intense exercise, such as during an active hunt.[46] The variation in HIIT beautifully mimics this, but it may be even more important for this group to be consistently active throughout the day.

E-WHAT? EWOT is an acronym that stands for exercise with oxygen training. This may be particularly helpful for those at risk of or with a history of vascular disease. Among many other benefits, EWOT improves circulation, peripherally and in the brain.[47] It's very important to use a specially designed EWOT mask, one that supplies a minimum of 8 to 10 litres (per minute) of pure (90–95 per cent) oxygen for the duration of the exercise period. Because it's impractical to carry oxygen with you, this type of exercise is better suited to use with a treadmill or stationary exercise bike. To locate an EWOT clinic near you, plug your post code into this site: https://www.ewot.com/apps/store-locator/. Depending upon your starting place, you may need to work up to fifteen-minute sessions, three days a week.

MOVE THROUGHOUT THE DAY. Indeed, having dedicated daily exercise time set aside is vital, *but it's equally important to increase your movement throughout the day.* You've probably heard the adage that sitting is the new smoking. It's sadly true, and one dedicated exercise session a day can't counteract our increasingly sedentary lifestyle. A new study revealed that every hour of light physical activity was associated with brain volume measurements equivalent to 1.1 fewer years of brain ageing.[48] Look for hidden opportunities to exercise in your daily schedule. Purposefully park your car as far away from your destination as possible so that you can incorporate a long walk while running your errands. Whenever you have the opportunity to take an lift or escalator, take the stairs instead. Reframe the way you look at your household chores. Rather than feeling overwhelmed by them, think of them as *opportunities* for increasing your activity level. Especially embrace your chores in the garden. Pulling weeds, spreading mulch, sweeping, raking, or shovelling snow all keep you active and make you stronger. Even household chores such as carrying laundry up and down the stairs, bending over to clean skirting boards, or mopping the floor help to keep your muscles strong.

WORK AROUND LIMITATIONS. Both yoga and Pilates are especially beneficial for anyone dealing with temporary or even long-term mobility restrictions. Much of the practice is done on a padded mat on the floor, so foot, ankle, knee, or hip issues needn't stop you. Qigong and tai chi are great slow-paced options. Seated exercise classes are another possibility for anyone recovering from an injury or dealing with mobility limitations. Specially designed chair workouts can offer decent exercise within a wide range of abilities. Your instructor can also offer modifications for any movement you have trouble performing due to injuries.

Remember, there are no FDA-approved medications (nor any in the pipeline) that come close to demonstrating the improvements seen with daily exercise. None. Exercise is free and accessible to everyone. Baby steps turn into exhilarating hikes through nature. The more active you become, the better you'll feel and the more you'll want to exercise.

CHAPTER 14

Sleep: Divine Intervention

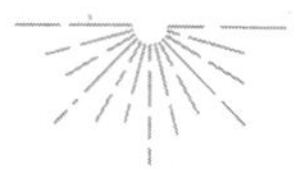

Sleep is God. Go worship.
—JIM BUTCHER

NYX, THE GREEK GODDESS of night, was so potent that even the all-powerful Zeus was afraid to enter her realm. Her son, Hypnos, was the personification of sleep, and he is turning out to be the most healing of all gods. An explosion of scientific discoveries in the last twenty years has shed new light on the fundamental role of sleep on our cognition and overall well-being. Sleep enriches our ability to focus, learn, memorize, and make logical decisions. It is critical for everyone at all stages of life. A lack of sleep affects our overall health and leads to obesity, diabetes, heart disease, increased inflammation, and a weakened immune system. All of these conditions are bidirectional and also impact brain health.[1] You'll recall that sleep is so important that we made it the foundation of the KetoFLEX 12/3 lifestyle. Indeed, restorative sleep is so vital that it would be very difficult to implement our entire protocol without this bedrock in place.

One of the most important roles of sleep is to help us consolidate memories. Throughout the day, our brains take in an enormous amount of information. These facts and experiences aren't directly logged and recorded in our brains. They first need to be processed, then stored. Many of these steps happen during restorative sleep. Bits and pieces of information are reviewed; some are discarded, but others are integrated and eventually transferred from our more tentative short-term memory to our more secure long-term memory—a process called consolidation.[2] Too little sleep or disturbed sleep has profound implications for many aspects of cognition, including our ability to focus, learn, form memories, and execute effective decision-making.[3]

While much of the biological necessity of sleep remains a mystery, some exciting new research reveals that our brain engages in critical restoration work as we sleep. The recently discovered glymphatic system, comprised of glial cells that act as a waste disposal system for the brain, plays an essential role in beta-amyloid clearance.[4] Research reveals that our glymphatic systems function most effectively during deep sleep, demonstrating a ten-to-twentyfold increased clearance rate. During deep sleep, glial cells shrink as much as 60 per cent, allowing a thorough cleansing and removal of toxic debris. Even one night of sleep deprivation reduces beta-amyloid clearance.[5] To facilitate glymphatic transport, you may want to try to sleep on your side, since a recent study demonstrated that this position most effectively cleared beta-amyloid.[6] If you naturally prefer sleeping on your back, you can experiment with using pillows to support side sleeping.

Obstructive sleep apnoea—and indeed, anything that reduces oxygen saturation at night—is emerging as an important risk factor for Alzheimer's disease.[7] This common type of sleep apnoea is caused by complete or partial obstruction of the upper airway, and is often associated with snoring. It is characterized by repetitive episodes of shallow or paused breathing during sleep and is typically associated with a reduction in blood oxygen saturation. If you or your partner snores, it's important to rule this condition out. In fact, oxygen desaturation is so common, and so important in cognitive decline, that it is critical for *everyone* with cognitive decline to check their oxygen saturation at night, which should be 96 to 98 per cent. You can start with a portable continuous pulse oximeter to check to see if you're getting too little oxygen throughout the night. (See "Tools for Success" in chapter 18 for details.) If this appears to be a problem, ask your doctor to refer you to a sleep specialist for a formal sleep study. The Royal Society for Public Health in the UK offers advice in the UK while in the US, the National Sleep Foundation provides information on how and when to seek help. Sleep studies are typically covered by medical insurance in the US and will determine the treatment plan, which may include a portable oxygen machine that provides continuous positive airway pressure, commonly called CPAP, to help treat this condition. It's very helpful to monitor oxygen saturation levels throughout the night periodically once you've begun using a CPAP, to ensure that the treatment is effective.

SWEET DREAMS ARE MADE OF THIS . . .

Too many people mistakenly assume that you can just lie down and you'll fall asleep. That's sadly not true for many of us, and this issue tends to become more bothersome as we grow older. You need to put some effort and preparation into your nightly sleep hygiene. The great news is that we can work to optimize sleep. Applying the strategies below will help improve both the quality and the quantity of your sleep.

- **Identify your unique circadian rhythm.** Our hunter-gatherer ancestors naturally went to sleep with the sunset and woke with the sunrise. Try to follow this pattern as your schedule and circadian rhythm permit. Each of us has a unique, inherent sleep-wake pattern that will dynamically change over the decades. Accommodating this cycle is a powerful way to promote restorative sleep, optimal cognition, and productivity.

- **Keep a regular sleep schedule.** Try to stick to a regular sleep schedule. This is not always possible because of family or work demands, but do your best to have a regular bedtime and time to wake up. Ideally, we should begin to wind down as the sun is setting.

- **Set a sleep goal.** Make seven to eight hours of sleep your goal. Research shows that adults getting less than six hours and more than nine hours are negatively impacted. The idea that older adults need less sleep is a myth.

- **To nap or not?** A lack of sleep can lead to the need for a nap, which can be helpful. Frequent napping, however, also has the potential to impair the quantity and quality of your restorative sleep.

- **Limit caffeine.** No caffeine (or other stimulating beverages or supplements) past noon. Work to identify which supplements are stimulating and be sure to include them in your morning stack.

- **Promote autophagy.** Eat your last meal of the day at least three hours before bed. This promotes autophagy, which cleans out cellular waste products. It's also much easier to sleep on an empty stomach.

- **Beware of nighttime hypoglycaemia.** Those who are insulin resistant should be aware that hypoglycaemic episodes can cause awakening in the middle of the night. A continuous glucose monitoring (CGM) system can be very helpful for becoming aware of this. As you become insulin sensitive with the KetoFLEX 12/3 lifestyle, this will resolve. Learn more in "Tips for Transitioning to a Longer Fast" in chapter 7 and "Tools for Success" in chapter 18.

- **Rethink a nightcap.** If you're struggling with sleep, this is another reason to refrain from alcohol. The seductive effect of alcohol may lead you to think that it's helping with sleep, but research shows that it powerfully disrupts our REM sleep cycle, impairing memory integration.

- **Exercise earlier in the day.** Don't exercise within three hours of bedtime. Exercise ramps up adrenaline and prevents sleep.

- **Reduce nighttime loo breaks.** Take your supplements about an hour before bed with as little water as possible.

While it's important to hydrate during the day, you don't want to have to wake up for a loo run.

- **Wind down.** Refrain from stimulating activities or conversations several hours before you plan to sleep.
- **Block blue light.** Wear your blue-blocking glasses three hours before bedtime, following our suggested guidelines for usage. See "A Sleep Hack to Enhance Melatonin Production" on page 224.
- **Your bedroom is for sleep.** Make your bedroom your sanctuary. Keep it clean and uncluttered, free from work and any other projects.
- **It's okay to sleep solo.** Sleep alone if you know you'll be interrupted at night. This is especially important if you and your partner have different sleep habits due to work or other demands.
- **No TV in the bedroom.** We know this is aspirational for many. If you must watch TV, learn how to set the sleep timer so that it will automatically turn off. Also, consider the use of a blue-blocking vinyl overlay that you can apply to your screen at night.
- **Minimize EMF exposure.** Minimize low-level radiation in the bedroom. Mounting evidence suggests that radiation from electromagnetic fields (including Wi-Fi) can impact overall health negatively. Make sure any electronic device in your room is turned off, placed as far from the bed as possible, or placed on airplane mode when you go to sleep.
- **Enjoy a bedtime story.** For those who read before bed, we know that the simple act of turning off your lamp can reawaken you, making it harder to fall asleep. And sleeping with the lamp on will disrupt your body's production of melatonin. For that reason, consider using either an eBook

or a tablet that lights up (set to the dimmest setting on airplane mode), with an automatic shutoff feature so that you don't have to turn off the lamp as you drift off to sleep. Be sure to pick a device with a blue-blocking programme, like Night Shift for iPad. If your model isn't compatible with a blue-blocking programme, you can use a blue-blocking vinyl that you can easily apply before bed. Another option is to listen to an audio book with automatic shutoff. If you prefer to read an actual book, consider an inexpensive red incandescent lightbulb or a blue-blocking LED lightbulb for your bedside lamp.

- **Keep your room dark.** Completely darken the bedroom or use a sleep mask. Any small bit of light at night will interfere with melatonin production.

- **Get hot.** Consider a warm shower, a bath, or even a sauna before bedtime. The juxtaposition of the cold temperature afterwards will help prepare you for bed.

- **Chill out.** Keep the bedroom cool. Research shows that keeping the temperature around 18 degrees Celsius, depending upon your preference, is optimal for sleep. If you tend to be cold, be sure to have a warm blanket to cover up. Also, consider sleeping in the nude to stay cool throughout the night.

- **Stay eco-cool.** If you feel wasteful cooling the whole house at night, consider using a mattress cooling pad. OOLER is one example that uses water to keep you cool, allowing you to place the electric temperature control unit away from the bed. Additionally, while the system can be controlled by Bluetooth, we encourage you to manually control your temperature to minimize Wi-Fi exposure. While this system is initially expensive, it may save money (and energy) in the long run. It's well suited to those who live in very warm climates or for rooms that can't be adequately cooled.

- **Get swaddled.** Try a weighted blanket. In the same way that babies who are swaddled sleep more deeply, some adults report a similar effect with a weighted blanket. This strategy is most effective for those who struggle to stay warm, although cooler versions are available for warmer weather.

- **Zone out noise.** Use a white-noise machine if you're regularly interrupted with extraneous noise from your heating system, air conditioner, outside traffic, neighbours, etc. Many have relaxing nature sounds (like rain, wind, or waves) that you can set to your desired volume to drown out bothersome noise. Be sure to place this as far from the bed as possible (with the volume optimized) to protect yourself from EMF.

- **Sleep clean.** Make sure your bed is as toxin-free as possible. Many mattresses, other bedding (mattress pads, pillows, sheets, blankets, etc.), and even pajamas are treated with harmful chemicals such as flame retardants. Exposure to these toxins can lead to serious health consequences, including neurological damage.[8] Look for organic or green products when it's time to replace bedding.

- **Consider aromatherapy.** Lavender essential oils have proven helpful in slowing heartbeat, relaxing muscles, and promoting slow-wave sleep. Put a few drops on a cotton ball near your bed to see how it affects you.

If you wake up in the middle of the night with stress or anxiety—mulling over a negative event in the past or feeling stressed about a future event—try a sensory mindfulness technique. Begin by simply focusing on the gentle natural rhythm of your breathing. Slowly breathe in and out. Gradually transition to focus on each of your five senses simultaneously. Feel the soft blankets against your skin, smell the lavender, listen to the sound of your breath, look at the subtle images behind your closed eyes, and taste the clean residue from your brushed teeth. By being fully present—*not thinking about the past or* future—you can relax and feel safe. With practice, you will find this very relaxing, and it will help you drift off to sleep. Regular daily meditation can also be very helpful in optimizing sleep.

Despite your best efforts, what if you simply can't fall asleep? Don't lie in bed, stressing about it. The last thing we want is for you to associate your bedroom with the stress of not sleeping, which can become a subconscious response pattern. Get up and go to another room; there, engage in a quiet activity such as reading in low light with your blue blockers. Return to your bedroom only when you begin to feel drowsy. If you have repeated problems falling and staying asleep and have already had a formal sleep study, consider using cognitive behavioural therapy for insomnia (CBT-I).

SLEEP DISORDER OR DEPRESSION?

We know that sleep quality and depression are often mutually antagonistic: a lack of sleep can cause depression, and people who are depressed often have trouble sleeping (or sleep in excess). A sense of pervasive sadness, a loss of interest in old hobbies, a change in appetite, a loss of energy, and trouble concentrating are tip-offs that you may be dealing with depression as opposed to a sleep disorder.[9] Many with type 3 (toxic) Alzheimer's patients present as having depression when the underlying cause is chronic inflammation caused by a toxic exposure.[10] If you feel this may be an issue for you, have a discussion with your functional medicine practitioner about finding the root cause of your symptoms. When possible, use natural strategies to improve both mood and sleep. Many antidepressants have anticholinergic properties and thus impede memory, since acetylcholine is centrally involved in learning and memory (the major Alzheimer's drugs, such as donepezil, or Aricept, prevent the breakdown of acetylcholine, thus *increasing* its concentration).[11] For many, simply restoring sleep quality and quantity may help with symptoms of depression. For others, finding and addressing root causes is imperative.

Isn't There a Pill for This?

Sleep medication might seem to help temporarily, but in the long run it may *increase* your risk for cognitive decline. Benzodiazepines taken for three to six months raise the risk of developing Alzheimer's by 32 per cent, and taking them for more than six months boosts the risk by 84 per cent.[12] Using benzodiazepines for longer than a year can result in cognitive impairment that can continue beyond cessation of the medication for up to 3.5 years.[13] The addictive qualities of these medications necessitate careful considerations for a slow tapering of dosage to prevent withdrawal symptoms. Common benzodiazepine sleep medications include, Prosom (estazolam) and Restoril (temazepam).

Non-benzodiazepine sleep medications and antihistamines have become increasingly common, but these, too, can negatively impair cognition by downregulating acetylcholine.[14] Anticholinergic medications have been found to correlate with an increased risk of dementia, the effect being proportional to the dose of the drug and the duration of use.[15] Common anticholinergic sleep medications include Ambien (zolpidem), Lunesta (eszopiclone), and Sonata (zaleplon), and antihistamines like Benadryl, paracetamol and ibruprofen.

Luckily, there are several supplements and medications that support the body, have neuroprotective properties, and naturally induce better quality sleep without negative side effects. Be sure to try one at a time and carefully record the effect. Be aware that if you decide to layer several at once, you may get a different effect. Tweak until you find a combination that's helpful.

- **Melatonin** Melatonin is a naturally occurring hormone that decreases with age. Supplementation has been shown to be effective in promoting better quality sleep, not by a sedative effect but rather through promotion of a healthy circadian rhythm, which is disrupted in Alzheimer's patients.[16] Melatonin can also improve mitochondrial function, reduce levels of tau, and have been shown to improve cognition in an Alzheimer's mouse model.[17]

- **Tryptophan** This is an amino acid that is naturally found in many foods, including milk, eggs, poultry, fish, and the seeds of pumpkin and sesame. Tryptophan is the precursor to 5HTP (5-hydroxytryptophan), and can be converted into serotonin (5-hydroxytryptamine), a neurotransmitter and key player in modulating the bidirectional gut-brain axis, linking cognition to the gastrointestinal tract.[18] Serotonin is also a precursor to the hormone melatonin, which helps your body regulate sleep and wake cycles. Tryptophan or 5HTP taken in the middle of the night may be particularly helpful for people who awaken and have trouble falling back asleep.

- **GABA** You'll recall that GABA is a neurotransmitter that blocks impulses between nerve cells in the brain and has a calming effect. GABA supplementation has been shown to effectively aid in sleep and has even been explored as a potential therapeutic target for Alzheimer's disease.[19]

- **Magnesium** Many people are deficient in magnesium, a mineral necessary for hundreds of biochemical reactions in the body and, most important, *critical for brain function*. Magnesium has sedative properties. Taken before bed, magnesium has been demonstrated to decrease circulating cortisol, increase melatonin, and improve sleep quality.[20] A more neurally bioavailable form of magnesium, magnesium threonate, has been shown to improve cognition in older adults.[21]

- **Ashwagandha** This herb commonly used in Ayurvedic medicine is an adaptogen that helps the body adapt to stress and exerts a normalizing effect upon bodily processes. Ashwagandha has demonstrated many health benefits, including stress reduction leading to improved sleep.[22] A recent study has found that triethylene glycol, found in the leaves of the plant, is responsible for a sleep induction effect.[23] Ashwagandha has also been found to improve memory in people with MCI as well as improving executive function, attention, and information processing speed.[24]

- **Bacopa monnieri** This is another Ayurvedic adaptogen that, among other effects, increases acetylcholine and improves cognitive performance.[25] It may be particularly helpful for those experiencing trouble sleeping due to stress. It can have a paradoxical energizing effect for some people. Be sure to initially experiment with a low dose (e.g. 100 mg) taken several hours before bed to test the effect for you.

- **Other options** Additional sleep options to consider include theanine, chamomile, lemon balm, valerian root, passionflower, lavender, and CBD oil.

- **Bioidentical hormone replacement therapy (BHRT)** Many women who use BHRT report improved sleep as a side effect. Progesterone, rather than having a true sedative effect, has been found to restore disturbed sleep in postmenopausal women, but women using oestrogen supplementation alone also report significant sleep improvement.[26] Carefully timed and judicious use of BHRT can also positively impact cognition.[27] Likely due to methodological issues, the effect of hormone replacement on cognition has been controversial, but a careful analysis of multiple studies reveals that it exerts a positive effect on cognition.[28] Indeed, women who undergo a removal of their ovaries prior to menopause are at greatly increased risk of cognitive decline without hormone replacement.[29] A search of the evidence suggests that the *type of oestrogen* matters: bioidentical oestrogen (same molecular structure as oestrogen in the body) correlated with a better cognitive outcome than conjugated oestrogen (made from the urine of pregnant horses and synthetic sources). Equally important is the *delivery method* of the oestrogen, with transdermal rather than oral showing the most benefit.[30] Women with a uterus must take progesterone with oestrogen to prevent an overgrowth of uterine cells that can lead to cancer. Those without a uterus may choose to do so for the sleep enhancement. Avoid a synthetic form of progesterone called progestin, which is correlated with an increased risk of breast cancer.[31] The role of progesterone on cognition is mixed, showing both benefit and detriment. Some studies demonstrate that chronic use actually has a negative impact on cognition, whereas intermittent use has a decidedly beneficial impact, especially on memory consolidation.[32] It may be best used for half the month, mimicking a women's natural cycle, preventing a buildup in fatty tissues, and thereby deriving optimal cognitive benefit. A "window of opportunity" hypothesis suggests that addressing hormonal decline early may best protect women's cognition, but a recent randomized controlled trial using BHRT on postmenopausal women *well beyond that window* (at 57 to 82 years), who were diagnosed with mild cognitive impairment, demonstrated preserved cognition compared to the control group.[33] Many women mistakenly assume that BHRT is extravagantly expensive, unaware that there are less expensive generic versions. A BHRT programme should always be initiated with the help of a hormone expert to weigh risk versus potential benefit carefully.

A SLEEP HACK TO ENHANCE MELATONIN PRODUCTION

Blue blocker glasses, with designer options, are gaining in popularity *because they work*. More and more people are donning these crazy-looking orange-coloured glasses several hours before bedtime to get the best sleep ever.

Let's dive into the science behind the trend. It has to do with a mismatch between modern civilization and our primitive biology. For hundreds of thousands of years, mankind awoke with the sun and fell asleep when it set. With the advent of fire, early man may have sat around a communal wood-fuelled bonfire for warmth and protection from animals, but even that light provided a gentle orange-red glow. Fast-forward to modern life, when people work around the clock. Fluorescent, LED, and incandescent lighting (all blue light) available twenty-four hours a day makes that possible, but it also throws our natural circadian rhythm (also known as our sleep-wake cycle) into a tizzy. Even worse is the strong blue light that comes from our electronic devices and televisions, especially right before we go to sleep.

Nature prepared us for sleep beautifully with gradual darkness, which automatically signals our pineal gland to produce melatonin necessary for falling and staying asleep. With indoor lighting and multiple electronic devices emitting a blue light that mimics daytime, our pineal glands are confused at best, thus underproducing this essential hormone that we need for sleep and more. Melatonin is also a powerful scavenger of free radicals and a wide-spectrum antioxidant protecting against mitochondrial oxidative stress while providing immunological benefits.[34] Its production naturally falls off as we age, but blue blockers enhance production.

Consumer groups have found that inexpensive versions of these glasses are just as effective as pricier designer options. Be sure to look for orange-tinted glasses (not medium or light yellow) designed to promote sleep. There are styles geared for those who wear glasses beneath blue blockers. See tips below to maximize effectiveness.

Wear them regularly—that is, each night if possible. They don't work like a sleeping pill, but over time they will induce restorative physiological sleep by increasing your own production of melatonin.

- If you already are supplementing with melatonin, you may have to decrease your dosage over time, since the blue blockers will be increasing your own production of melatonin.

(continued)

- Put them on approximately three hours before bed. You can easily wear them around the house, or they can serve as a hip conversational topic when you wear them to evening engagements.
- Choose a style that blocks all blue light. Wraparound versions are especially effective and specific styles can accommodate glasses beneath.
- Unless your bathroom is equipped with dim blue-blocking light (which is easy to do with a small lamp), be sure to perform any nightly face-washing ritual before donning your glasses. Otherwise, you'll be briefly exposed to harsh blue light right before you go to bed.
- Even with blue blockers on, try to minimize your exposure to electronic devices right before bed. Engage in other relaxing activities such as quiet conversation or reading.
- Once you're ready for sleep, ensure that your bedroom is 100 per cent dark or wear a sleeping mask to maintain the beneficial melatonin effect.
- Once you awaken in the morning, open your blinds to the full extent. Better yet, get outside as soon as possible. Exposing your eyes to blue light, especially in the morning, will help get your circadian rhythm back on track.

Poor sleep is a modifiable risk factor. Feel free to use a sleep tracker with the understanding that the majority are around 60 per cent accurate at best but can still provide a rough idea of how your sleep is trending. More expensive and accurate models are becoming available. (See more in "Tools for Success" in chapter 18.) By regularly employing all of these sleep optimization strategies, you can make bedtime a nightly ritual that you actually anticipate for the relaxation and restoration experience. Improving the quality of your sleep will also offer almost immediate benefits to your mood and overall cognitive performance. For more information about sleep, we highly recommend *Why We Sleep* by Matthew Walker, PhD.

CHAPTER 15

Stress: Trim Your Sails

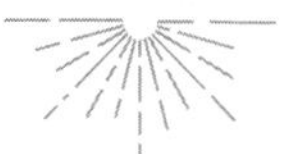

Adopting a positive attitude can convert a negative stress into a positive one.

—HANS SELYE

AS THE ORIGINAL STRESS guru, Professor Hans Selye pointed out, stress actually ages us. Therefore, preventing or managing stress—"trimming your sails" optimally for life's vicissitudes—has an anti-ageing effect, and clearly this is an important part of any optimal strategy to prevent or reverse cognitive decline. While our ultimate goal is to empower you to control your response to external stressors, in the short term, stress can be a very positive reaction, protecting us from harm. Furthermore, repeated *mild* stress, *with resolution*—such as that which occurs with exercise or fasting, for example—is *protective*. This is called *hormesis*. It is the chronic, unresolved, or severe stress that increases our risk for cognitive decline.[1] Understanding this dichotomy is helpful in dealing with the everyday stresses in our lives.

When we sense impending danger, neurotransmitters send information to the amygdala, a part of the brain that processes emotional signals, and a danger alarm is sent to the hypothalamus. The hypothalamus then acts as a switchboard, communicating with the rest of the body through the nervous system, activating the fight-or-flight response. From there, hundreds of involuntary bodily functions are activated. Adrenaline floods our body, increasing our heart rate and thereby contributing needed blood flow to our muscles and vital organs. We breathe more rapidly, small airways in the lungs open to flood our brain with oxygen. Our blood vessels are dilated, our blood pressure rises, and our senses are heightened. Glucose is released, supplying energy to all parts of the body, giving us the power we need to respond to the perceived threat. Without this exquisite built-in involuntary protective reaction, we wouldn't be able to run from mountain lions, escape from burning buildings, or rescue someone in need. The problem occurs when we can't turn this stress response off—when we begin to perceive relatively harmless exposures as bigger threats. As noted above, it's this chronic exposure to stress that can wreak havoc on our bodies, contributing to hypertension, heart disease, obesity, sleep disorders, and even changes in the brain.[2]

We're all exposed to stress from our home life and work demands. That's normal. What too many of us fail to understand is that our *response* to that everyday stress may be wired from very early or other traumatic experiences. When we learn as young children that the world is sometimes an unsafe place, this can set in place a negative feedback loop that colours our reaction to all future stress.[3] Very few of us get through childhood without some trauma. Researchers have created a questionnaire by means of which we can quantify those experiences, called Adverse Childhood Experiences (ACEs). Not surprisingly, people with higher scores are at risk for a multitude of coping and other related health problems; alcohol and drug abuse, obesity, depression, and sleep disorders. What has surprised researchers is that the biology of those with higher scores also appears to have changed, putting them at higher risk for chronic diseases such as diabetes, autoimmune disease, lung disorders, heart disease, and cancer.[4] In terms of cognitive health, those with higher ACEs scores show premature brain ageing, shortened telomeres, higher inflammatory biomarkers, and an increased risk for dementia and Alzheimer's.[5]

The good news is that we can change the way we react to stress. The first step is to simply understand that our current response is likely unhealthy. Most of us go through our daily lives constantly replaying critical or self-doubting chatter from our past. The further back this inner dialogue goes, the more hard-wired it may be. Many of us unconsciously replay early critiques, perhaps from our parents or schoolteachers. Or we may replay more recent conversations in which our partner, friend, or boss criticized us with statements like "You never pull your weight" or "You always let me down." Those who've also experienced more recent stressors—a physical or emotional assault; a car accident; the loss of a job, a loved one, or a relationship—can experience an even more heightened compounded response. Sometimes even when things are going well, we expect something bad to happen based upon our past experiences. This constant assault from the past can unconsciously affect us and our reactions to the world today. These past negative experiences can also cause us to worry excessively about the future. Intervening with a practice called mindfulness can create awareness, stop this negative feedback loop, and reset our response pattern.

MINDFULNESS This is the simple practice of being fully present in the current moment. When we are fully present, consciously aware of ourselves and the world around us, we aren't looking back and replaying negative self-chatter. We aren't worrying about the future. We are simply being, completely present in a non-judgemental and observant manner.

Mindfulness is being aware of the beauty of the sunrise as you drive to work; catching the eye of the supermarket checkout clerk and saying a kind word; eating slowly and consciously, feeling grateful for the nourishing food. *Unmindfulness*, on the other hand, is rushing to work not even noticing the sunrise; checking out at the supermarket, ignoring the worker who is serving you; mindlessly stuffing food into your mouth while watching TV. You can see how simply becoming mindful has the power to change the way you perceive the world. The more you learn to incorporate it into your daily practice, the more you'll become aware of how the past (or worry about the future) seeps into your subconscious if you aren't actively aware. Many people use mindfulness as an entrée into meditation.

Worried that mindfulness is touchy-feely nonsense without scientific research? Jon Kabat-Zinn, a molecular biology PhD from the Massachusetts Institute of Technology, who studied under Nobel laureate Salvador Luria, is largely credited with popularizing this practice. As a college student, he studied meditation with Buddhist monks and later went on to create an eight-week course called Mindfulness-Based Stress Reduction (MBSR) that ultimately dropped the Buddhist underpinning and instead put the practice into a scientific context.[6] Indeed, research shows that mindfulness lowers cortisol and blood pressure, improves sleep, and clinically reduces stress, depression, and anxiety while improving attention.[7] Most important, mindfulness powerfully protects middle-aged and older adults from the effects of stress on mental health.[8]

Try a mindfulness breathing exercise that can be used to address immediate feelings of stress. Deep breathing stimulates the vagus nerve, which helps to induce a relaxation response to stress. This exercise brings you to present awareness by simply focusing on and ultimately controlling your breath. It is a powerful technique that can be used at any time.

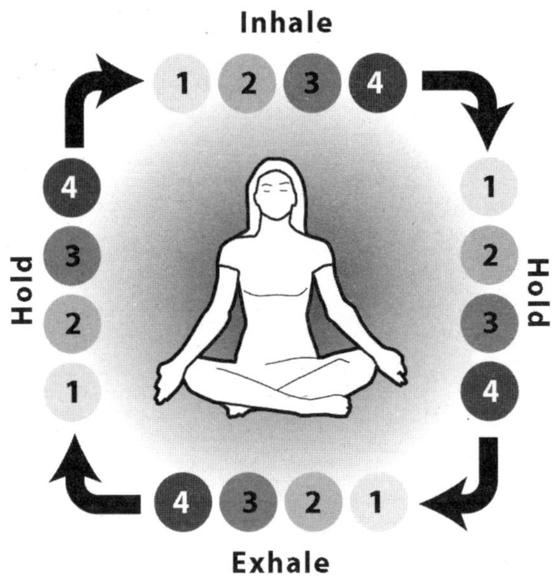

Square breathing

1. Sit upright and pay attention to your breathing.
2. Exhale slowly through your mouth to the count of 4. Hold to the count of 4.
3. Inhale slowly through your nose to the count of 4. Hold to the count of 4.
4. Repeat this pattern for several minutes.

There are hundreds of calming mindfulness techniques like this freely available on the Internet. There are also apps like Buddhify (free download with 200+ guided meditations with an optional £24-a-year subscription for more materials) or Calm (£30 a year, with a seven-day free trial) that offer guided mindfulness techniques, some of which segue into full meditation. There are many online and in-person options to learn MBSR, with the cost ranging from free to several hundred pounds.

MEDITATION When you're ready to take mindfulness to the next level, you may want to try meditation. Meditation is the practice of focusing on a specific word or thought, to clear and transform the mind to a calm and enlightened state. It has origins in numerous religious practices. The medical benefits of meditation are well documented and include sleep improvement, blood pressure reduction, pain relief, stress and anxiety reduction, and a decrease in depressive symptoms.[9] Meditation actually reverses the cytokine pattern seen in stress-induced depression.[10] Cytokines are small proteins involved in inflammatory and other types of cell signaling. Genes related to inflammation became less active in people practising meditation. A key protein that acts as an inflammation on-switch and increases amyloid production—called nuclear factor kappa B (NFκB)—is downregulated in meditators. This is the opposite of the effects of chronic stress on gene expression and suggests that meditation practice may lead to a reduced risk of inflammation-related diseases. Most important, meditation improves cognition, executive functioning, working memory, attention, and processing speed.[11] Still not convinced? There are dozens of studies demonstrating that meditation actually changes brain imaging. Meditation improves white matter connectivity and increases cortical thickness and grey matter concentrations in multiple brain regions.[12]

There are many different kinds of meditation. Some are focused exclusively on mindfulness while others, such as transcendental meditation (TM), use different techniques. The best form of meditation is one that motivates you to practise on a regular basis. Some people can get started with auditory-guided apps, others need visual online instruction, and still others do best with actual in-person training. A popular app called Insight Timer provides meditation instruction along with a huge library of guided meditations. The download is free (as are most features), with opportunities to purchase upgraded components or specific classes. Insight Timer has a motivational element: once you are logged in, you can see the number of people near you and all over the world who are meditating at any given time. Headspace is another app that gently leads you with instructive guided meditation. The annual subscription fee is around £45, along with a ten-day free trial to see if this learning style works for you.

If you're ready for a deeper dive, consider trying the Ziva meditation technique. This is an easily accessible, less expensive form of TM. Transcendental meditation was first brought to the United States by the Maharishi Mahesh Yogi in the 1950s and was popularized in the 1960s when the Beatles and other celebrities began to meditate. TM is a version of the ancient Hindu practice used by monks, translated for laypeople, called Vedic meditation. It involves the use of a mantra and is typically practised twice a day for 15 to 20 minutes.[13] TM has been widely criticized for the exorbitant cost of instruction (many classes cost nearly $1,000 [£800] or more), but the high price appears to be a purposeful tradition originating with the Maharishi Mahesh Yogi in an effort to limit access and add perceived value. Ziva has secularized the practice and geared it towards busy people with both online and in-person classes. Ziva is unique in that it ultimately moves you through mindfulness to remove current stress, on to meditation to remove past stress, and ultimately to manifestation to create goals for your future. The online programme includes fifteen lessons, extra sessions, and webinars, as well as a Facebook support group—all of which disappears after six months. Ziva is pricey (although still cheaper than traditional TM) with online courses starting at about $399 (£310).

PRAYER Every spiritual denomination uses prayer. Engaging in prayer has been shown to reduce stress.[14] Through unknown mechanisms, some research has also demonstrated that prayer can even positively affect outcomes.[15] We strongly encourage those who find comfort and peace using this process to utilize prayer instead of, or with, a meditative practice.

NEURAL AGILITY This audio download is part of the RevitaMind series and is different from meditation (which requires active participation) in that it's essentially a passive process. This may be best reserved for those who can't engage in a more active form of stress management. You simply slip on a headset and relax while listening to one of several audio clips, each lasting approximately thirty minutes. The science involves the synchronization of brain waves using specific audio beats, called *brain entrainment*, that encourage coordination towards the theta brain-wave range, which has been correlated with improved mood and memory.[16] This programme is $97 (£75) and offers a money-back guarantee if users fail to see a benefit after two months of regular usage.

DYNAMIC NEURAL RETRAINING SYSTEM (DNRS) Another programme to consider is DNRS, designed by Annie Hopper, a trained counsellor who healed *herself* after becoming chronically ill from a toxic exposure. Understanding that a traumatic brain injury was at the root of her symptoms, she used the science of neuroplasticity to identify methods to rewire her neural circuitry to heal. Hopper hypothesizes that many different types of very real brain traumas can cause the limbic system (which includes the amygdala and controls your stress response) to be reprogrammed: despite the passing of the initial threat, the limbic system remains hypervigilant and overresponds to non-threatening stimuli. After being in a heightened state for a long period of time, the immune system ultimately becomes depleted, leading to chronic and often debilitating illness.[17] DNRS focuses on retraining the limbic system, allowing the body to heal itself.

Hopper has successfully helped to heal many people suffering with toxic exposures, including multiple chemical sensitivity and mould, and also those with chronic fatigue syndrome, adrenal fatigue, autonomic dysfunction, fibromyalgia, Lyme disease, and many other chronic inflammatory states. The DNRS programme may be particularly helpful for those dealing with type 3 Alzheimer's or the pathology that leads to it.[18]

Hopper has worked with many reputable doctors, including Patrick Hanaway, MD, with the Institute for Functional Medicine, and is currently conducting research with the University of Calgary. You can learn more about her programme through her book, *Wired for Healing*. She offers an instructional DVD series for $249.99 (£192). To learn about additional options for healing, visit the Dynamic Neural Retraining System website.

HEARTMATH If you like data and are motivated by immediate feedback, HeartMath may be a good stress-relief tool for you to measure your progress. HeartMath is based upon the heart rhythm variability (HRV) science showing that greater HRV is associated with reduced stress, increased resilience, and an improved ability to adapt effectively to stress and environmental demands.

Higher HRV is associated with reduced biological ageing and better overall health—specifically psychological, cardiac, metabolic, and renal—and even with improved survival with cancer.[19] Those with a higher HRV also have better cognitive abilities, including executive function, attention, perception, working memory, and cognitive flexibility.[20]

HeartMath works by using either a wired or Bluetooth earlobe clip that transmits your real-time data to an app on your phone or tablet. You can see both your HRV and your *coherence* level. Coherence is a scientifically measurable state whereby psychological and physiological processes are aligned. Coherence is marked by a smooth sine-wave-like pattern in the HRV trace recording. It signifies a synchronization between the heart and brain, aligning the two branches of your nervous system towards increased parasympathetic (relaxation) activity, as well as harmonious balance between HRV, blood pressure, and respiration.[21] The goal is to achieve high HRV *and* coherence. The app provides you with real-time coaching tips as well as guided meditations to improve your numbers. The manufacturers recommend using it three to five times per day simply as a means of checking in to monitor your stress level. This information may help guide you when making dietary and exercise decisions throughout your day. For instance, if your HeartMath is showing a high level of discordance, it's probably not a good time to engage in intense exercise. The HeartMath system begins at about $129 (£100).

QIGONG AND TAI CHI Both qigong and tai chi, while different, are ancient Chinese practices that can be described as meditative movement used to align energy. Qigong is older, and the broader term, that includes a diverse number of practices that promote *qi*, or life essence, as described by the Chinese. Both qigong and tai chi use a wide range of slow meditative movements, standing or sitting meditation. Both practices incorporate the regulation of breath, mind, and body and are based upon traditional Chinese medicine principles.[22] Yoga is another great stress reducer, with a strong meditative element, that can also offer an athletic challenge. (See more about yoga in chapter 13.)

Qigong and tai chi are widely practised in China and are also gaining popularity in the West and throughout the world. Both practices have been correlated with many positive health outcomes, including improved cardiopulmonary markers, bone density, balance (fewer falls), sleep, and self-reported quality of life.[23] Additionally, both practices demonstrate an improvement in psychological symptoms including depression, stress, anxiety, and mood.[24] Most important, immune function and inflammation markers are improved with both qigong and tai chi interventions.[25]

It is best to learn either of these practices with a qualified instructor. Classes are offered in the UK, many outdoors when weather permits.

We encourage you to experiment and find several stress reduction strategies that appeal to you. Record the effect various practices have for you. Try to build stress reduction into your schedule by practising as often as possible, preferably daily. The benefits of stress reduction can become self-sustaining when practised regularly. In addition to these focused techniques, there are many strategies that we can all employ in our everyday lives to reduce stress.

- **Give yourself permission for self-care.** You are worthy. Allow time in your schedule to care for yourself. The pathology that leads to cognitive decline takes a decade or more. Even if you already have concerns about your cognition, by actively engaging in stress reduction *today*, you can change the way you respond to everyday pressures, creating a resiliency that confers long-term neuroprotection.

- **Don't overschedule.** Know your limits and set realistic boundaries. You needn't say yes to every social engagement, work opportunity, or family obligation. Decline opportunities that don't align with your priorities and goals.

- **Use lists.** We all have lots to get done every day. Start your day by writing down realistic goals and cross them out as you achieve them. This simple strategy can provide a sense of accomplishment, can help you stay focused and achieve more, and can reduce stress.

- **Unplug.** Many of us are old enough to remember when we communicated through occasional phone calls on our landlines or through actual letters in the post. Think of the enormous freedom that provided! We ran errands, performed our chores, and got through our workdays relatively uninterrupted. Now, with an explosion in technology, we're expected to be connected 24/7 through mobile phones, text messages, voice mail, fax machines, email, Facebook, Twitter, and Instagram. Constantly being on call and responding to everyone's demands drains you of energy, causing stress, anxiety, and even depression.[26] Most important, it doesn't allow you to focus on the task at hand. Limit your exposure to technology. The world will carry on without you. The psychological benefit goes way beyond the reduction in Wi-Fi and EMF.

- **Forget multitasking.** The ability to perform multiple tasks at one time is an overrated and newly prized skill, not in alignment with our still-primitive genomes. Science shows that our attention network performs best when we focus on one cognitive skill at a time. Constantly responding to multiple stimuli over time is draining, has a negative effect on our cognition, and can lead to feelings of stress.[27] Focusing on one thing at a time allows you to be present and mindful. It can also provide the opportunity for daydreaming, creativity, and problem solving. Give yourself permission to do one thing at a time and luxuriate in focusing on that single task.
- **Exercise.** In addition to all of the benefits we've already outlined, regular exercise is an excellent stress reducer. When you feel strong emotions, an invigorating walk can often provide a sense of clarity and calm.
- **Get adequate sleep.** Have you ever noticed how much easier it is to handle all of life's little stressors when you've had a good night's sleep? Science clearly demonstrates that adequate sleep improves our mood and ability to respond to stress.[28]
- **Reach out.** When situational or chronic stress affects your ability to enjoy previously pleasurable activities, eat normally, get adequate sleep, or simply feel happy, it's time to reach out to a helping professional. Reaching out for help is not a sign of weakness, but rather a sign of strength. A professional can help rule out other physical causes for your feeling of stress and work with you to identify coping techniques that work for you.

CHAPTER 16

Brain Stimulation: Upsizing

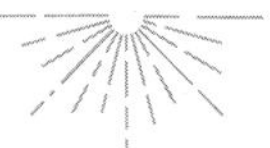

Never stop learning because life never stops teaching.
—EMMILY VARA

SCIENTISTS USED TO THINK that once brain function was lost, it was irretrievable. An explosion of research into the field of neuroplasticity is proving that this is not the case. Our brains continue to grow new neurons throughout our lives in response to social and mental stimuli as well as during healing from trauma or injury.[1] In 2000, the Nobel Prize in Physiology or Medicine was awarded to a team of scientists who used sea slugs to identify the molecular mechanisms of learning and memory. This was a crucial discovery for understanding normal brain function, but also for understanding how disturbances in this process can lead to neurological disease.[2] Moreover, this work provided irrefutable support for the notion that learning literally changes brain structure.[3]

Our brains can change throughout our lives, even in old age.[4] The brain's ability to grow and adapt is called neuroplasticity.[5] We all know that when we exercise, our muscles grow stronger. If we stop, our muscles atrophy. Even though the brain is not a muscle, the same principle applies. Challenging our brains provides the opportunity for growth. Our daily thoughts, habits, movements, and so forth can shape and rewire our brains whether we're aware of this process or not. It occurs both passively and actively. If we lead socially bereft, unstimulated lives, our brains will atrophy over time. Conversely, leading socially enriched, stimulating lives can protect our brains.[6] Evidence suggests that we can even consciously choose to heal and strengthen our brains after neurodegeneration has occurred from disease or traumatic injury.[7] You are the master of your fate; you are the captain of your *brain.*

CREATE YOUR TRIBE. The strength and breadth of your social interactions play a huge part in how well you're likely to age and even how long you're likely to live. Research found that those with strong social bonds were 50 per cent less likely to die than those with a weaker social network.[8] Social connectivity is as important as other accepted risk factors, such as diet, exercise, and sleep for healthy ageing.[9] Additionally, those who are married, exchange support with family members, have contact with friends, participate in community groups, and engaged in paid work are 46 per cent less likely to develop dementia.[10]

It's worth noting that social connectedness is a subjective experience. Some with few friends or family members can be perfectly content, while others with a broader support system can still feel lonely. It's your perception that colours your experience.

- **Take stock of your feelings of loneliness or isolation.** Do you have someone to call on if you are sick, are having a financial crisis, or simply want to hang out? If not, you may want to spend some time and energy expanding your social network. The ability to create a "tribe" has nothing to do with the size of your family or their geographic closeness. You needn't lament the fact that you're an only child, don't have children, or live far away from family members. The people in your life—your friends, co-workers, and neighbours—can become your tribe.
- **Connect to the people you're exposed to every day.** That's how friendships are born. Don't wait for others to reach out

to you. Reach out to them. Ask questions. Be interested in their lives. Offer to help them. Join a book club or exercise class. Volunteer for a social cause. Having a shared goal or interest can create the basis for a stronger relationship.

- **Prioritize actual meet-ups, as opposed to connecting through social media.** Statistics show that the average American is devoting almost eleven hours a day to screen time.[11] As people spend time on social media, their social lives are shrinking, and they feel lonelier than ever. The neuropeptide oxytocin, the "love hormone" that plays a powerful role in social bonding, is released during actual human interaction.[12] Cortisol, the stress hormone, is reduced when we connect.[13] Our brains are stimulated and engaged in positive ways that aren't present when we communicate through text or email.[14] Human interaction may be even more important as we age. A rich social life can offer meaningful protection against cognitive decline.[15]

- **Create meetings that promote a healthy lifestyle.** We all have friends who like to meet for a late-night supper or for cocktails or dessert—*none of which support your new healthy lifestyle.* Feel free to suggest alternative options. Suggest meeting for morning coffee, a healthy cookery class, or a walk instead. These activities may encourage your existing group of friends to become healthier with you, or you may naturally drift towards a new set of friends who share your new goals. It's important to surround yourself with people who make it easy for you to adhere to your new healthier way of living.

- **Consider co-habitating with like-minded friends.** As we become less capable of accomplishing all of the tasks associated with independent living and home ownership, it's tempting to automatically consider moving in with family or to an assisted living facility. Of course neither of these is automatically the wrong choice. But a growing number of seniors are choosing to live together in a communal arrangement to pool resources. Imagine the TV show *The Golden Girls* with a healthful twist—sharing organic veggies instead of cheesecake! Living with like-minded friends can also offer a host of social benefits and extend your functional independence.

FIND YOUR PURPOSE. Your life may depend upon it. Research has found that having a purpose in life is a strong determinant of both overall health and mortality. This holds true across our life-spans, providing the same benefit for every age group. Having a passion, an overall set of values and drivers, may be even more important as we age. Adults who leave the workplace and seek organization in their daily schedule may benefit the most from having a greater sense of purpose.

Evidence shows that older adults who have a strong sense of purpose display the same physical brain changes as their less purposeful counterparts, *but score much higher on cognitive testing*.[16] Nurturing what excites you offers powerful neuroprotection. Whether it's volunteering at your local humane society, writing poetry, or mentoring young people, go for it. Having a passion, especially later in life, can extend your health span and your brain.

NEVER STOP LEARNING. The amount of education one has is emerging as a predictor of cognitive decline. Those with more education are less likely to develop dementia.[17] This may have to do with a concept called cognitive reserve. This refers to the idea that those who have greater exposure to education may be more resilient to the natural brain changes that occur with ageing.[18] Does that mean you're doomed if you had a limited amount of education? Absolutely not! Evidence suggests that everyone can derive cognitive benefit from learning at all stages of life.[19]

Building reserve may require a reframing of our current mindset. Too often, when faced with a challenging task, such as setting up new technology, we're tempted to turn it over to a professional (or young person), especially as we age. No more. Look at these everyday challenges as *opportunities* for you to expand your neural connections and build up your cognitive reserve. This is a part of creating a growth mindset as we age as opposed to a mere conservation (or even worse, downsizing) mindset. Actively look for ways to expand your cognitive reserve.

- **Take a class.** Many seniors may not have had the opportunity to enroll in post-secondary education, but it's never too late. There may even be benefits to taking a college course later in life. Seniors typically don't have to worry about SATs or entrance essays. Some universities even offer tuition waivers for older students. The University of the Third Age is a UK-wide movement that brings together people in their "third age" to develop their interests and continue their learning in a friendly and informal environment. Many community colleges tailor classes specifically for seniors. These classes may not be free but are usually discounted. You might even be eligible for a tax benefit from enrolling in higher education. You could consider auditing a class, which simply means that you get to enjoy the benefit of attending lectures without paying for the class or having the stress of turning in assignments and taking tests. There are also many online opportunities for continuing education. Additionally, many local libraries and senior community centres also offer educational opportunities. Learning later in life can reduce gaps in earlier education history and help to build cognitive reserve.[20]
- **Learn a foreign language.** Lifelong bilingualism may increase cognitive reserve and delay onset of dementia between four and five years.[21] The number of languages you speak could even offer added protection.[22] These findings have been mixed, however, suggesting that education and cultural differences may be playing a part in the varied conclusions.[23] Nonetheless, imaging consistently shows that bilingual seniors have more grey matter in the executive function and language processing regions of the brain.[24] Learning an additional language later in life also appears to offer

neuroprotection. A small study using a one-week-long intensive Gaelic language intervention found a significant cognitive improvement in attention switching for all age groups that was maintained even nine months later, but only for the participants who practised five hours a week or more.[25] A study that controlled for intelligence by performing an IQ test at age 11 and then again at age 70 found that learning a second language led to significantly better cognitive abilities even if that language was acquired in adulthood.[26] It's especially fun and meaningful to learn a new language prior to travelling to a foreign country. Many people report enhanced learning simply by being immersed in the new language and culture. One-on-one or group lessons are widely available (depending upon the language), and online options are gaining in popularity, with Rosetta Stone and Babbel among the programmes earning top marks.[27] We also know that it's extraordinarily powerful to combine interventions. Why not plug in your earbuds and use a language-learning app to learn Spanish during your power walk? ¡No hayproblema!

- **Learn to play a musical instrument.** Thank your parents if you learned to play a musical instrument as a child. Research shows that those who did have a reduced risk of developing cognitive decline as they age.[28] The number of years one studied even plays a part—the more years, the greater the reduction even if the lessons occurred more than forty years ago.[29] Those lucky enough to have begun playing before age seven created more white matter connectivity that serves as a scaffold upon which ongoing experiences can build.[30] Even if you never had the opportunity to play an instrument as a child, you can still benefit by learning now. A study using twins to control for other genetic factors found that the twin with musical knowledge *in older adulthood* was 36 per cent less likely to develop dementia.[31] Evidence suggests that music stimulates the brain and enhances memory in older people.

In one study, adults aged 60 to 85 without previous musical experience showed improved processing speed and verbal fluency after a few months of weekly piano lessons.[32]

If you're inspired to start playing, choose an instrument that aligns with the type of music you enjoy. A good way to find a competent instructor is to visit a retail shop where musical instruments are sold. As this trend of embracing musicianship later in life grows, many establishments offer classes specifically for older adults. Group lessons and ensemble playing also offer an opportunity to add a fun social component, increasing the benefit.

- **Do puzzles.** Challenge your brain for fun! A recent study found that the more people over the age of fifty engaged in challenges like sudoku and crosswords, the better their brains functioned. In fact, those who did these types of puzzles were found to have brain function equivalent to ten years younger than their age, with speed and accuracy showing the greatest gains.[33]

LISTEN TO MUSIC. Even if you're not quite ready to begin playing an instrument, simply listening to music may offer some cognitive benefits. A recent study using functional brain imaging showed that dementia patients who were exposed to music that they had previously enjoyed demonstrated much higher levels of functional connectivity in several regions of the brain.[34] Music stimulates deep neural connections that activate many regions of the brain, including the medial prefrontal cortex (regarded as a region of the brain that supports self-referential processes) and the limbic (known to be associated with emotions). This may help explain why listening to music evokes feelings connected with prior experiences and awakens memories from the time period when you last heard a particular song. Familiar music, even from decades ago, in essence provides the soundtrack for the replay of forgotten memories.[35]

A Finnish study has shown that listening to classical music

positively affects gene expression profiles. The activity of genes involved in dopamine secretion and transport, synaptic function, learning, and memory was enhanced by simply listening to Mozart's Violin Concerto No.3.[36] One mechanism by which music may provide neuroprotection is through the induction of neurogenesis through hormone optimization. Listening to music has been demonstrated to reduce cortisol levels and enhance oestrogen and testosterone levels.[37]

Turn off the TV and listen to music instead. Music can enhance your exercise, household chores, or even work experience. You can always use earbuds or headphones when you're in close proximity to others or to simply improve the listening experience. Choose music to suit your mood and activity. Invigorating rock and roll or rousing classical music is great for working out. There are even apps such as RockMyRun and GYM Radio that curate specially chosen music to enhance your workout. Pzizz is another app that offers music specifically created to help you focus, concentrate, and de-stress, as well as sleep.

DANCE. There's a surprising amount of evidence that suggests dancing offers cognitive benefit. We're not talking about putting on your favourite music and rocking out, although that's great exercise, but rather about learning and performing specific dances with a partner. The combination of physical exercise (which on its own is neuroprotective) plus the cognitive element of learning and remembering a new dance, integrated with the social aspect of coordinating with a partner and responding to his or her cues, appears to offer enhanced neuroprotection. Memorizing the steps alone is not enough to challenge the brain; it's the novelty of responding to your partner and creating your unique combined artistic expression that appears to promote new neural pathways. Dancing integrates multiple brain functions, simultaneously expanding neural connectivity. Indeed, a recent study imaged the brains of seasoned ballroom dancers compared to novices and found the dancers to have elevated neural activity in sensorimotor regions and functional alterations demonstrating higher levels of neuroplasticity.[38]

A study published in *The New England Journal of Medicine* examined the leisure activities of a group of senior citizens over a period of several decades and found that dancing provided the greatest risk reduction (76 per cent) of any activity studied, cognitive or physical.[39] Another recent study using a group of seniors compared the benefits of a six-month intervention of conventional rigorous exercise versus a challenging dance programme with novel and increasingly difficult choreography. Those who engaged in the dance intervention demonstrated larger volume increases in multiple brain regions as well as an increase in BDNF levels.[40] Need more evidence? A group of adults over age 60 with mild cognitive impairment (MCI) were randomized to either a control group or a twice-weekly challenging dance intervention. After forty-eight weeks, the dancers showed significant improvements in multiple cognitive assessments.[41]

Consider changing up date night and dusting off your dancing shoes. Learning the fox-trot, tango, and rumba is not only fun but may also provide the perfect combination of athleticism, cognitive challenge, and social interaction to promote neuroplasticity.

TRAIN YOUR BRAIN. Several recent studies suggest we can actively challenge our brains at any age to create neuroplasticity by using online brain-training programmes. BrainHQ from Posit Science has the most scientific research supporting its efficacy. The IMPACT study, with 487 cognitively normal participants aged 65 or older, was the first large-scale clinical trial to examine whether cognitive exercises can make a difference in memory and processing speed. Participants were either randomized to engage in forty hours of six auditory exercises chosen from among the BrainHQ repertoire or watch forty hours of educational DVDs with quizzes afterward to test knowledge. Auditory memory and attention was significantly greater in the brain-training group, as were multiple secondary measures. More impressive was the comparison from baseline for those who engaged in the brain-training intervention. Auditory memory improved an equivalent of ten years, auditory processing speed was increased by 131 per cent, and most important, the intervention spilled over into their daily lives, with 75 per cent reporting positive changes.[42]

That last finding is key to understanding whether or not computerized cognitive training is spilling over into daily life. Critics suggest that brain games make players smarter only in the trained domain.[43] Proving that acquired skills actually have an effect on daily life and thus contribute to preventing or remediating cognitive decline is more difficult. Three out of four of the IMPACT study participants who took part in the computerized training reported improvements ranging from remembering a shopping list without having to write it down, to hearing conversations in noisy restaurants more clearly, to being more independent and feeling more self-confident, to finding words more easily and having improved self-esteem in general. These are impressive findings, but considering that the intervention was only eight weeks long, it doesn't establish evidence that this type of intervention can have an effect on onset of cognitive decline with this study.

The ACTIVE study, one of the largest studies to examine cognitive training effects, took a longitudinal look at the evidence. They used a data set of more than 2,800 people, between 74 and 84, with limited (if any) cognitive decline, spread across six different sites in the United States. Folks were randomized into one of four interventions: memory instruction, reasoning instruction, a speed intervention using a computer game, and a control group with no intervention. Interventions occurred in small groups, led by a trainer in ten 60- to 75-minute sessions over a five- to six-week period. Some of the participants received periodic booster sessions. The participants had their cognitive and functional capabilities tested during the first six weeks of the study and then again after one, two, three, five, and finally ten years.

The most dramatic improvement was seen using a speed of processing computerized exercise focusing on increasing the player's useful field of view. Gamers briefly saw a car in the centre of the screen with a road sign somewhere in the periphery. They were tasked with correctly identifying the car and noting where the sign appeared. As the player's proficiency increased, the game became increasingly more difficult, with the time the car and sign were shown decreasing while multiple distractions were introduced. The risk of developing dementia was 29 per cent lower for participants who engaged in this speed of processing training than for those who were in the control group. Additionally, the benefits of the training were stronger for those who underwent booster training. The memory and reasoning training interventions also showed benefits for reducing dementia risk, but those results were not statistically significant.[44]

BrainHQ has replicated this game, called Double Decision, and now offers it as a part of their online training. It is one among several other speed exercises designed to enhance cognition. Other areas of focus include attention, memory, people skills, intelligence, and navigation. You can pick a specific area that you want to work on or randomly work in multiple categories. The creators of the site recommend that you try to get ninety minutes in every week. Many people aim for three or four thirty-minute sessions per week, but each exercise is broken up into two-minute bites so that you can easily squeeze it into your daily schedule. You're able to track your progress and compare your results to age-matched peers. Be careful not to get too competitive with yourself so that you increase your stress level. The amount of sleep you've had, a virus, your general stress level, and many other factors can affect your performance. Keep it fun and note trends over time as opposed to changes in your scores over one or two days. BrainHQ is an excellent way to monitor your progress.

RESIST DOWNSIZING; UPSIZE INSTEAD! We've outlined many different ways that you can challenge your brain, everything from staying socially engaged to finding your passion to pursuing lifelong learning, using the arts (music and dance) as well as computerized brain training. Pick a few strategies and incorporate them into your everyday life. The most important thing is to reframe your perspective on ageing. Resist looking at getting older as a time of retirement or mental downsizing; instead consider it a time for growth. So much of our lives are spent fulfilling obligations: caring for family, earning a living, and so forth. Our responsibilities typically lighten as we get older. This is the perfect time to focus on all of the areas of interest that you may not have had a chance to pursue. Meet new people, learn new things, embrace music and dance, follow your passion. Doing so will not only enrich your life but may also increase your health span. For those who wish to further explore this topic, we recommend *The Brain That Changes Itself* by Norman Doidge.

CHAPTER 17

Oral Health: The Whole Tooth and Nothing but the Tooth

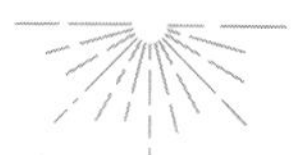

Every time you get the world by the tail,

you gotta remember there are teeth on the other end.

—SHARON LEE

ALTHOUGH IT MAY SOUND strange, in a sense you can think of Alzheimer's disease as a success story, albeit a temporary one—by the time you receive a diagnosis of Alzheimer's disease, your brain has been protecting itself quite effectively for a few decades. If it had not done so, your cognition would very likely have been damaged much earlier by the insults to which you are exposed. As I described earlier, the insults may come from several different sources, such as insulin resistance due to sugar intake, or leaky gut, or toxins from specific moulds such as *Stachybotrys* (toxic black mould) or *Penicillium*. However, what is emerging as one of the most important sources for the insults associated with cognitive decline is—you guessed it—your mouth. Sustenance flows in, and loving words flow out, but unfortunately, while providing such critical functions, your mouth and lips also harbour multiple contributors to cognitive decline: (1) mercury amalgams[1]; (2) *Herpes simplex* (the virus of "cold sores"[2]); (3) periodontitis[3]; (4) gingivitis[4]; (5) root canals (although this potential contributor remains controversial); (6) the oral microbiome.[5]

Let's take a look at each of these and determine how to address each one in order to prevent or reverse cognitive decline.

MERCURY AMALGAMS Here we are talking about the old-fashioned silver fillings, which contain approximately 55 per cent mercury. Each amalgam filling releases about 10 micrograms of mercury into your circulation each day. Unlike the mercury from seafood, which is organic mercury, the mercury from dental amalgams is inorganic mercury (although it may be converted to organic mercury in the gut). You can distinguish these two forms by evaluating urine, blood, and hair, and that is what is done with the Mercury Tri-Test from Quicksilver. However, both organic and inorganic mercury can contribute ultimately to cognitive decline, so it is important to test for mercury toxicity. One of the confusing aspects of mercury toxicity related to dental amalgams is that there is no simple linear relationship between how many amalgams you have in your mouth and how much mercury leaks from the amalgams, since some leak more than others. Rather, it is the surface area of the amalgams that correlates better with leak.

Therefore, it is recommended that anyone with a high inorganic mercury level, or with cognitive decline, have his/her amalgams removed. This is not as simple as it might sound. During the removal process, you may be exposed to an increased level of mercury, and therefore, the best approach is to have the amalgams removed by a special biological dentist who has experience with the prevention of mercury exposure during amalgam removal. Furthermore, it is best to have only one or two amalgams removed at a sitting, then to wait a few months before removing the next one or two, and repeat this until all have been removed, so that any exposure is minimized and your body has time to excrete any mercury that accumulates at the time of removal.

COLD SORES These are typically caused by *Herpes simplex* type 1 (HSV-1), although they may also be from HSV-2. Cold sores are extremely common, and their recurrent appearance indicates that the *Herpes* virus is living in our nerve cells in the trigeminal ganglion, which is the group of nerve cells that provides feeling to our faces. Fortunately, this does not seem to cause any long-term damage to our nerve cells; unfortunately, these same ganglion cells have two arms, the one that reaches our lips and faces, and another that reaches up into our brains, thus providing access to our brains for these same viruses—literally, the virus can "climb down" one arm of the cell to get to our lips, or "climb up" the other arm to get to our brain.

Dr Ruth Itzhaki has spent her career studying this important potential relationship between *Herpes* viruses and Alzheimer's disease, and has pointed out that *Herpes* treatment should be considered in patients with Alzheimer's disease. A very compelling study from Taiwan found that people who had recurrent outbreaks of *Herpes* had a markedly lower level of nearly 80 per cent in their development of dementia if the outbreaks were treated. Therefore, suppressing these outbreaks may very well be helpful in the overall plan to minimize dementia, and there are several ways to do this.

The use of acyclovir or valacyclovir is one very effective way to prevent outbreaks, as well as treating outbreaks once they occur. These drugs have minimal toxicity and are generally well tolerated, and therefore some people take them for months or even years. Typical doses are 500 mg or 1000 mg orally, once or twice per day.

Other people prefer to suppress with a non-pharmaceutical approach, such as taking lysine, humic acid, or fulvic acid. However, a complementary approach is to enhance your immune system, supporting the natural antiviral effects of your immune system. There are numerous compounds that support immunity, such as *Tinospora cordifolia*, AHCC (active hexose correlated compound), propolis, Manuka honey, berberine (which also reduces glucose and is often used to treat type 2 diabetes), low-dose naltrexone, thymosin alpha-1, and Transfer Factor PlasMyc.

PERIODONTITIS This is the term for inflammation around the teeth, with associated gum retraction, and it is caused by infections with different bacteria, such as *Porphyromonas gingivalis* (*P. gingivalis*), *Treponema denticola*, *Fusobacterium nucleatum*, and *Prevotella intermedia*, among others. When your teeth and gums are healthy, these pathogenic bacteria are minimized, but when your teeth and gums are unhealthy, these damaging species can set up residence and invade.

And here's the shock: although these bacteria had always been thought to be confined to the mouth, they are turning up all over the body, in surprising associations with several different diseases, including the plaques of cardiovascular disease, the proliferating cells of cancers, and the brains of patients with Alzheimer's disease. These findings suggest that the oral bacteria are gaining access to our bloodstreams and finding their way to our blood vessel cells, thus contributing to cardiovascular disease; to our organs, thus contributing to cancer; and to our brains, thus contributing to cognitive decline. These realizations are fuelling a whole new field of oral-systemic care and expertise, as pointed out by Dr Charles Whitney—just as in our studies of Alzheimer's disease and its relation to our overall systemic health, we must consider our oral health in relation to our chronic systemic diseases as well.

Therefore, when you are taking care of your dentition, you are helping to prevent cognitive decline. Please consider these steps to give yourself the best chance for cognitive success:

- Talk to your dentist about a test for these pathogenic bacteria (*P. gingivalis* et al.), such as OralDNA. This will tell you whether you have high levels of these dangerous bacteria, and will give you an idea about your overall oral microbiome.
- If you do find high levels of the pathogenic bacteria, you may wish to use Dentalcidin toothpaste and mouthwash to reduce these, and also talk to your dentist about steps to reduce these microbes.
- Using a water flosser and an electric toothbrush helps to improve overall oral health.
- You may want to try oil pulling, which is easy—you swish coconut oil between your teeth for about ten minutes each day, and this also helps to reduce bacteria associated with tooth decay.
- If you have root canals, these may be sources of chronic infection, so please talk to your dentist about evaluation and potential removal.

- If you have gingivitis—inflammation of your gums, often associated with bleeding gums—and this continues after you have treated your pathogens, then your gingivitis may be due to mouth breathing.
- Just as there are benefits to optimizing your gut microbiome, there are also benefits to optimizing your oral microbiome, such as reducing the pathogenic bacteria, and there are now oral probiotics available, such as *Streptococcus salivarius*.

These steps should minimize your pathogenic oral bacteria, reduce periodontitis and gingivitis, improve your oral microbiome, prevent tooth decay, enhance the look of your teeth and gums, and minimize the access of oral pathogens to your brain, thus helping to prevent cognitive decline.

CHAPTER 18

Translating Data into Success

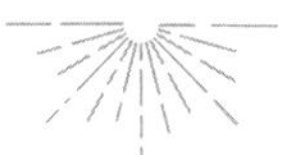

It's never too late to be what you might have been.
—GEORGE ELIOT

FINDING YOUR TEAM

1. **Become your own health advocate.** Simply by reading this book, you have taken great strides to protect your brain health by becoming educated about the many factors that can influence it. With this education, you can become your own health advocate. You have learned about the importance of avoiding insulin resistance, nutritional and hormonal deficiencies, inflammation, toxins, and more. You know the optimal biomarker goals you need to achieve and are able to track and tweak them as you progress on your health journey.
2. **Find a like-minded tribe.** Those who are working on prevention or who are becoming concerned about minor cognitive changes may be able to work within a supportive online community such as that offered by the non-profit ApoE4.Info. Most of the subscribers to this website carry one or two copies of the ApoE4 gene and are proactively using individualized protocols that follow the model we describe. Members include ordinary people of all ages and cognitive abilities,

academics, scientists, doctors, and other healthcare professionals. Their common goal is that everyone is focused upon cognitive health. They regularly share their N-of-1 experiments, analyze the latest medical research, and generally support one another on their health journeys. Many of the members order their own medical tests and regularly track and tweak their biomarkers. (See "Tools for Success" on the next page to find direct-to-consumer laboratory testing options.)

3. **Partner with a traditional healthcare professional.** Ideally, you'll be able to find a local doctor who is willing to partner with you (if you live in the UK you may have to seek out a private practitioner and pay for the consultations). It's often best to approach doctors with whom you've already established a respectful and trusting relationship. Some patients report sharing a copy of *The End of Alzheimer's* and receiving a positive reaction. Indeed, there are many smart, compassionate, and caring doctors, doctors' assistants, and nurse practitioners who may be willing to partner with you. It's often helpful to bring a partner or friend with you when making this initial outreach. Simply having a supportive person with you shows your level of concern and adds to the gravity of your request. Many of the biomarker tests we recommend are very easy for traditional healthcare professionals to order and are reimbursable by medical insurance (this may not be the case in the UK).
4. **Consider partnering with a functional medicine practitioner.** If you're unable to find a traditional GP to partner with you, you may want to consider using a functional medicine practitioner. These are licenced medical professionals in their specialities (including some medical doctors, naturopathic doctors, osteopathic doctors, chiropractic doctors, nurse practitioners, or physician assistants) who take additional course training that focuses on finding the root cause of disease within a patient-centred integrative science-based healthcare approach. Additionally, licensed nutritionists,

dietitians, health coaches, mental health professionals, and others can also receive functional medicine certifications. It may be helpful to use the advanced search engine to include a speciality on which you'd like to focus. Initial appointments are typically an hour or more in length, as opposed to a standard seven- to fifteen-minute allopathic doctor's visit. The longer appointments enable the practitioner to obtain a complete patient history to guide treatment. Many functional medicine practitioners often partner with health coaches and nutritionists who can also help to guide you. The downside of working with a functional medicine practitioner is that many insurance providers either won't cover these practitioners or require a separate deductible that you have to reach before covering their service. Some functional medicine practitioners do work with patients to get as many tests as possible covered through their traditional medical insurance policies. Less commonly, some accept traditional medical insurance, even Medicare in the US. It's best to communicate with their offices directly to make inquiries about billing so that you can properly anticipate the expense.

5. **Consider using the services of Apollo Health (www.apollohealthco.com).** This group offers a "cognoscopy" directly to patients and has created a brain health community that offers new information on best treatment of cognitive decline, brain training, cognitive assessment, nutritional information, and other support. If your results reveal areas of concern or you are interested in prevention, you can join their subscription service, which connects you with a doctor who's been trained by Dr Bredesen, as well as many other supportive features.

TOOLS FOR SUCCESS

Integral with this approach is the ongoing data collection that quantifies your progress. We want you to collect data along your journey to help you optimize your health continuously to protect your cognition. You needn't just *hope* that you're on the right track. We want you to track and tweak your choices based upon real-time feedback and periodic laboratory and cognitive testing. We list everything from very basic tools to extravagances. Some tools, such as the dual glucose and ketone meter, are initially important for assessing your baseline but will become less important as your journey progresses. Don't worry about getting everything on our list. We encourage you to read the handbook first and thoughtfully think about the tools you already have, those that will be most helpful to you initially, those you can put off, and others you simply don't need. We recognize that everyone is coming to this programme at different stages. Some of you will already be practising some (or even many) of the strategies outlined in the handbook. Kudos! Focus on the tools that you think will enhance your journey. Be aware that your need for various tools will evolve as your journey progresses.

JOURNAL We strongly encourage you to use a journal that will allow you to track the many changes you'll be making on your journey. Regardless of the pace at which you adopt your new lifestyle, you (or your spouse or caretaker) need to become your own *principal investigator,* a term used for scientists conducting clinical trials. It's helpful to track your *before* and *after* while applying each intervention. A journal allows you to track positive and negative side effects to various strategies and also to identify *confounders,* other influences that may be playing a part in how you react. Journaling enables you to track your progress and to make adjustments as necessary.

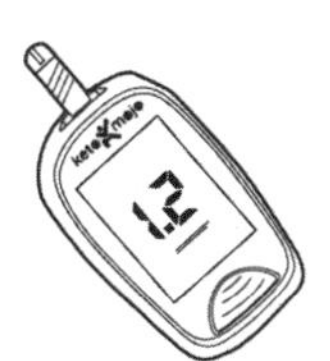

DUAL-PURPOSE METER TO MEASURE GLUCOSE AND KETONES This is a small handheld device that uses a drop of blood obtained by a *lancet* (a penlike instrument with a tiny spring-loaded needle on one end) to test your glucose level and ketone level by using separate paper strips. It's important to use a system that accurately measures both glucose and ketones (especially low levels of BHB). The Precision Xtra and the Keto-Mojo blood glucose and ketone monitoring systems both work well. The testing strips for the Keto-Mojo system are considerably less expensive, but similar prices can be found for the Precision Xtra strips by searching the Internet for bargains. You'll find the use of your dual glucose/ketone meter is extremely helpful initially to assess your numbers and to help you keto-adapt. After this period, you'll need to use it only periodically for check-ins or when something feels different. (Pro tip: When compared to blood testing, urine ketone testing strips are *not* accurate for measuring low levels of BHB. Breath ketone meters measure acetone, another type of ketone, but can be skewed by methane from some carbohydrates like resistant starch and/or alcoholic beverages, providing inconsistent results.)

How to use glucose measurements

- If you're diabetic and taking medication to reduce your blood sugar, enlist the help of your doctor *before* beginning this programme. The KetoFLEX 12/3 programme will ultimately reduce or eliminate the need for your medication, but your doctor needs to instruct you on how to reduce your dosage as your blood glucose levels improve.
- Record your blood glucose measurements so that you can track your progress. Measuring your glucose provides you with real-time data to track how your body is responding to a given food or meal.
- Always follow manufacturer's instructions for how to perform a glucose test. Glucose testing strips are inexpensive and widely available.
- It's helpful to test fasting morning glucose before coffee, supplements, or medications. Your goal is a reading between 70 and 90 mg/dL (3.89–5.00 mmol/L).
- If your reading is within that range, you are likely insulin sensitive. You needn't perform postprandial (after-meal) checks at *every* meal unless you want to check your response to a specific food. Continue testing fasting morning blood glucose for a week or two to see if you continue to stay in

range. If you have occasional lapses, move on to postprandial checks.

- If your reading is higher than the recommended range, perform regular postprandial checks after each meal so that you can identify the foods that are causing your glucose spikes and make adjustments to your diet.
- A postprandial test is typically performed at one hour, then at two hours after finishing a meal. Some people experience delayed glucose elevation, so it's often a good idea to do the second test even if the first one is within range.
- One hour after finishing a meal, your blood glucose should be 90–125 mg/dL (5.00–6.94 mmol/L). Two hours after a meal, your goal is 90–110 mg/dL (5.00–6.11 mmol/L). Five hours after a typical meal, your blood glucose should return to the fasted range of 70–90 mg/dL (3.89–5.00 mmol/L).
- If your readings are higher than the stated goals, it's helpful to identify the foods that are causing the hyperglycaemic response. Obvious culprits are anything with glucose or fructose, even "healthy" sweets like fruit. Starchy carbohydrates such as white potatoes, rice, oats, pasta, and bread are common triggers. Even sweet potatoes can cause a spike; hence, they are recommended for use only in small quantities. Other typical culprits are resistant starches, such as legumes, and quinoa. Additionally, the macronutrient context of your meal can contribute to higher readings. Carbohydrates or even protein in excess should be suspected.
- Try replacing the suspected trigger with healthy fats (EVOO, olives, avocados, nuts, and seeds) or non-starchy vegetables at your next meal. Repeat your postprandial testing and record your body's response.
- Be aware that *everyone* has a different glycaemic response to the same food, one based on genetics, general state of health, gut microbiome status, stress levels, and myriad other factors. You may even have a variable response to the same food due to extraneous contributors, such as stress, poor sleep,

hormone status, and multiple other factors. Identifying and addressing your triggers will help you to heal.

- Once you've keto-adapted—that is, switched from burning primarily glucose to burning fat—your fasting morning glucose may rise a bit over time. Concurrently checking ketones can offer you reassurance. Their presence (>0.5 mM) indicates that this is likely of little consequence, especially if your haemoglobin A1c and fasting insulin levels remain within range.
- After you've been keto-adapted for weeks, you may wish to transition to a glucose-burning state for a day each week by adding more approved carbohydrates so that your body maintains metabolic flexibility. The ability to transition back and forth seamlessly from a glucose-based fuel to a fat-based fuel is called metabolic flexibility and is a sign of optimal health. You may notice a cognitive fogginess that accompanies this transition out of ketosis. Be sure to track this cognitive change in your journal and switch back to your typical ketogenic diet at your next meal.
- Your blood glucose may be elevated temporarily following exercise. Your liver responds to the energy demands of exercise by releasing more glucose. This is typically inconsequential and will quickly drop down to your pre-exercise level or even lower.

How to use ketone measurements

- You may not generate your own ketones (this is *endogenous* ketosis, the long-term goal) very well until your fasting glucose falls within the goal range of 70–90 mg/dL (3.89–5.00 mmol/L), which may take weeks to months depending on your level of insulin resistance. Using ketone supplements (coconut oil, MCT oil, or ketone salts or esters) before this time (*exogenous* ketosis) is an excellent transitional option and will temporarily put you into ketosis, but you will not be keto-adapted at this stage.

- Measuring blood ketone levels can provide you with real-time data to help determine whether you are burning glucose or fat as your primary source of fuel—ketones indicate that you are burning fat.
- Be sure to follow the manufacturer's instructions. Ketone testing strips are more expensive than glucose strips. Once you've become keto-adapted, you will learn to feel the difference and will no longer need to test on a regular basis. You may want to record the changes in your cognition, mood, and energy with different BHB levels.
- When your fasting blood glucose is in range, you can begin checking your fasting ketone level at the same time that you check your fasting morning glucose. You can often use the same finger stick if you act quickly. This might be difficult at first but will become easier over time. Be aware that this is when BHB is typically at the *lowest* level, for a variety of reasons. Any level >0.5 mM is in range for a fasting morning test.
- *For the purpose of healing insulin resistance and improving cognition, your goal is to maintain a ketone level between 0.5 and 4.0 mM.* The higher end of this level may ultimately be necessary for those with more advanced symptoms, 1.0–4.0 mM. Lower levels may be more appropriate for those at risk or working on prevention. Your response will help you find levels that are right for you.
- As you extend your fast, your BHB level will rise even higher. When glycogen stores are depleted, those who are metabolically flexible will begin creating ketone bodies as an alternative fuel.
- You may want to test BHB prior to breaking your fast. It should be higher than your fasting morning level and may even be at the peak for the day.
- When you exercise, your BHB levels may temporarily drop due to the extra glucose released by the liver to meet the demand of exercise. This is temporary and inconsequential. Exercise ultimately puts you into a higher level of ketosis after recovery.

- Eating a diet that is low in carbohydrate, with adequate protein and lots of healthy fats, as described in the Brain Food Pyramid, will help you to sustain and increase your BHB levels throughout the day.
- If your BHB levels drop after eating, it may indicate that you are eating an excess of carbohydrates or protein and not enough healthy fat.
- For some, depending on your metabolic health, fasting, exercise, and eating schedule, testing ketones at the end of the day yields the highest BHB level because you've had an opportunity to apply all three KetoFLEX 12/3 strategies: fasting, exercise, and diet.
- Once you've been keto-adapted for a while, pay attention to anything that feels different: a sense of being hungrier than usual, a dip in cognition or energy, or a change in mood. These may be clues that you've shifted out of ketosis and back to burning glucose.
- Being hungrier than usual may also be a sign of weight loss. Use your body weight scale to check. If you are losing too much weight, follow our "Strategies for Gaining Weight" outlined in chapter 8.
- Many other factors, such as poor sleep, stress, or illness may affect ketone levels. If you suddenly have difficulty getting into ketosis, go back to the beginning of these guidelines to readapt. It's usually fairly easy once your body has become used to burning fat as fuel. Some find it helpful to use small amounts of coconut oil or MCT transiently during the re-adaptation process.

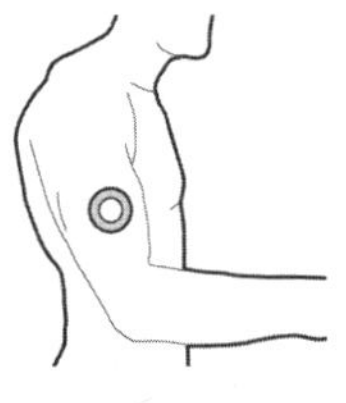

CONTINUOUS GLUCOSE MONITORING (CGM) This is a system that can offer valuable insight for everyone. It allows you to track glucose every 1 to 10 minutes for up to fourteen days. A tiny sensor is placed under your skin (as a relatively painless patch on your arm) that transmits data to your reader, smart phone, or watch, providing real-time data so you can see the effect a specific food is having on your glucose. CGM also enables you to monitor your glucose while you sleep, often alerting you to hypoglycaemic episodes. CGM is relatively inexpensive but requires a prescription from a doctor. It is often covered by insurance, including Medicare in the US. This is not widely available in the UK under the NHS; seek out a private practitioner if you are interested in trying this device.

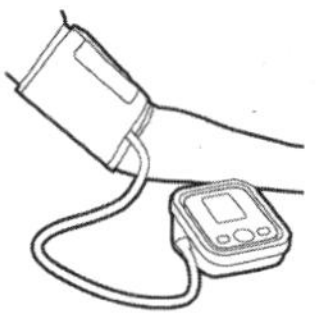

ACCURATE BODY WEIGHT SCALE You needn't spend a lot of money. Just be sure that your scale is accurate by validating it against the scale in your doctor's office. Be sure to weigh yourself in the same clothes (around the same time of day) on their scale and yours. It's very easy to lose weight with the KetoFLEX 12/3 lifestyle. If that's a goal, terrific. If it's not (or you've already achieved your optimal weight), see "Strategies for Gaining Weight," page 98, for tips on how to maintain or even gain weight. Too much weight loss, a BMI <18.5 for women and <19 for men, can actually be counterproductive to your cognitive health.

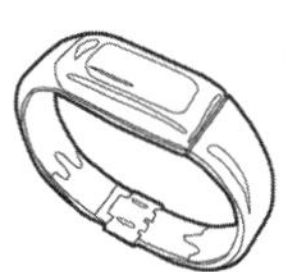

PEDOMETER A pedometer is a small portable device that helps you measure your activity level by counting every step you take through the motion of your walking (or running) cadence. Pedometer instructions will often tell you to calibrate the device for accuracy. Do so using the stride that is most common for you. We recommend a very inexpensive non-Wi-Fi unit to protect against electromagnetic field exposure while you exercise. It's very tempting to use popular high-tech versions, and it's fine to do so, but just remember that they do expose you to small amounts of radiation.

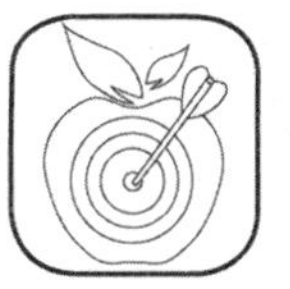

CRONOMETER Cronometer is a free online food diary that offers a variety of helpful features, including the ability to track macronutrient ratios. (Macronutrients are simply foods we require in large quantities—proteins, fats, and carbohydrates.) See the "Tracking Macronutrient Ratios" section for instructions. This can be helpful for those who are initially trying to reach ketosis.

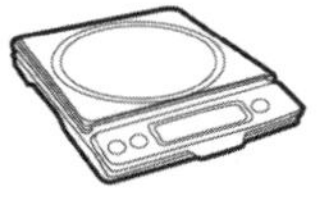

DIGITAL FOOD SCALE If you decide to track your macronutrient ratios, you may wish to invest in a good-quality food scale. You'll save a lot of time rather than trying to measure food the old-fashioned way. These are relatively inexpensive, less than £15, and well worth the expense. Most will allow you to change the unit of measurement—for example, grams or ounces—to match Cronometer. You also have a tare function that enables you to pre-weigh your container, and with the subsequent measurement, the scale will automatically subtract it, thus directly providing the weight for the food.

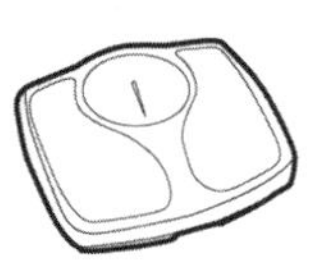

BLOOD PRESSURE MONITOR An automatic home blood pressure monitor can be helpful to track your progress. Blood pressure monitors may also be available at most pharmacies. This is important for those who are taking medication for *hypertension* (high blood pressure) and also for those who experience *hypotension* (low blood pressure). Accurate automatic home blood pressure monitors are inexpensive and widely available. The KetoFLEX 12/3 lifestyle will reduce your blood pressure, ultimately negating the need for medication. If you begin the programme taking medication to reduce your blood pressure, combined with the KetoFLEX 12/3 approach, it may drift *too* low. Symptoms include light-headedness and fatigue. Carefully monitor to see when you need to discuss a reduction in medication with your doctor. If you already have low blood pressure, be aware that it may drop even lower. Ensuring that you have an adequate amount of sodium in your diet can easily alleviate symptoms.

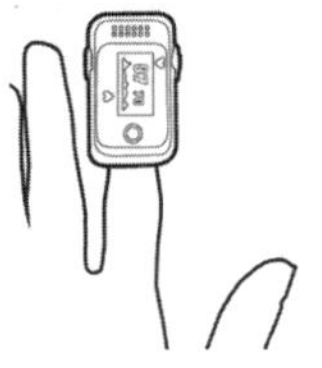

IHEART PULSE WAVE VELOCITY MONITOR iHeart offers personal heart monitoring with a small portable device that allows you to track the elasticity of your arteries by simply clipping a pulse oximeter onto your finger, which transmits data to an app on your phone or tablet. The information is correlated against an algorithm that provides your biological age. It's a good way to track the effect the KetoFLEX 12/3 changes are having on your heart health. It has decent scientific validation, but the downside is that it's pricey at about $195 (£150).

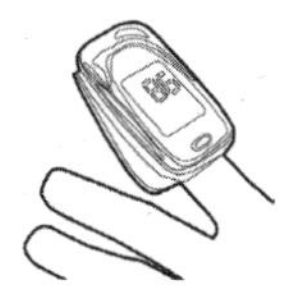

CONTINUOUS PULSE OXIMETER This is a small portable device that will allow you to rule out sleep apnoea (and other conditions) that can lead to nighttime oxygen desaturation, which is strongly associated with cognitive decline. You can purchase a continuous pulse oximeter system. There are two products we like because of their medical grade accuracy. The first is the Innovo 50F Plus (about £120 or $149.99), which is a snug-fitting wristwatch that provides continuous monitoring of oxygen saturation and pulse rate with 24-hour data collection and analysis. You can use either Bluetooth or a cable to download the collected data to your personal computer via Windows. You can also easily use this device during the day to monitor your oxygen levels. The only downsides are that the Innovo 50F Plus isn't compatible with Apple or Android devices, and some people find it difficult to sleep with a tight-fitting watch. Another option is the Beddr SleepTuner (about £120 or $149), which is both Apple and Android compatible. Beddr uses a small optical sensor that adheres to the middle of your forehead to measure your blood oxygen levels and heart rate throughout the night. Beddr provides a detailed report that you can see on your smartphone or tablet. The only downside to this device is that it's only practical for nighttime use. More information can be found in chapter 14.

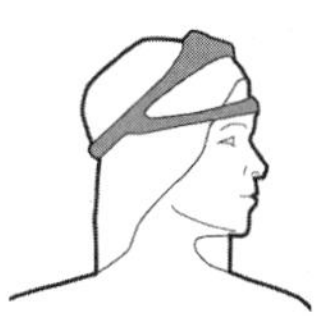

SLEEP TRACKING Sleep tracking devices, which can be worn on your finger or wrist, placed on your bedside table, or even under your sheet or mattress, can provide some information about the quality and duration of your sleep, both of which can aid in the transport of beta-amyloid. Because sleep trackers use a combination of inputs (movement, heart rate, respiration) as opposed to directly measuring brain waves, they are inherently inaccurate and are best used to get a rough estimation of sleep duration and quality. Those who are serious about monitoring their sleep may want to consider Dreem 2, an FDA class II medical device that straps onto your forehead during sleep and actually measures brain activity, along with respiration, heart rate, and movement, to provide an accurate and detailed sleep report via an accompanying app. This product also offers sleep coaching, with tips on how to improve your sleep quality. The downside is its price at around $499 (£390).

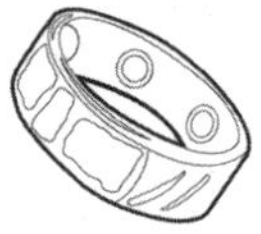

OURA RING For the reader who likes to geek out with data collection, the Oura Ring may be for you. It looks like a stylish ring but is actually a high-tech physiological quantification device. It measures sleep, heart rate, heart rate variability, activity, body temperature, movement, respiration, and more without exposing the wearer to Wi-Fi. As you might expect, it's expensive, with prices starting at around $299 (£230).

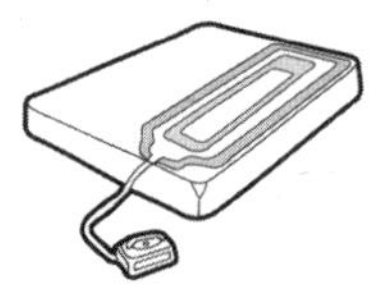

CHILIPAD AND OOLER These are mattress cooling pad systems that help you get restorative sleep without cooling the whole house at night. They recirculate cooled water throughout the mattress pad, with the electronic temperature control unit placed at least 45 centimetres (or more) from the bed, minimizing direct EMF exposure. ChiliPAD is the first generation, with the newer OOLER now available. The systems are pricey, starting at around $499 (£390). While this is initially expensive, it may save money (and energy) in the long run. It's well suited to those who live in very warm climates or for rooms that can't be adequately cooled.

DIRECT-TO-CONSUMER LAB TESTING Throughout much of the United States (excluding New York, New Jersey, California, and Rhode Island) consumers can order their own laboratory testing. Some providers in this marketplace include Health Testing Centers, Life Extension, Walk-In Lab, and DirectLabs. This is very helpful when you are trying to track the effect the various strategies are having upon your health. You can see our full updated list of labs and goals for a cognoscopy (a cognitive wellness evaluation) in Table 1 in chapter 1. It would be ideal to get them all done, but we understand that not everyone needs or can afford that full panel of testing that is now available directly to the consumer at mycognoscopy.com. If you live in the UK, you will need to seek out a private medical practitioner who will prescibe these tests for you for a range of fees.

DIRECT-TO-CONSUMER GENETICS TESTING Many companies are now offering direct-to-consumer genetic testing, providing health and ancestry information. 23andMe is one provider that offers health information, including ApoE4 status, which can be helpful in determining your risk for Alzheimer's disease. Other providers include Genos, FamilyTreeDNA, and AncestryDNA.com. (Do *not* rely on Ancestry.com for ApoE status.)

PROMETHEASE Promethease, recently acquired by MyHeritage, offers access to a wiki-style curated interpretation of your raw genetic data from many direct-to-consumer genetic testing providers, including 23andMe. For a moderate fee, Promethease offers results from many genes beyond the limited health information.

GENETIC GENIE Genetic Genie is a free (donations accepted) online service that uses your raw genetic data from 23andMe to interpret your methylation and detoxification pathways. Those with impaired methylation are at risk for higher homocysteine levels, implicated in Alzheimer's pathophysiology, and those with impaired detoxification pathways are at risk for type 3 (toxic) Alzheimer's. Knowledge of both risks can help you tweak your approach.

FOUNDMYFITNESS GENETICS REPORTS Dr Rhonda Patrick of FoundMyFitness offers a variety of regularly updated health reports based on the raw genetic data from 23andMe and AncestryDNA, ranging in price from a donation of your choice to $10. We discuss her comprehensive report outlining vitamin D and omega-3 fatty acid metabolism, vitamin B_{12} absorption, and more in our "Using Genes to Guide Your Dietary Choices" in chapter 12.

MONTREAL COGNITIVE ASSESSMENT (MOCA) The MoCA is a cognitive screening test that you can use to assess and track the effect various strategies are having upon your cognition. There are versions that can be self-administered and others that require a partner to provide simple instructions. This screening tool, which takes approximately ten to twelve minutes, can be repeated as often as every month, using a different version each time, to avoid a learning effect. Note that the MoCA may not be sensitive enough to detect the earliest cognitive changes—it is best for those with MCI or Alzheimer's—so for those interested in prevention or early reversal, you may wish to use a more sensitive test such as CNS Vital Signs (accessible on the Apollo Health website).

BRAINHQ BrainHQ is a subscription-based online brain-training service that uses scientifically proven methods to enhance cognition. It's designed to be helpful at many different levels of cognitive performance, and constantly adjusts to your improved performance by offering more challenging games. BrainHQ also offers an updated cognitive assessment of your skills in attention, brain speed, memory, people skills, intelligence, and navigation as compared to your age-matched peers. You can use your performance as a means of tracking your overall cognition. (See more in chapter 16.) You can subscribe for £9 a month or £66 a year.

Please note that this list is not exhaustive, and additional tools can be found in the various chapters outlining specific strategies.

PART THREE

THE HANDBOOK SECTION 2: More Silver Buckshot

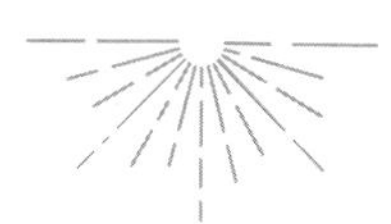

CHAPTER 19

Dementogens: Swimming in the Alzheimer's Soup

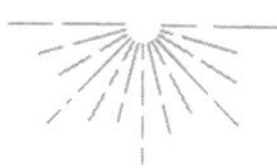

Something is rotten in the state of Denmark.
—WILLIAM SHAKESPEARE, *HAMLET*

THE HIGHEST RATE OF dementia-related death in the world is in Finland, and it has been suggested that one of the main reasons for this may be mould-produced mycotoxins.[1] Thus, as Shakespeare might have said, something is rotten in the state of Finland. But this is not just a Finnish problem, this is a global problem—we are all exposed to toxins like never before in history. We inhale the air pollution that increases risk for Alzheimer's.[2] We eat mercury-laden fish such as tuna and swordfish. We prepare vegetables laced with glyphosate (from Roundup, the weed killer). We build our homes and colonize our sinuses with neurotoxin-producing moulds. We burn paraffin candles that fill the room with benzene and toluene. We drink water tainted with pesticides and arsenic. We marinate in the mercury spewn from coal burning even thousands of miles away. In short, we are swimming daily in an Alzheimer's bouillabaisse. Therefore, our ability to detoxify on an ongoing basis is absolutely critical, and a breakdown in detoxification increases risk for cognitive decline.

We are all familiar with carcinogens—chemicals that cause cancer—and thanks to Professor Bruce Ames and the Ames test he developed to detect carcinogens, we can detect these in our food, water, beauty products, and other agents to which we are exposed. However, there is currently no analogous test for *dementogens*—chemicals that cause dementia—yet they are everywhere, and we are exposed daily. We can break these poisons down into three groups: metals and other inorganic chemicals; organic chemicals such as toluene and pesticides; and biotoxins, which are toxins produced by living organisms such as moulds.

> Celeste is a 60-year-old woman who, at the age of 57, began to have problems with concentration, compromising her work. She developed difficulty with organizing and then began to lose her memory. Although this was initially attributed simply to worry over her family history of Alzheimer's disease, it became clear that it was far more than that when her MRI showed a severely atrophied hippocampus, with a size less than the 1st percentile for her age. Two mycotoxins were discovered in her urine—ochratoxin A and gliotoxin—and a diagnosis of type 3 (toxic) Alzheimer's disease was made. She started on the ReCODE protocol and improved. On several occasions, she was re-exposed to moulds when water leaks occurred in her home, and each time she declined, but improved once again when the exposure was removed and she continued her protocol. However, she developed a kidney stone and had a very traumatic day: the stone caused severe pain and required surgery, and thus she was given anaesthesia and narcotics. The following day she had declined once again, and did not improve for weeks thereafter.

Celeste illustrates a critical point regarding dementogens: their effects tend to be additive, so that anything that increases the overall toxic burden—such as anaesthetic agents or re-exposure—or reduces ongoing detoxification—such as stress, sleep loss, a reduction in glutathione, or liver or kidney damage—tips the balance back in favour of decline. Furthermore, as long as the exposure exceeds the detox process, decline will continue, and this may occur for years. However, once the balance is tipped in the positive direction, with reduced exposure and augmented detoxification, improvement may once again proceed.

Therefore, after identifying the toxin or toxins contributing to cognitive decline—and typically there is more than one, just as there was for Celeste—the most important recommendation is to do everything possible to minimize exposure and maximize breakdown and excretion. Two excellent recent books offer important insights into the processes of detoxification: *The Toxin Solution* by Dr Joseph Pizzorno is most helpful for chemotoxins (chemical toxins) such as pesticides, mercury, and anaesthetics, whereas *Toxic* by Dr Neil Nathan is most helpful for biotoxins such as the mycotoxins to which Celeste was exposed.

So the first step in dealing with dementogens is simply to determine your exposure:

- You can check your exposure to **metal toxins** easily, using blood or urine or even hair. Several different laboratories perform these tests. (Quick: What do chicken, groundwater, rice, and angry lovers have in common? Arsenic!) Quicksilver has an excellent mercury test called the Tri-Test, since it evaluates blood, urine, and hair. It reports not only how much mercury exposure you have, but also how much is inorganic mercury—which comes from your dental amalgams (the old-fashioned "silver fillings")—and how much is organic mercury—which comes from eating seafood, especially fish high in mercury such as tuna, swordfish, and shark (and any large-mouthed, long-lived fish, since these are the ones that accumulate the most mercury). Quicksilver also offers an all-metals test that includes other metals such as iron, aluminium, lead, and arsenic. One important caveat to remember is that seafood should not be eaten for one week before testing for arsenic, since it may lead to a false positive result, due to the presence of non-toxic arsenic in seafood (the arsenic is bound up by protective molecules in the seafood—kind of reminds you of Alzheimer's amyloid, doesn't it?).

Metals such as mercury appear not just in the blood and urine, but also collect in the organs, including the brain, liver, and skeleton. Therefore, many practitioners prefer to give a binding agent before urine collection, in order to pull some of the metals from the body and get a better idea of the overall load. One such test is offered by Doctor's Data.

The simplest test for toxic metals is to measure them in blood, so it is common to evaluate blood samples for mercury, lead, arsenic, cadmium, iron, copper, and zinc. Iron, copper, and zinc are actually important for health in the right amounts, but can be toxic when the body is overloaded.

> Lillianna is a 60-year-old woman who developed difficulty in the recognition of objects, which progressed. After a PET scan and spinal fluid analysis, she was diagnosed with Alzheimer's. She had zero copies of the common Alzheimer's risk gene allele, ApoE4; however, she was found to have very high levels of mercury and arsenic. In addition, her testing indicated an exposure to biotoxins. It was suspected that she had developed type 3 (toxic) Alzheimer's due to heavy exposure to the World Trade Center cloud, and this suspicion was confirmed when she developed a cancer that is highly associated with World Trade Centre cloud exposure.

The cloud emitted from the 9/11 tragedy at the World Trade Center was a smorgasbord of toxins—from the jet fuel of the crashed planes to the metals from the computers and building structure to the moulds and bacteria in the buildings to the asbestos and glass particles from the insulation to the dioxins from the burning plastic to the PCBs (polychlorinated biphenyls) from the electrical transformers. It was as if a lifetime of serious toxic exposure had been concentrated into a few hours and days. Many of us recall that serious pulmonary disease, and in some cases cancers, developed in so many of the first responders, as well as those in the surrounding area. The toxic manifestations did not stop there, however: within fifteen years, 12.8 per cent of the responders had already developed cognitive decline.[3] It is not yet known what the long-term effects will be on the many residents of New York City who had less exposure than the first responders but were nonetheless enveloped by the expanding cloud, but this remains a significant concern.

In Lillianna's case, she had high levels of both mercury and arsenic, as well as probable mycotoxin exposure. Of all of the metal exposures, mercury is the one that is most commonly associated with Alzheimer's disease. However, since the Alzheimer's amyloid and its parent, APP, are actually specialized to bind metals,[4] it's not surprising that the protective downsizing response we refer to as Alzheimer's disease can be incited by metal exposure. Furthermore, the overall detoxification process can be stressed by exposure to multiple metals, such as lead, cadmium, iron, copper, and the metalloid arsenic. Aluminium has also been implicated in Alzheimer's disease, and although this remains controversial, it will not be surprising if aluminium does indeed turn out to be another metallic risk for Alzheimer's disease.

- You can check your exposure to **organic toxins** by getting a toxin test from Great Plains Laboratories (GPL-TOX) or any other laboratory that does testing for such toxins. It is a good idea to include the test for glyphosate (the main active chemical in Roundup), since there is increasing evidence that this is not only a carcinogen but also a neurotoxin.[5] In addition, all of these various organic toxins can add to your overall toxic burden, as noted above, reducing your glutathione (a major cellular detoxicant and antioxidant) and interfering with your body's ability to detoxify, thus increasing your exposure to all of the many agents that you might otherwise have resisted.

Isla is a 50-year-old "multi-tasking wonder woman" executive who began to have difficulty with word finding and language at the age of 48. The symptoms progressed, and she was evaluated with a PET scan, an amyloid

> PET scan, and a spinal tap, all of which confirmed that she had Alzheimer's disease as the cause of her primary progressive aphasia (PPA). Although her standard dementia testing was negative, her toxin testing revealed very high levels of benzene, formaldehyde, and mercury. Further discussion with her husband disclosed the fact that she had worked in the presence of burning paraffin candles for many years; he even pointed out that the smoke was so irritating that he had had to avoid visiting her at work.

Isla's testing mirrored the very toxins present in paraffin candles. These candles are quite toxic, so if you like to burn candles frequently, please use beeswax candles rather than paraffin!

The recent designation of glyphosate (the active ingredient in the herbicide Roundup) as a probable carcinogen by the World Health Organization[6] may be accompanied at some point by its designation as a neurotoxin as well. Glyphosate, in use since 1974, has three major mechanisms. First, it binds metals such as manganese, copper, and zinc, thus altering all sorts of enzymatic pathways that require these metals.[7] Second, it blocks the shikimate pathway required by plants to make key amino acids—which is why it is a good weed killer—but unfortunately this pathway is also required by bacteria! Yes, the very bacteria that we depend on, as our gut microbiome, to metabolize, synthesize, and protect us. So—no surprise—blocking this critical pathway damages your microbiome, throwing the critical bacteria of your gut into disarray. Third, glyphosate, which is essentially glycine methyl phosphate—in other words, it looks a lot like our simple amino acid glycine—has been suggested to substitute for glycine in some proteins, interfering with their normal function.[8]

Therefore, although the jury is still out on whether glyphosate will prove to be a neurotoxin or not, the combination of theoretical, epidemiological, and anecdotal evidence suggests that we should know whether we have high levels of glyphosate, and if we do find such exposure, we should at the very least undergo detoxification to reduce its carcinogenic effect.

- You can check your exposure to **biotoxins** by checking urinary mycotoxins, and there are two different tests in common use: GPL urinary mycotoxins and RealTime Labs urinary mycotoxin test. You can also get an idea about whether you have been exposed by checking your immune system's response: those with biotoxin exposures often have elevations in C4a, TGF-beta-1, MMP-9 (matrix metalloproteinase-9), leptin, and reductions in vascular endothelial growth factor (VEGF) and melanocyte-stimulating hormone (MSH). You can also check your visual contrast sensitivity (VCS), a test that looks at how well you can distinguish fine shades of grey. You tend to lose this ability with biotoxin exposure, and testing can be done at your doctor's office or online. (In the UK you may have to seek out a private practitioner and pay for these tests.)
- You can check your ability to detoxify by evaluating your diet and lifestyle, biochemical testing, and genetic testing for detoxification pathways. If you are not getting at least 30 grams of fibre per day, your detoxification is likely to be suboptimal; if you are not sweating and using non-toxic soap, if you are not drinking filtered or reverse osmosis water, if you are not eating crucifers and other detoxifying foods (as described in the first section of the Handbook), then your detoxification is likely to be suboptimal. For biochemical testing, you want to know your glutathione, homocysteine, vitamin C, liver function (GGT, ALT, AST), and kidney function (BUN, creatinine). For genetic testing, there are several tests available, such as the one from IntellxxDNA, which determines whether your genome includes mutations associated with reductions in detoxification, such as in glutathione peroxidase. These genetic tests are very helpful in planning optimal treatment, especially for those of us who are ApoE4-negative, since we often have reduced detoxification as a contributor to cognitive decline, especially in type 3 (toxic) Alzheimer's.

PREVENTION AND TREATMENT OF DEMENTOGEN EXPOSURE

The most important concept in the prevention and treatment of dementogen exposure is to recognize that this is a dynamic process. In today's world, it is impossible to avoid dementogens completely, so a combination of minimizing exposure and optimizing detoxification is the best approach. Please remember that you are constantly excreting toxins—in sweat, urine, breath, and stool—as well as disarming them biochemically and sequestering them in fat, bones, brain, and other organs, so you are using multiple mechanisms to minimize your ongoing toxic burden. However, we each have a limit to what our body can deal with, and when this is exceeded, we develop toxin-related illnesses such as Alzheimer's disease, Lewy body disease, Parkinson's disease, and ALS (amyotrophic lateral sclerosis, also called Lou Gehrig's disease). As you can well imagine, with the multiplicity of dementogens to which we are exposed, virtually any toxin can contribute to exceeding the threshold, and thus the overall toxic burden is important, not just a single major toxin exposure.

The first step is to *minimize exposure* to dementogens. These toxins may enter when you breathe (air pollution, the World Trade Centre cloud, the mould toxins and inflammagens from water-damaged buildings) or eat or drink (the mercury from tuna, high-glycaemic foods, or inflammatory gluten or dairy products) or when your skin comes in contact with them, such as some health and beauty aids. These may also be produced within your body, such as the mycotoxins produced by moulds that may reside in your sinuses or GI tract, or be absorbed from dental or surgical procedures, or be released from sites of sequestration, such as the release of mercury as we near menopause or andropause and enter the earliest stages of pre-osteoporosis.

In order to minimize your exposure to dementogens, therefore, you can do the following:

- Purchase a HEPA filter, such as IQAir or another model. It's best if it filters both particulates and toxic gases. Since HEPA filters can be noisy, you may wish to run it when you are out of the house, but many find it helpful to run continuously.

- Avoid smoking and second-hand smoke.
- Avoid air pollution to the extent possible. This includes not only automobile exhaust but also the pollution associated with fires, such as the California wildfires that have become so common in the past few years, destroying air quality. This also includes the smoke from candles, especially paraffin candles, which emit numerous toxins such as benzene and toluene. Since the small (2.5 micron) particles of air pollution are particularly damaging, the use of N95 masks or P100 masks, fitted snugly and using straps both above and below the ears, is important. Your brain will thank you.
- Avoid prolonged mouth breathing, since your nasal passages also provide a filter for particulate matter. Mouth breathing also increases risk for gingivitis, lowers oxygen absorption, and fails to warm the air the way nose breathing does, which may lead to lung irritation.
- Check your ERMI score,[9] and if it is over 2, consider remediation to remove mould exposure. If you do decide to remediate, please stay out of the house during the remediation process.
- Especially if your house shows any signs of mould, spend more time outdoors and away from air pollution.
- Use a water filter, such as a reverse osmosis filter. Filters are available for water jugs, under the kitchen taps, and whole house systems. We use an AquaTru because it includes both a carbon filter and reverse osmosis, but there are many other makes. Tap water often contains bacteria, viruses, multiple metals, organic toxins, traces of various drugs, and other contaminants, so using a filter is an excellent method to minimize dementogen exposure. Furthermore, avoid contaminated water near fracking sites.

- Eat organic fruits and vegetables, especially for the Environmental Working Group's Dirty Dozen, which represent the greatest exposure: strawberries, spinach, kale, nectarines, apples, grapes, peaches, cherries, pears, tomatoes, celery, and potatoes. In contrast, the Clean Fifteen are less of a concern for pesticide exposure because they have more protection than the Dirty Dozen and are therefore not as important to buy organic: avocados, sweet corn, pineapples, frozen green peas, onions, papayas, aubergines, asparagus, kiwi, cabbages, cauliflower, cantaloupes, broccoli, mushrooms, and honeydew melon.
- Avoid toxins in health and beauty aids. You may wish to use the app Think Dirty to give you an idea of what toxins are in each product. You may also wish to consult the Environmental Working Group for its recommendations.
- Avoid eating fish high in mercury. These are the long-lived, large-mouthed fish, such as tuna, shark, swordfish, marlin, orange roughy, tilefish, bluefish, grouper, and king mackerel. Choose instead the small, low-mercury SMASH fish—salmon (not farmed), mackerel (not king), anchovies, sardines, and herring.
- Avoid dental amalgams due to their high content of inorganic mercury. If you already have dental amalgams, and especially if your inorganic mercury is high, you may wish to have these removed. As noted in chapter 17, this should be done by a biological dentist, trained to minimize your exposure to mercury during removal. This should also be done deliberately, one or two at a time rather than many at once, then repeating every few months until all have been removed.
- Avoid food-associated dementogens. In addition to the mercury from fish such as tuna, and the pesticides and herbicides (including glyphosate) from non-organic fruits and

vegetables, there are many other sources of toxins in some foods, such as the arsenic in some chicken and in some rice, antibiotics and hormones in some meats, bisphenol A (BPA) in tinned foods, trans fats in many fried and baked foods, nitrates in sausages and other processed meats, sulfates in processed foods, preservatives, and dyes. Of course, the most common dementogens in food are sugar, high-fructose corn syrup, and other simple carbohydrates.

- How you cook your food is important! Unfortunately, cooking is an efficient way to produce dementogens. Advanced glycation end products (AGEs), which bind directly to a brain receptor called RAGE that increases Alzheimer's pathology; polycyclic aromatic hydrocarbons (PAHs); heterocyclic amines; and acrylamide, a neurotoxin particularly high in French fries and chips—all are formed with high-temperature cooking. AGEs and PAHs are formed when meat is blackened or charred. Trans fats are present in products such as shortening. Cooking with vegetable oils releases toxic aldehydes. Oils that have been heat-treated are deficient in antioxidants, and therefore cold-pressed oils such as olive oil are preferable for low-temperature cooking, while heat-resistant fats such as avocado oil, butter, or ghee are preferable for higher-temperature cooking. Please see the cooking suggestions in part 2.

- Plastics provide a source for multiple toxins, such as bisphenol A (BPA) and other endocrine disrupters, phthalates, dioxins, vinyl chloride, ethylene dichloride, lead, and cadmium, among others. Therefore, to the extent possible, please use other storage vessels such as glass.

- Machine-printed receipts also contain BPA, so please minimize handling of receipt paper.

- Avoid the lead that is in some paints (for example, on some coffee mugs) and old plumbing.

The second step is to *optimize detoxification*. The good news is that our bodies are constantly detoxifying, through metabolism and excretion in urine, stool, breath, and sweat. The better news is that we can support this process in a number of ways. The bad news is that even after we lessen our exposure to toxins, those that have accumulated in our organs over years can leach out, continuing our exposure. However, as long as the dynamic balance is towards detoxification, we are going in the right direction, provided that the detoxification process is not so aggressive that we are re-exposed to high levels of toxins as they once again course through the bloodstream on exit.

Let's start with the basics that we should all be doing to keep a healthy level of detoxification.

- Drink filtered water, from one to four litres per day.
- Eat fibre, both soluble and insoluble, preferably from foods such as celery and lettuce (and many others such as avocado, Brussels sprouts, kale, dark chocolate, prunes, etc.), but many of us like to supplement with organic psyllium husk or konjac root (e.g. PGX). The goal is to exceed 30 grams of fibre per day (recognizing that our ancestors consumed about 100 to 150 grams per day!), which will help you with toxin elimination.
- Sweat! Whether you prefer to work up a sweat with exercise or the sauna or other activities, this will remove toxins, and you can follow up with a shower with non-toxic soap such as Castile, in order to ensure that the exiting toxins do not re-enter your body. A Finnish study on saunas found a dramatic reduction of more than 50 per cent in risk for dementia in those who took saunas multiple times per week.[10]
- Spend time outside the house! Tip the balance towards detoxification rather than further accumulation of toxins, especially if your home has an ERMI score >2 or new, off-gassing furniture or other volatile organic compounds.

- Heal your gut if it is leaky (as discussed earlier), then include probiotics (such as fermented foods) and prebiotics (such as Mexican yam or Jerusalem artichoke, or as supplements) in your diet. Some like to support the gut with Triphala, an Ayurvedic combination of Amalaki, Bibhitaki, and Haritaki that has multiple mechanisms of action such as microbiome enhancement and immune supportive effects.

- Ensure that your own endogenous detoxicants, such as glutathione, are optimized, by taking N-acetylcysteine (500 mg twice per day) or liposomal glutathione (250 mg twice per day) or S-acetyl glutathione (200–300 mg twice a day), sulforaphane, and cruciferous vegetables.

- Support your liver, the most important detoxification organ. Many like to take milk thistle, and there are many liver cleanse products that feature milk thistle. Many other foods and supplements also provide liver support, such as curcumin (which is also an anti-inflammatory and a beta-amyloid binder), tauroursodeoxycholic acid (TUDCA), organic apples (which contain pectin, a toxin-binding agent), walnuts, avocado, free-range eggs, sardines, cruciferous vegetables, salad greens, artichokes, and fish oil.

- Support your kidneys, another critical detoxification organ system. This includes enhancing blood flow to your kidneys with beetroot juice (240 ml twice per day), blueberries (100 g per day), ginkgo biloba (60 mg twice per day), gotu kola (100 mg twice per day), and magnesium citrate (500 mg per day); and reducing kidney-damaging foods such as those high in nitrogen (in other words, make meat a condiment, not a main food), phosphate (such as processed cheese), and salt (such as baked beans and salty soups).

- Consider massage, since this may also enhance detoxification and improve lymphatic flow.

- Minimize and manage stress. We have observed that patients with type 3 (toxic) Alzheimer's tend to be hypersensitive to stress, declining markedly with lack of sleep, viral infections, and other stressors, whereas they often respond very positively to meditation, restorative exercise (avoid marathons), sauna, and optimization of hormone levels.

The third step is the *targeted treatment of specific dementogens.* This is a major field unto itself, so if your testing has revealed evidence of mycotoxin exposure, heavy metal toxicity, or organic toxicity (e.g. with high levels of glyphosate, toluene, or pesticides), please set up an appointment with a practitioner who specializes in detoxification and, beyond that, one who specializes in chemotoxicity (for metals and organics) or one who specializes in biotoxicity (for biotoxins such as mycotoxins), since these are often distinct subspecialists. It is important to note that detoxification may take months or even years, may be complicated, may lead to increased toxicity if it is overly aggressive (and therefore must be managed carefully), but can be absolutely lifesaving for those with cognitive decline due to dementogens, especially those with type 3 Alzheimer's disease or pre-Alzheimer's disease.

For those with metal toxicity such as mercury, some specialists prefer chelating agents, such as DMSA for mercury and EDTA for lead, or chlorella for multiple metals, whereas others prefer the use of Nrf2 activation, as utilized by Quicksilver's Qube product. The basic detoxification outlined above in the second step should be continued as well.

Kay is a 61-year-old woman who complained of difficulty with organization and completing tasks. Her executive function was scored at the 1st percentile for her age, and overall cognitive score at the 33rd percentile for her age. Her ApoE genotype was 3/3 and her PET scan showed reduced glucose metabolism in her temporal lobes, compatible with cortical atrophy. Her mercury level was high at 14 micrograms per litre. She was treated with chelation and after seven months felt much better. Her mercury had dropped to the high-normal range, her cognitive scores improved from the 1st percentile to the 77th percentile in executive function, and her overall cognitive score increased from the 33rd percentile to the 79th percentile.

For those with chemical toxicity due to organic toxins such as benzene or toluene, the detoxification outlined in the second step should be followed, and in addition, vasodilation with niacin may be helpful, but this should be carried out only with a doctor's guidance. Although any of these toxins may damage the gut microbiome, one in particular—glyphosate from the weed killer Roundup—is a direct microbiome toxin, and therefore detoxification should include not only a product like Restore (now called ION*Gut Health) or Cleardrops zeolite, which help to heal the gut, but also probiotics and prebiotics.

For those with biotoxins such as mycotoxins (e.g. trichothecenes, ochratoxin A, gliotoxin, aflatoxin, or others), the expert practitioner who evaluates and treats you will likely utilize some variation on the protocol developed by Dr Ritchie Shoemaker.[11] Some using the Shoemaker Protocol add antifungals such as itraconazole or amphotericin B, since moulds can colonize sinuses or the GI tract and thus continue to produce mycotoxins within your body (for example, see Dr Neil Nathan's book *Toxic*); however, Dr Shoemaker's recommendation is to avoid antifungals, since these may lead to antimicrobial resistance, and focus instead on the detoxification and other aspects of the protocol, the main points of which are summarized below.

- Virtually all experts in biotoxin treatment agree that the most important factor in the treatment of biotoxin illness is removal of the source—as you might well imagine, patients rarely improve as long as there is continued exposure. As noted above, exposure can be reduced by the use of HEPA filters. If the ERMI score of your home or workplace is 2 or greater, remediation may be required before improvement can occur. During remediation, it is critical to be away from the house, and in the worst cases—such as those with toxic black mould (*Stachybotrys*) and its dementing trichothecenes—you may want to consider moving to another, less toxic home permanently.

Dr Ritchie Shoemaker has written an excellent book, *Surviving Mold: Life in the Era of Dangerous Buildings*, which I recommend wholeheartedly for anyone interested in mould-related illness.

- Treatment of the microbes producing the biotoxins is the next step. Deep nasal cultures often reveal bacterial biofilms, which are like igloos that protect the bacteria from antibiotics, making it difficult to eradicate them. The biofilms often contain MARCoNS, which are *Staph* bacteria that are resistant to multiple antibiotics. These may be treated with Biocidin or BEG spray—Bactroban (mupirocin) 0.2%, EDTA (edetate disodium) 1%, and gentamicin 3%—or colloidal silver. This may be combined with SinuClenz and Xlear to reduce burning and help healing. In addition, better results may be achieved if 15 per cent mucoadhesive polymer gel (MAPG) is added to the spray. For mould species, these are sometimes treated with itraconazole (as noted above), but some find that immune enhancement with guduchi (*Tinospora cordifolia*) works just as well.

  Inactivating and excreting the pathogen-associated biotoxins is critical, and there are several techniques to achieve this. Intravenous glutathione may be associated with a rapid improvement in mental status, and although this is transient (typically lasting several hours), twice-weekly infusions may lead to sustained gains. Increases in glutathione may also be achieved with oral S-acetyl glutathione or liposomal glutathione or N-acetylcysteine. Next, intranasal VIP (vasoactive intestinal peptide) provides trophic support to the brain, and is typically administered once MARCoNS cultures are negative. These administrations are frequently associated with cognitive improvement.

  As noted earlier, certain foods enhance detoxification, such as coriander, cruciferous vegetables (cauliflower, broccoli, various types of cabbage, kale, radishes, Brussels sprouts, turnips, watercress, kohlrabi, swede, rocket, horseradish, maca, rapini, daikon, wasabi, pak choi, and related vegetables), avocados, artichokes, beetroots, dandelions, garlic, ginger, grapefruit, lemons, olive oil, and seaweed. Toxin elimination is enhanced by binding with cholestyramine, Welchol, bentonite clay, charcoal, zeolite (e.g. Cleardrops), or Guggul; by sweating in a sauna followed by showering with a non-toxic soap (e.g. Castile) to emulsify and remove the sweat-associated toxins; and by urination following hydration with filtered water. Finally, patients with biotoxin-associated illness often improve most when their protocols include hormone optimization, and this may be because of the association of adequate progesterone levels with optimal detoxification.

- After treatment, just as we want to benefit from an optimal gut microbiome, we also want to restore an optimal sinus, nasal, and oral microbiome. Probiotics with *Lactobacillus sakei* may be used, or ProbioMax ENT, or other sinus probiotics. The point of this is the same as optimizing your gut microbiome—the protective microbes prevent the reappearance of the damaging microbes. Without this step, the MARCoNS may recur more readily.

One class of dementogens deserves special mention: anaesthetic agents. It is very common to hear that a patient's cognitive decline began after general anaesthesia and the associated surgery, especially if the time under anaesthesia was prolonged or there were multiple episodes. General anaesthesia contributes to cognitive decline by multiple mechanisms. First is the overall burden of toxicity, with reduction of glutathione and stress on the detoxification systems (although it should be noted that anaesthetic agents also have some neuroprotective effects).[12] Second is the hypoxia (poor oxygenation) and hypotension (low blood pressure) that occur commonly while under general anaesthesia, thus compounding the toxicity from the anaesthetic agents. Third is the severe stress that occurs with surgical procedures. Fourth is the common use of antibiotics associated with surgical procedures, which alters the microbiome and may increase gut permeability. Fifth is the inflammation that occurs with surgery and in general with healing. Thus general anaesthesia and its associated surgical procedures represent a potent dementing programme, associated with a doubling of the risk for dementia.[13]

Therefore, if you are contemplating or require general anaesthesia, you may wish to consider:

- Talking with your surgeon ahead of time. Is general anaesthesia necessary? Is it possible to use local anaesthesia? How long is the anaesthesia likely to be used? Surprisingly, spinal anaesthesia has been shown to be no better than general anaesthesia, and possibly even worse, in its risk for the subsequent development of dementia.[14]

- Talking with your anaesthetist ahead of time. It is common to allow blood pressure to drop during general anaesthesia, and sudden drops can reduce critical blood flow; therefore, your anaesthetist can ensure that your pressure does not suffer a rapid drop during your procedure, and that it remains optimal. Your anaesthetist can also choose shorter-acting anaesthetic agents, ones that will be cleared rapidly following your surgical procedure. Also, make sure to discuss any medications you are taking with your anaesthetist.

- The strategy to prepare yourself for general anaesthesia is to optimize your detoxification in preparation for the exposure to anaesthetic agents so that these can be cleared rapidly, with minimal organ damage. This can be achieved by combining the detoxicants glutathione (which can be taken as the precursor N-acetylcysteine 500 mg twice per day or as liposomal glutathione 250 mg twice per day or as S-acetyl glutathione 300 mg twice per day), milk thistle 70 mg three times per day, choline 1 gram per day, and methionine 1 gram per day, along with a high-potency multivitamin that includes vitamin C (at least 500 mg) and B vitamins. These should be taken for a minimum of one week prior to surgery and two weeks post-operatively.

- Supplements to avoid (typically one week) before surgery (and please discuss with your surgeon) include fish oil, acetyl-L-carnitine, vitamin E, garlic, gingko, and ginger due to their blood-thinning effects. Other supplements, such as St John's wort and valerian root, should be avoided several days before surgery as they may prolong the effects of anaesthesia. Make sure that your surgeon has a full list of your supplements and medications. Inquire well ahead of the surgery date which ones you need to stop taking and when you can resume.

- In addition, consider an anaesthesia-clearing diet (as soon as your gut is working again, of course) for a few weeks after surgery (such as KetoFLEX 12/3): Start with bone broth for easy digestibility and to provide your body with the extra protein and collagen necessary for repair and wound healing. Then include a diet high in fibre, high in crucifers such as broccoli (preferably cooked for easy digestibility), low in alcohol, and including filtered water, one to four litres per day. Many of the anaesthetic medications are fat soluble, so resuming mild ketosis with healthy fats will keep you in fat-burning mode to aid in detoxification and reduce inflammation. Sauna-induced sweating followed by washing with Castile soap several times per week for the same time period is also recommended.

CHAPTER 20

Of Microbes and Microbiomes

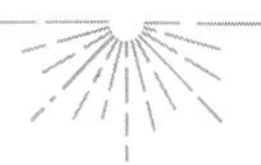

It seems improbable that enough infective matter or vapour could be secluded around the fingernails to kill a patient.

—NINETEENTH-CENTURY "EXPERT" SCEPTICAL THAT DOCTORS' FAILURE TO WASH THEIR HANDS COULD KILL AN OBSTETRIC PATIENT BY CAUSING INFECTION

JUST AS THE NINETEENTH-century experts were sceptical of germs as a cause of disease, today's experts are sceptical that cognitive decline can be reversed, and sceptical that functional medicine approaches are superior to monotherapeutics, despite increasing evidence to the contrary. In an intriguing recent experiment, scientists exposed mice to *Candida*, a common yeast, by injecting it into the bloodstream.[1] The initial assumption was that the yeast would be kept out of the brain by the well-known blood-brain barrier, which excludes most proteins and other large molecules—which are still far smaller than yeast organisms—from the brain. Surprisingly, however, the yeast entered the brain readily despite their large size, and induced an inflammatory response that resembled, pathologically, the earliest stage of Alzheimer's disease. This is yet another experiment that implicates treatable infections, and the brain's response to infections, as one of the potential contributors to the development of Alzheimer's disease. Moreover, it is a particularly relevant one, because the brains of Alzheimer's patients have indeed been demonstrated to harbour *Candida* in at least some cases.

Our exposure to the very organisms that have the potential to engender cognitive decline is ceaseless, since it has become increasingly clear over the last few decades that humans are not the discrete individual organisms we imagined ourselves to be. Rather, we are part of a village—over 1,000 different organisms (bacteria, viruses, phages, yeasts, moulds, spirochetes, and parasites—oh my!) inhabit our guts, skin, sinuses, mouths, and other bodily parts. These affect our very thoughts, moods, sense of self-preservation, and disease processes.

Thus we are not truly individuals, but complex collaborations among these many organisms, and when these collaborations break down, especially as we age, they lead to some of the most common illnesses that plague us today, including Alzheimer's disease, depression, inflammatory bowel disease, and type 2 diabetes.

For those of us with cognitive decline, or at risk for cognitive decline, the status of our gut microbiomes—the makeup of the various bacteria and other microbes in our intestines—is critical, since the human gut microbiome plays an important role in virtually *all* of the major risk factors and drivers of cognitive decline: inflammation, autoimmunity, insulin resistance, lipid metabolism, obesity, nutrient absorption, amyloidogenesis, neurochemistry, sleep, stress response, and detoxification. As one of many examples, specific bacteria, *Lactobacillus* and *Bifidobacteria*, are involved in the production of the neurotransmitter GABA from glutamate, and an imbalance in this ratio occurs in Alzheimer's disease.[2] Furthermore, our gut and our brain talk to each other incessantly, both chemically and electrically!

When we look at the gut of someone with Alzheimer's disease, what do we see? A *change* in the composition of the bacteria, so that the distribution looks very much like someone with obesity or type 2 diabetes.[3] What happens if we "fix" the microbiome? Laboratory experiments are very promising in this regard, since altering the gut bacteria in Alzheimer's-model mice ("Mouzheimer's") can improve or exacerbate the problem, correlating with which microbiome is created.[4] In another study using probiotics in a Mouzheimer's mouse,[5] cognitive decline was reduced, inflammatory mediators were inhibited, and normal protein processing was restored. Probiotic treatment was shown to activate the SIRT1 pathway, which is an important longevity and anti-Alzheimer's pathway.[6] Furthermore, healing our gut and optimizing our microbiome has wonderful effects on many factors, from inflammation to nutrient absorption to neurotransmitters to insulin resistance, so this represents a truly promising part of the overall therapeutic protocol for cognitive decline.

So since the microbiome is "messed up" in Alzheimer's, what messed it up? Caesarean birth (since the mother's microbiome is not passed on to the newborn as it is with natural childbirth), stress, antibiotics, alcohol, reduced fibre consumption, refined carbohydrates, ageing, inflammation, and parasites are among the many factors that can affect the intestinal microbiome.[7] On the flip side, probiotics, prebiotics, gut healing, and faecal transplants all offer promise as potential therapeutics for the beneficial manipulation of the gut microbiome. Therefore, when we take antibiotics for an infection, it's a good idea to remember that we have altered our gut microbiome, and therefore we should return it to normal with the aid of probiotics and prebiotics.

Indeed, the care and "feeding" of our microbiomes is critical to keeping our best cognition! This is true not just for avoiding inflammation, supporting nutrient absorption, and providing critical metabolites, but also for detoxification.[8] Prebiotic feeding of the microbiome affects transit time and excretion of toxins. As you might well imagine, if your gut is slow, the removal of toxins through the gut is correspondingly slow, so we do better with rapid transit (less than 24 hours) than slow. In a reciprocal fashion, specific toxins alter our microbiome, such as triclosan, pesticides, glyphosate (the nearly ubiquitous weed killer), plasticizers, heavy metals, and some drugs (e.g. antibiotics, proton-pump inhibitors, and synthetic oestrogens).[9]

Beyond the metabolic, immunological, and toxic effects of the microbiome and its effects on cognitive decline, the microbes of the gut may actually produce their *own* amyloids, and these may impact our own beta-amyloid production, degradation, and clearance.[10] It has been suggested that bacterial-derived amyloids may indeed deposit in our brains and affect the overall production of amyloid.[11]

Therefore it is clear that, to prevent and reverse cognitive decline, we certainly want to include supporting and optimizing our microbiome. In a generic sense, we do this with probiotics, prebiotics, and avoidance, if possible, of the agents that damage our microbiome. In a more specific sense, what is on the horizon is exciting: as we begin to tease out, from the many different types of bacteria, those that exert the major effects on key cognitive features, we should increase the precision and efficacy of "fixing" our microbiome. For example, in one study, an increase in brain-derived neurotrophic factor (BDNF) was associated with one particular species of *Bifidobacteria*.[12] In another study, a response against one bacterial species, *Mycobacterium vaccae*, was associated with a reduction in the stress response and microglial activation, inducing an anti-inflammatory response in the central nervous system.[13] Given the large number of potential species, there are almost limitless opportunities for therapeutic neurochemical and immunological effects in neurodegeneration, so please stay tuned!

INFECTIONS AND COGNITIVE DECLINE

Of course, in addition to the many microbes that make up the gut microbiome, we are exposed to infectious agents from many different sources. For years, suspicion has been visited on these infectious agents regarding Alzheimer's disease, but the smoking gun has been missing. However, recently the suspicion has turned into an indictment[14] as more and more evidence links chronic infections, and the inflammatory responses that result, to cognitive decline. In contrast, acute infections such as pneumococcal pneumonia or urinary tract infections are common exacerbators for those who already suffer from cognitive decline, and common reasons for setbacks in those whose cognition is otherwise improving on treatment.

In theory, any infection that activates the innate immune system may be associated with Alzheimer's disease; however, specific organisms have been implicated repeatedly. *Herpes* family viruses such as HSV-1, which produces cold sores and inhabits the major nerve supplying sensation to our face—called the trigeminal nerve—are likely to be important players in Alzheimer's risk. Indeed, suppressing outbreaks of *Herpes* is associated with reduced risk for dementia.[15] There are several ways to accomplish this, and it is often helpful to try a few different ways and determine which works best for you. You can take lysine or, alternatively, you can take valacyclovir or acyclovir. These are well tolerated, and some people take these for years without any major side effects. You can also take humic acid or fulvic acid. You can also talk to your doctor about the possibility of using Transfer Factor PlasMyc, especially if you have symptoms in the setting of active viral infection.

Organisms associated with poor dentition—most notably the bacterium *P. gingivalis* but also others such as *Fusobacterium nucleatum*, *Treponema denticola*, *Prevotella intermedia*, *Eikenella corrodens*, and others—have been implicated in periodontitis-associated risk for Alzheimer's.[16] Therefore, for anyone with poor dentition, it is worth discussing treatment with a functional dentist. Oral probiotics, including such organisms as *Streptococcus salivarius* and *Lactobacillus sakei*, are increasingly available, and these hold promise in minimizing the periodontitis-associated organisms, and by extension in reducing periodontitis-associated risk of cognitive decline.

Tick-borne organisms are commonly associated with long-term infections and cognitive decline. More than half of those who contract *Borrelia burgdorferi*, the Lyme disease organism, are co-infected with other organisms carried by ticks, such as *Babesia*, *Bartonella*, *Ehrlichia*, or *Anaplasma*. *Babesia* is the most common organism that occurs along with the Lyme *Borrelia*, and it is a parasite that infects red blood cells and is related to the parasites that cause malaria. *Bartonella*, *Ehrlichia*, and *Anaplasma* are all bacteria carried by ticks, and all are treatable with appropriate antibiotics as well as natural treatments. However, these chronic infections are often difficult to eradicate without persistent treatment and careful follow-up evaluation.

Fungi—moulds such as *Aspergillus* and yeast such as *Candida*—are also potential contributors to cognitive decline, not only because of their mycotoxin production and their potential for direct infection, but also because they often interfere with the immune response. Indeed, *Candida* has been identified in the brains of patients with Alzheimer's disease,[17] as have other yeasts and moulds.[18] The major moulds associated with toxin production in patients with chronic inflammatory response syndrome (CIRS) and type 3 Alzheimer's disease are *Stachybotrys* (the toxic black mould), *Penicillium*, *Aspergillus*, *Chaetomium*, and *Wallemia*. The water-damaged buildings that harbour these moulds also expose us to fumes from volatile organic compounds, various bacterial fragments, spores, and other inflammatory agents—truly a dementing soup.

Patients with type 3 Alzheimer's disease are affected not only by mould-produced mycotoxins but also often by biofilms, which are like igloos protecting bacteria. These biofilms make the ensconced bacteria much harder to treat with antibiotics. The most common bacteria identified in these biofilms are MARCoNS, which are Staph bacteria that reside deep in the nasopharynx and are resistant to multiple different antibiotics. MARCoNS may be treated with BEG spray, Biocidin, or colloidal silver.

In summary, the organisms that live within us—those that constitute our holobiome (the sum total of microbiomes of our gut, skin, sinuses, etc.) and those that invade and infect us—are critical determinants of our cognition, risk for cognitive decline, and progression of cognitive decline. The beta-amyloid that is so strongly associated with Alzheimer's disease is elaborated as an antimicrobial (among its other effects), and thus consideration and treatment of the complex interactions between the immune system, the various microbes, and the nervous system are important to produce the best therapeutic outcomes.

CHAPTER 21

Supplements: My Kingdom for a Source

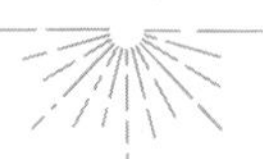

Either you are driven by what helps your patients or by what helps your career.

—R. F. LOEB

Someone who doesn't believe in a new treatment because he hasn't seen the results is simply uninformed; someone who doesn't believe despite seeing results is an "expert."

—R. F. LOEB

From a recent email:

> My wife, who is 69 years old, started showing signs of memory loss about a year ago, and was diagnosed as having Alzheimer's. As you can imagine we were devastated learning of this news. My wife's sister died of Alzheimer's just a few years ago and her mother died from Alzheimer's, so it runs in her family. Her doctor told her to take Aricept but there was no cure and her health would only decline.
>
> My wife could not carry on even a simple conversation, she was not a "functioning person," and it was so sad.
>
> My son called me in October after you told him about the Bredesen Protocol. I was very sceptical and it sounded "too good to be true."
>
> In November of 2018 we met with Dr Deborah Cantrell to do the blood work, an MRI, and the ApoE test. The ApoE was 3/4. We received a list of vitamins, probiotics, turmeric, and sublinguals to take. She started taking these in January and she is 95% better!!!! Everyone that knows my wife saw her decline and now these same people see her today and ask, "Is she

> cured of Alzheimer's??" My simple answer is, "The regimen of vitamins and other things she has taken has turned her life around."
>
> I cannot tell you HOW MUCH my wife, myself, my son, and my grandchildren appreciate your introducing us to the Protocol and Dr Cantrell, and my wife has her life back.

Are supplements "worthless" when it comes to cognitive decline, as some have claimed?[1] Well, first of all, as their name implies, they are *supplementary*. Numerous patients have tried avoiding the various other parts of the protocol and following only the supplement recommendations, and few have shown much improvement. The whole point of the protocol is to use all available methods to change the brain's biochemical signalling away from the synaptoclastic signalling of Alzheimer's disease and towards the synaptoblastic signalling of normalcy. Thus the point here is not about whether supplements work or don't work; it is about what we can employ to bring about the critical changes in neurochemistry that are necessary for prevention and reversal of cognitive decline, given the specific contributors for each person. Since Alzheimer's disease is a very serious illness, we must pull out all of the stops in what amounts to an emergency situation, and high-quality supplements targeted to the specific needs of each patient, as part of the overall protocol, have proven effective time and time again. Moreover, we have had numerous examples of those who discontinue their supplements—for example, in preparation for a surgical procedure or while travelling or running out—and note clear decline in the ensuing weeks. These observations suggest that supplements are indeed important as part of an optimal personalized protocol.

Since the underlying contributors to cognitive decline are many, and since they vary from person to person, the arsenal of supplements is accordingly large and personalized. For example, if as doctors purporting to offer treatment for cognitive decline we fail to evaluate and treat insulin resistance, then we are providing suboptimal care. If we fail to evaluate and treat systemic inflammation, we are providing suboptimal care. If we fail to evaluate and treat gastrointestinal hyperpermeability (leaky gut), we are providing suboptimal care. If we fail to evaluate and treat Alzheimer-associated pathogens (such as *Herpes simplex* or *Porphyromonas gingivalis*), then we are providing suboptimal care. If we fail to evaluate and treat mycotoxin exposure, then we are providing suboptimal care. If we fail to evaluate and treat chemotoxin exposure, we are providing suboptimal care. If we fail to evaluate and treat sleep apnoea and other causes of oxygen desaturation, we are providing suboptimal care. If we fail to evaluate and treat microbiome abnormalities, we are providing suboptimal care. If we fail to evaluate and treat hormonal deficiency, we are providing suboptimal care. If we fail to evaluate and treat nutritional deficiencies, we are providing suboptimal care. If we fail to evaluate and treat vascular disease, we are providing suboptimal care. If we fail to evaluate and treat methylation defects, we are providing suboptimal care. Therefore, since supplements are available to address all of these critical contributors, they represent an important part of the overall armamentarium.

So let's look at the various supplements available by examining the biochemical goals—what are we trying to achieve in order to improve cognition? As we go over each of these, please remember that identical biochemical goals can often be achieved with specific foods and lifestyle changes, and indeed, when you have a choice, it is preferable to minimize the supplements. The most natural way you can reach a biochemical goal is the best way to do it. As an example, you can support your microbiome by taking probiotics from fermented foods such as kimchi or sauerkraut, or you can take a probiotic capsule—it's your choice. In this case, new supplements offer specific strains of bacteria with desirable effects, bacteria that survive the digestive process better than those from fermented foods, and specific colony counts, so the fermented foods and probiotic capsules are actually complementary. However, there are times when food may not supply a needed nutrient—for example, vegetarians are often deficient in vitamin B_{12}, and thus high in homocysteine, an important risk factor for Alzheimer's disease, so in such cases, supplements are critical.

A note on sourcing: there are many high-quality sources for herbs and supplements, and using a trusted source is important. For herbs, Banyan Botanicals, Gaia Herbs, Natura Health Products, Metagenics, and Cytoplan are all highly recommended (which is not to say that others do not provide high-quality herbs, only that these are trusted and among those reproducibly high in quality). These are available online in the UK. For supplements, Pure Encapsulations, Garden of Life, LifeSeasons, Metagenics, Cytoplan, and Thorne, among others, are trusted brands.

With these points in mind, what are the goals of the supplements that are helping to provide synaptic support? Here are the key questions that these address.

- **How can I lower my homocysteine?**

Optimal homocysteine is below 7 micromolar, and this may require vitamin B_{12} (as methylcobalamin, S-adenosylcobalamin, and/or hydroxocobalamin) at 1 mg per day, methylfolate at 0.8 mg per day (although some use this up to 15 mg), and pyridoxal-5-phosphate (P5P) at 20 mg per day (beware of high doses of pyridoxine over 150 mg, since these may cause nerve damage, making your feet feel numb and making it difficult to walk). Some add trimethylglycine 500 mg (up to 3 g) if high homocysteine persists. Adequate choline is also helpful, and this can be obtained from your diet (e.g. egg yolks, liver) or via supplementation with citicoline, GPC choline, or lecithin.

- **How can I reduce systemic inflammation?**

For most of us following the KetoFLEX 12/3 diet described in the first section of the Handbook, the anti-inflammatory effects of the diet will prevent systemic inflammation. However, for those of us whose hs-CRP is still over 0.9 mg/dL, reducing inflammation is critical, and thus supplementation is important. This is a three-step process: (1) Determine what is causing the inflammation, be it leaky gut or chronic infection or metabolic syndrome or some other cause. (2) Resolve the inflammation, which can be accomplished with specialized pro-resolving mediators (a product called SPM Active has been produced by Metagenics, following the seminal research of Professor Charles Serhan; 2 to 4 capsules per day for one month can be taken to resolve ongoing inflammation) or with omega-3 fats such as DHA and EPA, at a total dose of 1 to 3 grams of omega-3 fats. (3) Prevent further inflammation with curcumin 1 g per day, and/or omega-3 1 g per day, and/or ginger 1 to 3 g per day, and/or boswellia 300 to 500 mg twice per day, and/or cat's claw (*Uncaria tomentosa*) 250 to 350 mg per day (cat's claw has multiple additional effects, such as reduction of beta-amyloid). If possible, avoid the gastric and kidney damage associated with aspirin and the liver toxicity associated with acetaminophen.

How do I achieve insulin sensitivity?

Just as with inflammation, the diet and lifestyle described in the first section of the Handbook should relieve insulin resistance and create insulin sensitivity for most of us. However, again, this approach can be supplemented with several very effective compounds that are readily available over the counter: (1) berberine 500 mg three times per day is very effective in glucose control; (2) zinc picolinate (or other forms of zinc) improves insulin release and action. It is important for those who are zinc deficient, which includes one billion people globally, many of whom have taken PPIs (proton-pump inhibitors) for GERD, which is gastric reflux, or heartburn. Zinc picolinate can be taken at dosages of 20 to 50 mg per day; (3) cinnamon ¼ teaspoon each day; (4) chromium picolinate 500 mcg twice per day; (5) alpha-lipoic acid (or, preferably, R-lipoic acid) reduces AGEs by increasing the protective enzyme glyoxalase and through its antioxidant effect, among other mechanisms, and is typically taken at a dosage of 100 to 500 mg per day; (6) bitter melon and aloe vera are also both used as supplements for their modest effects on haemoglobin A1c; (7) as noted earlier, high-fibre diets and supplements improve glucose control.

■ How can I achieve ketosis?

Just as for insulin sensitivity, most of us will be able to achieve ketosis with the KetoFLEX 12/3 diet, exercise, quality sleep, and avoidance of stress. This endogenous ketosis is preferable. However, for some, this may not lead to a sufficient level of ketosis (at least 0.5 mM BHB, and preferably 1.0–4.0 mM BHB); in which case MCT oil, from 1 teaspoon to 1 tablespoon three times per day, is often helpful. Start at 1 teaspoon and work up over a few weeks in order to avoid diarrhoea.

You can also take ketone salts or ketone esters to achieve ketosis in the same range. You can use the Precision Xtra ketone meter or the Keto-Mojo or Keto Guru to measure the ketone level. Alternatively, although measuring ketones in the urine (which measures acetoacetate) or with a breathalyzer (which measures acetone) is not as accurate, at least it will get you started.

■ How can I increase neurotrophic signalling?

Neurotrophins are growth factors that support the neurons by binding to specific receptors on the neurons. For example, brain-derived neurotrophic factor (BDNF) is increased by exercise, and exerts an anti-Alzheimer's effect. Similarly, nerve growth factor (NGF) supports the brain's cholinergic neurons, which are important in memory formation. Not only do exercise and ketones increase BDNF, but so does whole coffee fruit extract (WCFE), also called NeuroFactor, which seems to be most effective when taken in the morning or evening, at 100 or 200 mg. This can be obtained from LifeSeasons or Garden of Life or other sources.

Another approach is to take 7,8-dihydroxyflavone, which binds to the BDNF receptor and increases signalling. The optimal dosage is not yet known; it may be best to start with 25 mg each day for three days, then twice each day for one week, then three times per day.

Pterostilbene 50 mg per day also increases BDNF, as well as boosting dopamine. Lithium orotate 5 to 10 mg twice per day also increases BDNF, among its other salutary effects.

ALCAR (acetyl-L-carnitine) transports fatty acids into mitochondria to utilize for energy, and has been shown to increase NGF (nerve growth factor). A typical dose is 500 to 1000 mg one to three times per day.

Hericium erinaceus, which is lion's mane mushroom, also called Yamabushitake, has been shown to increase NGF, reduce inflammation, and improve cognition in patients with MCI.[2] A dosage of 250 to 500 mg three times per day with meals is typical. Some like to make a tea with this mushroom.

Beyond these supplements and herbs, there is tremendous potential in the use of intranasal trophic factors, and I hope that we will see increasing access to these in the years to come. For some, such as insulin and NGF, there is excellent brain penetration when administered intranasally, while for others, such as netrin-1 (which binds to APP itself), there is not. However, for those with poor penetration, often using a small active fragment (peptide) that has good penetration is enough, so whether using full-length insulin or NGF, or active fragments of netrin-1 or other poor penetrators, these contribute important potential to the overall armamentarium. All of these—insulin, NGF, BDNF, ADNP, netrin-1, GDNF, and others—exert potent signalling and supportive effects on neurons, enhancing survival, outgrowth of processes (called neurites), and synapse formation and retention. We must be careful not to flood the system—for example, we do not want to make insulin resistance worse with high levels of insulin. Nonetheless, these represent powerful allies in the overall programme for cognitive decline, and hopefully these will be available in the near term.

How can I increase my focus and attention?

A common complaint from those with cognitive decline is the lack of ability to keep focused and maintain attention. This is a first step in memory formation—it is critical to focus and assign importance to new information, since unimportant details are preferentially forgotten. Caffeine is a well-known enhancer of focus and attention.

Pantothenic acid 100–200 mg is also helpful, although due to its stimulating effect, it should be avoided late in the day. Gotu kola 100–500 mg once or twice per day is also effective. Taurine has both effects on anxiety reduction and on enhancing focus, and is taken at 500–2000 mg per day; lemon balm 300–600 mg also reduces anxiety and enhances focus. Some prefer to sniff peppermint, which also enhances focus and improves mental clarity. ALCAR 500 mg also enhances focus.

How can I improve my memory?

Memory is the brain's quintessential function, a complex and truly remarkable property, one that is affected by many different parameters. Learning and memory are affected by focus and attention, neurotransmitters (especially acetylcholine, glutamate, and for the positive feedback of reward, dopamine), trophic factors (e.g. NGF and BDNF), signals from cyclic AMP, the reading of DNA to produce memory-associated proteins, synapse formation and strengthening, hormones, nutrients, and genetics. All of these processes (except your underlying genetics) can be modulated by various nutraceuticals and herbs.

As noted above, focus and attention can be enhanced by numerous agents, from caffeine to theanine to taurine to pantothenic acid to ALCAR to lemon balm (not to mention a good night's sleep, exercise, ketosis, and the avoidance of insulin spikes); acetylcholine can be increased with citicoline (CDP-choline) 250–500 mg twice per day, GPC choline (500–1200 mg), phosphatidylcholine (400–1500 mg three times per day), huperzine A (50–200 mg twice per day), Bacopa monnieri (250 mg with meals), centrophenoxine 500–1000 mg, DMAE (dimethylaminoethanol) 50–200 mg, saffron 25–30 mg per day, or maca (from the Andes; beware imitations from elsewhere) 0.5–5 g per day; dopamine can be increased with precursors such as tyrosine and phenylalanine, cofactors such as pyridoxine, precursors such as the L-dopa found in *Mucuna pruriens*, or inhibitors of dopamine breakdown such as the drug selegiline or oat straw extract (800–1600 mg per day).

Cholinergic and glutamatergic signalling can be enhanced by a group of nutraceuticals called racetams, including piracetam (250–1500 mg three times per day), aniracetam (375–750 mg twice per day), oxiracetam (250–500 mg three times per day), and phenylpiracetam (100 mg twice per day). Some include creatine 200–5000 mg per day for energy support when using any racetam. Shankhpushpi 100–400 mg produces some similar effects to the racetams.

Neurotrophic factors, as noted on page 301, can be increased with ALCAR, *Hericium erinaceus* (lion's mane mushroom), whole coffee fruit extract, pterostilbene, or 7,8-dihydroxyflavones, among others.

Cyclic AMP signalling can be enhanced by caffeine (50–100 mg) and L-theanine (200 mg; often combined in order to minimize the rapid heart rate induced by caffeine alone), as well as forskolin (150–250 mg per day), or by artichoke extract 500 mg, which contains luteolin. Synapse formation is supported by DHA (docosahexaenoic acid, an omega-3 fat) 1 g per day, along with citicoline 250–500 mg twice per day.

Magnesium threonate 2 g (which includes 144 mg of magnesium), which can be taken in the evening or as 667 mg three times per day, supports synaptic transmission, as does phosphatidylserine 100–300 mg per day. Benfotiamine 150–300 mg twice per day may support memory formation in those deficient in thiamine (vitamin B_1), a vitamin critical for learning and memory formation.

■ How can I support my mitochondrial function?

Mitochondria are the "batteries" of our cells, and their compromise plays a crucial role in neurodegeneration. They may be compromised through damage to their own DNA, or through a failure in the normal turnover, or through damage to their membranes or components. Just as the autophagy that we activate at night while we sleep helps to remove damaged cell components, the mitophagy that chews up damaged mitochondria and allows the production of new ones supports optimal neuronal function.

Coenzyme Q (CoQ) or its reduced form, Ubiquinol, is frequently used, at a dosage of 90–200 mg. PQQ (pyrroloquinoline quinone) is used to increase mitochondrial number, and is taken at a dose of 10–20 mg. NAD+ (nicotinamide adenine dinucleotide) is a critical energy source for mitochondria, and also activates SIRT1, which increases the synaptoblastic signals we want for cognitive support. Nicotinamide riboside 200–300 mg per day increases NAD+; an alternative mechanism to activate SIRT1 is to take resveratrol 150–500 mg.

Protection of mitochondria typically includes R-lipoic acid 100 mg, vitamin C 1–4 g, mixed tocopherols and tocotrienols 400 IU, and energetic support includes ALCAR 500 mg, Ubiquinol as above, nicotinamide riboside as above, and creatine 200–5000 mg per day.

▪ How can I support my adrenals?

The chapter on minimizing stress offers the best way to reduce, avoid, and manage stress. However, supplementary adrenal support is often helpful, and Rhodiola rosea 300–600 mg (for 1% rosavin; if 2% is used, reduce to 150–300 mg) is commonly utilized for this purpose, along with Schisandra 1–3 g per day with meals, and holy basil 200–600 mg three times per day. These are often combined with licorice root (deglycyrrhizinated) 0.5–5 g per day.

For those with low pregnenolone or DHEA, supporting with low doses starting at 10–25 mg per day is often helpful while returning your own adrenal function.

▪ How can I improve detoxification?

This is discussed in chapter 19.

▪ How can I heal my gut?

The use of bone broth to heal the gut is discussed in chapter 9. There are multiple other supplements used for this purpose as well, such as L-glutamine, cabbage juice (which contains L-glutamine), ProButyrate, deglycyrrhizinated licorice, slippery elm, Triphala, and lignite extract (Restore, now called ION*Gut Health). After gut healing, which may take a month or two, these can be discontinued or taken on an intermittent basis.

■ How can I optimize my microbiome?

As noted earlier there are about 1,000 different species in the gut microbiome (ignoring for the moment the rest of the holobiome, such as the skin microbiome, the sinus microbiome, and the vaginal microbiome), and although general patterns have been identified in association with conditions such as Alzheimer's and type 2 diabetes, fine details are as yet unknown. Therefore, the best we can do currently is to provide genera such as *Lactobacillus* and *Bifidobacteria*, and then to feed these bacteria with prebiotics such as those found in Mexican yam or Jerusalem artichoke.

Food is the best choice for probiotics and prebiotics, as described in chapter 20 earlier. However, these are also available as supplements. Some like VSL#3 (which has been used successfully in inflammatory bowel disease), others prefer one of the Garden of Life probiotics, whereas others prefer probiotics from Schiff or LifeSeasons or any of several others. *Saccharomyces boulardii* 250–500 mg two to four times per day is a common adjunct, especially for those with gut infections such as *Helicobacter pylori* or *Clostridium difficile*. If you are on antibiotics and thus have damaged your microbiome, taking sporebiotics (derived from spores rather than live probiotics) is also supportive, prior to the reintroduction of probiotics after the discontinuation of antibiotics.

Some suggest the use of goldenseal, which inhibits bacterial drug-resistance pumps, as a method to destroy some of the more pathogenic bacteria and select for more microbiome-friendly species.

As noted in chapters 9 and 20, our microbiomes need nutrition, which can be provided by high-fibre diets or resistant starches, or by supplemental prebiotics such as organic psyllium husk or konjac root (which is in PGX).

▪ How can I support my immune function?

The beta-amyloid associated with Alzheimer's disease is a part of the innate immune system response, and multiple pathogens have been identified in the brains of patients with Alzheimer's, such as spirochetes, oral bacteria, *Herpes* viruses, and fungi. Therefore, immune support represents one strategy to reduce the overall need for chronic activation of the innate immune system, with its associated amyloid-beta production. One combination used by Ayurvedic doctors for many centuries is Amalaki (500–1000 mg twice per day), *Tinospora* (300 mg three times per day), and ashwagandha (500 mg with meals). In addition, basic nutritional support such as vitamins A, D, and zinc also support the immune system.

Humic acid and fulvic acid provide immune stimulation and are often used for those with chronic viral infections such as *Herpes simplex* or *Cytomegalovirus*, or other chronic infections such as Lyme disease. Another approach to patients with chronic infections is Transfer Factor PlasMyc.

Multiple herbs and supplements provide immune support, including AHCC (active hexose correlated compound, a mushroom extract, typically taken at 3–6 g per day), Avemar, Astragalus, beta-1,6-glucan, licorice root, black elderberry, echinacea, olive leaf, propolis, and oregano.

▪ How can I optimize my vitamin D level?

Optimal vitamin D levels are controversial. On the one hand, it has been argued that vitamin D level simply reflects time outdoors, rather than any mechanistic effect on health parameters; on the other hand, vitamin D mediates the transcription of hundreds of genes, by which it affects critical processes such as neuroplasticity, the immune system, tumour formation, cardiovascular disease, and calcium regulation.

To reach an optimal vitamin D level, the "hundreds rule" is easy to use: subtract your level from your target level and multiply by 100 to determine your approximate dosage. For example, if your target is 60 (and I recommend a target of 50–80 ng/ml) and your current level is 25 (which is fairly typical), then 60 − 25 = 35, which means you would take 3500 IU of vitamin D. Please remember to include vitamin K_2 at least 100 mcg, in order to mobilize the calcium and prevent its deposition in arterial walls, and take your vitamins D and K with some good fat (e.g. avocado or nuts) for best absorption. Overall vitamin D dosage should be kept lower than 10000 IU to avoid toxicity, and serum levels below 100 ng/ml—and please try to get at least some of your vitamin D from sunlight!

- **How can I improve blood flow to my brain?**

When we evaluate the brains of those who have died with dementia, the most common finding is Alzheimer's disease, and the second most common finding is vascular dementia. Furthermore, vascular disease is common in Alzheimer's, and omnipresent in type 5 Alzheimer's. Therefore, improved cerebral blood flow may be very helpful, and there are numerous products to support that: nitric oxide, which causes dilation of blood vessels, is increased by rocket, beetroot extract, Neo40 1 tablet one to two times per day, L-arginine 3–6 g one to three times per day, ProArgi-9 at 1 scoop (5 g of L-arginine) in water each day, pine bark extract (Pycnogenol) up to 100 mg three times per day, so any of those products may be used. Alternative approaches include ginkgo 40–120 mg three times per day, nattokinase 100 mg one to three times per day, vinpocetine 5–20 mg three times per day, or Hydergine 1–3 mg three times per day. Finally, those with a vascular contribution to cognitive decline may wish to consider a vegan or vegetarian diet, and may consider EWOT (exercise with oxygen therapy).

- **How can I achieve neuroprotection?**

Unfortunately, the term *antioxidant* has been conflated with protectant, when in fact too much antioxidant activity may interfere with cellular processes such as fighting infections. Thus getting the optimal amount of antioxidant activity, rather than the maximal amount, is the goal. This includes protection of membranes with vitamin E (mixed tocopherols and tocotrienols 400 IU), as well as vitamin C 1–4 g per day, the many protective phytonutrients in vegetables (discussed in chapters 4 through 12), and glutathione (a key antioxidant, detoxicant, and cellular protectant), as basics. A mitochondrial-targeted antioxidant, mitoquinol, has been developed for potential use in neurodegenerative diseases.[3] TUDCA (tauroursodeoxycholic acid) also shows promise as a neuroprotectant,[4] and is typically given at a dose of 300–1000 mg per day.

There are multiple approaches to enhancing glutathione: N-acetylcysteine (500–600 mg one to three times per day) is a precursor of glutathione. Since glutathione itself is absorbed poorly, one can take it as liposomal glutathione 250 mg twice per day, or S-acetyl glutathione 100 mg twice per day, or as inhaled glutathione or intravenous glutathione.

Beyond these basics, there are dozens of pathways and hundreds of compounds that provide neuroprotection, so the form of neuroprotection that is best for you will depend on your subtype—whether you have ongoing inflammation or trophic loss or toxin exposure or vascular damage or traumatic history. Vitamin D is a good anti-inflammatory, as are curcumin, omega-3 fats, and others listed on page 299 and minimizing inflammation is critical to neuroprotection. Oestradiol is another neuroprotectant, and protective neurosteroids such as pregnenolone and DHEA can be purchased over the counter.

Neurotrophins, discussed earlier, are some of the most powerful neuroprotectants. In fact, one of the protective effects of ketones is via the upregulation of BDNF. However, for their optimal effects, inflammation should be minimized and glutamate balanced with GABA.

CHAPTER 22

Troubleshooting: If at First You Don't Succeed

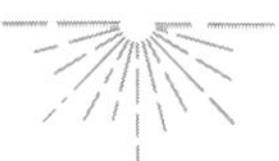

Problems are not stop signs, they are guidelines.
—ROBERT H. SCHULLER

THIS IS WHAT GETS me up in the morning:

> I wrote to you to tell you how much my wife, who had been diagnosed with Alzheimer's in January of 2018, had made amazing progress since starting the ReCODE Protocol. Today I want to tell you that she has continued to make GREAT improvement. The protocol saved her life. I have my wife back, and our children and grandchildren have their mother and grandmother back.

And this is what keeps me up at night:

> I am SO discouraged because my husband does not show any marked signs of improvement despite all our good efforts.

How do you know if things are going as they should? How do you know if you are on the right track? Well, typically it takes a few weeks to get all of your lab results and get started on the protocol, and then a few months to get the various parts of your personalized programme optimized. When that is done—and please remember that the underlying degenerative process of Alzheimer's may be ongoing for ten or even twenty years before diagnosis, so it should come as no surprise that it takes some time to impact this process—people typically note improvements in three to six months. We have seen improvements in four days and in more than a year, but three to six months is typical.

> Betsy is a 79-year-old woman who first developed memory loss after anaesthesia for a hysterectomy at age 66. She was diagnosed with Alzheimer's disease at age 74 and placed on Aricept, which was then discontinued because it did not help and caused her to be aggressive. Even after significant lifestyle intervention for diabetes, her dementia symptoms continued to progress, including sundown syndrome at age 75, in which she would become confused and very agitated starting about four P.M. and would pack her suitcases to move back with her mother (who had been deceased for several decades). This went on for three years until she was evaluated by Dr Wes Youngberg, who ordered the comprehensive Bredesen Protocol labs. In spite of her extremely low cognitive scores (MoCA 0/30 and mini-mental status of 1/30), she began to exhibit a dramatic turnaround when her husband started giving her specific nutritional supplements to address a very high homocysteine of 15 and a previously undiagnosed autoimmune condition. The greatest improvement occurred after adding lithium orotate 10 mg daily. After having been unable to read for three years, she regained the ability to read words on TV, headlines in newspapers, and road signs. To her husband's great relief, after she had been following this new strategy only one month, Betsy's sundown syndrome resolved, with only an occasional mention of her mother once or twice per week. This major challenge had resolved through careful attention to the areas of the protocol that had not been fully addressed previously.

The most common cause of poor response is lack of compliance. Please give yourself a break—it is challenging to do the multiple parts of the programme, and indeed, we are trying to simplify it, but the underlying disease process is unfortunately complicated. The good news is that you don't necessarily need to follow every step to see improvement, because what is important is that there is a threshold you need to exceed to get going in the right direction. There is no way to measure this threshold directly, so you just need to keep tweaking until improvement begins.

The second most common cause of poor response is failure to identify and target a contributor, such as an infection or leaky gut or toxin exposure. Therefore, please don't give up only a few weeks after the initial tests—please keep optimizing your responses and keep working with your practitioner and health coach.

In addition to compliance and missing a contributor, there are several more key points to review to make sure you have the best chance for improvement:

- **Are you checking ketones, and are you typically in the range of 1.0 to 4.0?**

This is the level associated with best improvement. Those who are down around 0.2 to 0.5 (measured in millimolar beta-hydroxybutyrate, or mM BHB) don't typically do as well. You may need to use MCT oil or ketone salts or esters to achieve this level, and you may want to cycle off once per week with some sweet potato or something like that, but achieving this range of ketosis is associated with the best chance for improvement.

- **Is your score on BrainHQ or MoCA stable, declining, or improving?**

For most people, subjective improvement such as noticing memory improvement or more engagement in discussions or better organization is associated with objective improvement such as higher scores on MoCA or BrainHQ or CNS Vital Signs. In other words, these usually go hand in hand. However, sometimes people don't realize how much better they actually are, so it's helpful to look at your scores to see how you are doing. Please remember that the natural history of Alzheimer's is for relentless decline, so even modest improvements or stability represent a very good sign that you are headed in the right direction.

- **Did you rule out sleep apnoea? Did your oximetry show no desaturation events at night?**

One of the most common and usually unrecognized contributors to declining cognition is sleep apnoea—when we stop breathing for periods at night, and our oxygen is reduced. We usually think of this as occurring in men who are overweight and snore, but it turns out that both men and women, at any weight, snoring or silent, may actually reduce their oxygen at night (with or without sleep apnoea) so it is critical to know whether this is a contributor to your cognitive decline, even if your cognition is "normal." It is easy to do, and your doctor may lend you an oximeter for a few nights to check, or you can purchase one. You'd like to see that you remain with 96 to 98 per cent oxygen saturation at night, without dips down below 94 per cent. You'd also like to know that you have fewer than five apnoeic (non-breathing) events per hour—this is called an AHI (apnoea-hypopnoea index) of less than 5—and preferably 0.

- **Did you heal your gut, then take probiotics and prebiotics (in food or as supplements)?**

The good news here is that it is relatively easy to heal your gut and improve your microbiome, and this will help you in many ways, from nutrition to immunity to detoxification to improving your mood. The bad news is that most doctors ignore your gut status, so if this hasn't been checked and your cognition is not improving, then please address this important area. The target is no leaky gut (you can check this with Cyrex Array 2, for example) and no dysbiosis (abnormal gut flora).

- **Are you exercising at least four times a week? Doing both cardio and strength training?**

As noted in chapter 13, exercise has multiple mechanisms to improve cognition, from increasing the brain support BDNF to improving insulin sensitivity to improving blood vessel status. If you have been exercising minimally or not at all, then stepping it up may be helpful. Perhaps try a trainer and see if you like that, but however you do it, exercising for at least 45 minutes at least four times per week is very helpful.

- **Do you have a health coach who can help keep things optimized? (Or a spouse or significant other who can do the same?)**

One patient named Ken said to me, "I need a dominatrix!" I told him that he was talking to the wrong person, but I understood his point—some people need the carrot/incentive approach, while others do better with the stick/disincentive approach, so knowing your own proclivities and preferences is helpful. Some do well with a personal health coach, others with group coaching; some like in-person coaching, while others prefer telemedicine coaching; and some prefer their spouses to do the coaching—whatever works best for you. By the way, Ken ended up with a weight trainer and some occasional health coaching, and he is doing very well.

- **Do you have a health practitioner who understands this approach?**

This can be very important, especially if your practitioner is not ordering the right tests, is not addressing the critical contributors to cognitive decline, or is overly pessimistic. You have probably heard about the placebo effect, but you may not have heard about the nocebo effect. This is the negative effect on health that occurs with negative expectations, and such expectations are common when your doctor or other person of authority tells you that you have an untreatable illness.

- **Are you using the KetoFLEX 12/3 diet (or something similar)?**

The many different effects of this diet—ketosis, autophagy, insulin sensitivity, nutrient support, mitochondrial support, immune support, detoxification—are all designed to improve cognition and prevent cognitive decline, so if you are still not following this diet, you may be scuttling your chances for cognitive improvement.

- **Have you optimized biochemical parameters?**

Is your hs-CRP <0.9, fasting insulin 3.0–5.0, haemoglobin A1c 4.0–5.3, vitamin D 50–80? Hormones and nutrients optimized? Homocysteine $\leq$7? B_{12} 500–1500? RBC Mg >5.2? Optimizing these metabolic parameters is critical to providing the synaptoblastic signalling we need to counter cognitive decline, so if you are still suboptimal with any of these, getting to the right range is likely to be important.

- **If these parameters are optimized, have you had a trial of WCFE?**

WCFE is whole coffee fruit extract, and its effect is to increase BDNF (brain-derived neurotrophic factor, which supports neurons) markedly. If you have optimized your metabolic status, healed your gut, and resolved your inflammation, you should be able to rebuild your synapses, and BDNF is a key contributor (along with vitamin D, oestradiol, testosterone, thyroid hormone, citicoline, DHA, and others). In addition, Dr Keqiang Ye from Emory University has identified a compound called 7,8-dihydroxyflavone (also available over the counter) that binds to the BDNF receptor, thus providing a similar effect.

- **Have you identified and treated all pathogens?**

If you are chronically infected by *Borrelia*, *Babesia*, *Bartonella*, or other pathogens, these should be treated—if possible, without using antibiotics (or if antibiotics are used, monitor cognition carefully, and if there is a decline, move to a non-antibiotic approach). Pathogens may reside in the blood, sinuses, mouth (e.g. with periodontitis), gut, brain, skin, or other organs. Beyond destroying pathogens, restoring the optimal microbiome to these various sites provides important support for best cognition.

- **Have you identified and treated toxins (metallotoxins, organic toxins, and biotoxins), optimizing the rate of detoxification?**

The umbilical cord blood of today's newborns contains hundreds of toxins—we are exposed to a panoply of toxins like never before in history. These often contribute to cognitive decline. The good news is that we can identify these toxins—which can be metals such as mercury, organics such as toluene or formaldehyde, or biotoxins such as trichothecenes—and remove them over time. One critical tip is that detoxification that is overly aggressive may actually worsen symptoms, so it is important to work with your doctor—preferably a detox expert—to adjust the rate of detoxification. There are some excellent books on detoxification that have appeared recently, such as *The Toxin Solution* by Dr Joseph Pizzorno—which is particularly helpful for chemical toxins such as benzene, fluoride, bisphenol A (BPA), and phthalates—and *Toxic* by Dr Neil Nathan—which is particularly helpful for biotoxins such as mould-produced toxins such as trichothecenes.

- **If you have mycotoxins, have you been treated with cholestyramine (or other binding agents such as Welchol or**

clay or charcoal or zeolite)? Had intranasal VIP? Cleared MARCoNS? Is your C4a back to normal? MMP-9 back to normal?

If you have exposure to mycotoxins (which can be determined by a urine sample), reducing this exposure and excreting these toxins are likely to be important for optimizing your cognition. Not only can these mould-produced toxins damage your brain directly, but they can also compromise your immune system, the very thing you want to avoid in Alzheimer's disease.

- **Is your glutathione level optimized?**

Glutathione is like a great parent—it protects you against many enemies. It's critical for detox and a key antioxidant. You really want your glutathione to be optimal—in fact, low glutathione is common with chronic toxin exposure, since you are literally exhausting your cleanup mechanisms. Therefore, please ensure that your glutathione level is optimal—target a minimum of 250 mcg/ml, which is 814 micromolar. You can increase your glutathione by taking its precursor, NAC (N-acetylcysteine), or taking liposomal glutathione, or S-acetyl glutathione, or intranasal glutathione, and some with severe toxicity take intravenous glutathione or inhaled glutathione. In addition, there are many other contributors to help detox, as described in chapter 19, such as sulforaphane, diindolylmethane, and ascorbate.

- **Have you included brain stimulation?**

It has turned out that optimal results are often associated with the inclusion of a form of brain stimulation—whether this is accomplished by light stimulation such as Vielight, defocused laser stimulation, magnetic stimulation such as MeRT (magnetic e-resonant therapy), or another approach. Of course, brain training represents a form of brain stimulation, but including at least one of these physical modalities with the overall protocol, especially in the presence of optimal biochemistry, may be complementary.

- **Is it time to consider stem cells?**

If everything has been addressed and optimized, and improvement has not occurred or a plateau has been reached, you may wish to consider stem cells. Please beware—when it comes to stem cells, there are many charlatans out there. However, there are ongoing trials of stem cells for Alzheimer's disease, and there are good groups in Dallas, Panama, New York, and several other sites.

If we all adopt the guidelines outlined in the Handbook, start as early as possible, continue to optimize, and use the troubleshooting approach outlined here, we should be able to reduce the global burden of dementia. We should be able to make Alzheimer's a rare disease, as it should be. And we should be able to bring a virtual end to Alzheimer's disease with the current generation.

EPILOGUE

The Triumph of Twenty-First-Century Medicine

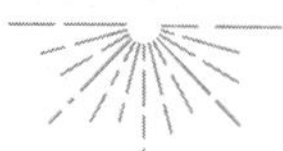

I knew her before she was a virgin.
—OSCAR LEVANT, regarding DORIS DAY

YOU MAY OR MAY not remember Doris Day—she was a leading actress and singer in the 1950s and 1960s who projected such a wholesome image that she was labelled the "World's Oldest Virgin." The mordant pianist Oscar Levant pointed out that he had known her prior to the adoption of that image, and therefore had known her "before she was a virgin."

Though this may sound like a non sequitur, that is the way I feel about medicine. Yes, as bizarre as it may seem, I knew medicine before it was about health! Before it was about addressing what actually causes disease. It is hard to believe now the horribly unhealthy things doctors did to themselves and to their patients, things that, sadly, many are still doing. Doctors not only smoked frequently, they actually did television commercials to sell cigarettes! They often did not exercise and routinely grew obese and developed early cardiovascular disease; they regularly adopted horrible nutrition habits and told their patients that nutrition is unimportant in disease treatment; they often dispensed with sleep despite their need for discerning judgement; they ignored evaluation of the very processes causing the diseases they were attempting to treat; they treated chronic complex illnesses with ineffective drugs; and many focused less on what was needed by the patients and more on what hospital profit-driven policy demanded or what the sales rep pushed on them.

When I was taught medicine, we studied, we practised, and we taught end-stage medicine—we learned and looked for signs of cancer metastasis and heart failure and dementia that were years down the road from when we should be identifying and treating the associated conditions.

As I look back on all of this, it is discomfiting to recall how bad it was. It was like training for years to be a meditation instructor, then yelling at your trainees constantly—it just made no sense. Worst of all, these antiquated practices have been passed on to each class of new doctors: as one education leader said, "We know we are lying to the medical students, but they keep believing our lies, so we keep telling them." Not a very progressive approach, to be sure!

I grew up in the 1960s, a time of societal upheaval. A time when the president having an extra scoop of ice cream was not considered news. A time when grassroots movements were changing social structures, music, art, and wars. We need such a movement now to effect a tectonic shift in health—the way we think about it, learn it, practise it, and benefit from it.

Thankfully, changes are beginning to occur, at least in some practices. Indeed, twenty-first-century medicine, focused on disease causes and contributors, using programmatic treatment instead of monotherapy, represents a paradigm shift from twentieth-century medicine. These changes are bringing about better results than ever before—for cognitive decline, type 2 diabetes, hypertension, rheumatoid arthritis, lupus, depression, leaky gut, autism spectrum disorders, and other chronic illnesses. To the detriment of us all, however, the changes are being adopted only begrudgingly—despite the improved results, medical schools have resisted teaching this twenty-first-century medicine. Therefore, the vast majority of practitioners still practise in-n-out, prescription-pad medicine that ignores the physiology underlying the disease processes. Because of these practices, the ongoing medical revolution, although it has been relatively unadvertised and little discussed to date, is arguably the bloodiest revolution in history, one that will continue to claim the lives of the billions with chronic illness until we modernize and optimize our practices, until medicine and technology are seamlessly integrated, until medicine and health become one, and until practitioners and patients—indeed, until all of us—take responsibility for global health.

Just as the twentieth century saw the virtual end to the scourges of polio, syphilis, and leprosy, the twenty-first century will see the virtual end to the scourges of Alzheimer's, Parkinson's, Lewy body disease, multiple sclerosis, autism, schizophrenia, rheumatoid arthritis, lupus, ulcerative colitis, and other complex chronic illnesses. These diseases will be recorded historically as twentieth-century diseases, increased dramatically by a lethal combination of undiagnosed chronic pathogens, a toxin smorgasbord unlike anything in history, a non-physiological food supply, immune system compromise, chronically stressful lifestyles, and overall, the futile attempt that nearly our entire species has made to pursue a life that deviates significantly from our evolutionary design capacity.

Thus the road map is clear. We know what to look for in each person, we know how to identify the contributors, we know how to deal with each one. Now we need to enact it, perfect it, and scale it. Fixing cognition will become as routine as straightening teeth.

Our daughter was married this year, and I could not help thinking about the world in which she had grown up—a world of emails, social networks, tweets, smart phones, search engines, e-commerce, and cloud storage. Such a different world from the one in which I grew up. She will raise her children in a world in which, thankfully, Alzheimer's disease is not the scourge it has been for my generation.

Each one of us is a unique, N-of-1 experiment. May your experiment be successful, fulfilling, joyous, and lasting.

Acknowledgements

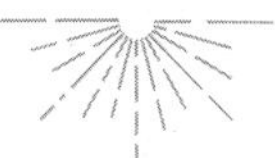

First and foremost, I thank my wife, Aida, who is always focused on improving patients' lives, and our daughters, Tara and Tess. I thank Julie Gregory and Aida for their critical contributions to the book. I am grateful to Phyllis and Jim Easton, and to Diana Merriam and the Evanthea Foundation, for their commitment to making a difference for people with Alzheimer's disease. I am also grateful to Katherine Gehl, Jessica Lewin, Wright Robinson, Dr Patrick Soon-Shiong, Douglas Rosenberg, Beryl Buck, Dagmar and David Dolby, Stephen D. Bechtel Jr., Gayle Brown, Lucinda Watson, Tom Marshall and the Joseph Drown Foundation, Bill Justice, Dave Mitchell, Josh Berman, Marcus Blackmore, Hideo Yamada, and Jeffrey Lipton.

I am grateful for invaluable training from Professors Stanley Prusiner, Mark Wrighton (Chancellor), Roger Sperry, Robert Collins, Robert Fishman, Roger Simon, Vishwanath Lingappa, William Schwartz, Kenneth McCarty Jr., J. Richard Baringer, Neil Raskin, Robert Layzer, Seymour Benzer, Erkki Ruoslahti, Lee Hood, and Mike Merzenich.

I am also grateful to the functional medicine pioneers and experts who are revolutionizing medicine and healthcare: Drs Jeffrey Bland, David Perlmutter, Mark Hyman, Dean Ornish, Ritchie Shoemaker, Neil Nathan, Joseph Pizzorno, Ann Hathaway, Kathleen Toups, Deborah Gordon, Jeralyn Brossfield, Kristine Burke, Ilene Naomi Rusk, Jill Carnahan, Sara Gottfried, David Jones, Patrick Hanaway, Terry Wahls, Stephen Gundry, Ari Vojdani, Prudence Hall, Tom O'Bryan, Chris Kresser, Mary Kay Ross, Edwin Amos, Susan Sklar, Mary Ackerley, Sunjya Schweig, Sharon Hausman-Cohen, Nate Bergman, Kim Clawson Rosenstein, Wes Youngberg, Craig Tanio, Dave Jenkins, Miki Okuno, Ari Vojdani, Elroy Vojdani, Chris Shade, health coaches Amylee Amos, Aarti Batavia, and Tess Bredesen, and the over fifteen hundred doctors from ten countries and around the United States who have participated in and contributed to the course focused on the protocol described in this book; and courageous individuals such as Kristin, Deborah, Edna, Lucy, Frank, and Edward, who are, through their discipline and commitment, helping so many others with cognitive decline. In addition, I am grateful to Lance Kelly, Sho Okada, Bill Lipa, Scott Grant, Ryan Morishige, Ekta Agrawal, Jane Connelly, Lucy Kim, Melissa Manning, Gahren Markarian, and the team at Apollo Health, for their outstanding work on the ReCODE algorithm, coding, and reports; to Darrin Peterson and the team at LifeSeasons; to Taka Kondo and the team at Yamada Bee; and to Hideyuki Tokigawa and his documentary team.

None of what is described in this book would have been possible without the outstanding laboratory members and colleagues with whom I have worked over the past three decades. For the fascinating discussions, the many whiteboard sessions, the countless hours of experimentation, the patience to repeat and repeat experiments, and the unflagging dedication to enhancing humankind's health and knowledge, I am grateful to Shahrooz Rabizadeh, Patrick Mehlen, Varghese John, Rammohan Rao, Patricia Spilman, Jesus Campagna, Rowena Abulencia, Kayvan Niazi, Litao Zhong, Alexei Kurakin, Darci Kane, Karen Poksay, Clare Peters-Libeu, Veena Theendakara, Veronica Galvan, Molly Susag, Alex Matalis, and all of the other present and past members of the Bredesen Laboratory, as well as to my colleagues at the Buck Institute for Research on Aging, UCSF, the Sanford Burnham Prebys Medical Discovery Institute, and UCLA.

For their friendship and many discussions over the years, I thank Shahrooz Rabizadeh, Patrick Mehlen, Michael Ellerby, David Greenberg, John Reed, Guy Salvesen, Tuck Finch, Nuria Assa-Munt, Kim and Rob Rosenstein, Eric Tore and Carol Adolfson, Akane Yamaguchi, Judy and Paul Bernstein, Beverly and Roldan Boorman, Sandy and Harlan Kleiman, Philip Bredesen and Andrea Conte, Deborah Freeman, Peter Logan, Sandi and Bill Nicholson, Mary McEachron, and Douglas Green.

Finally, I am grateful for the outstanding team with which I have worked on this book: for the writing and editing of Corey Powell and Robin Dennis; figures by Joe LeMonnier; manuscript review by Deirdre Moynihan; literary agents John Maas and Celeste Fine of ParkFine; and editor Caroline Sutton, publisher Megan Newman, and Avery Books at Penguin Random House.

Visit endofalzheimersprogram.com to see every reference in this book.

Index

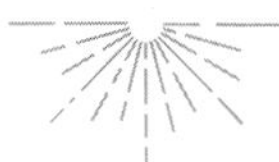

Note: Page numbers in *italics* refer to illustrations or graphs.

Also by Dr Dale Bredesen:

The End of Alzheimer's

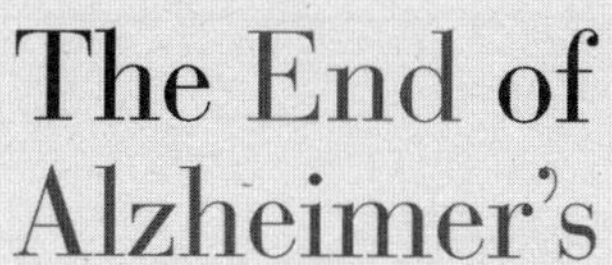
The End of Alzheimer's
The First Programme to Prevent and Reverse the Cognitive Decline of Dementia
Dr Dale Bredesen
'This phenomenal book tackles the most important health issue of our time...a must read'
Dr Rangan Chatterjee

The first proven plan to reverse Alzheimer's Disease.

In *The End of Alzheimer's* Dr Dale Bredesen rewrites the science of Alzheimer's Disease. He reveals the 36 affecting metabolic factors and outlines a proven programme to rebalance them, offering real hope to anyone looking to prevent and even reverse cognitive decline.

"Dr Dale Bredesen's research is some of the most exciting work that I have seen in years and tackles the most important health issue of our time . . . This is a masterpiece and a must-read book."
Dr Rangan Chatterjee, MRCP, MRCGP, author of *The Four Pillar Plan*

" . . . a masterful, authoritative, and ultimately hopeful patient guide that will help you prevent and reverse Alzheimer's disease, whether you have the ApoE4 gene or not. My patients fear Alzheimer's more than any other diagnosis. This is the book to transmute fear into action."
Dr Sara Gottfried, author of the *New York Times* bestseller *The Hormone Cure*

"This book represents a major turning point in our approach to Alzheimer's disease. For the first time ever, patients and families affected by Alzheimer's—as well as those at high risk for this devastating disease—truly have a reason to be hopeful."
Chris Kresser, MS, LAc, author of the *New York Times* bestseller *The Paleo Cure*